COMPLETE REPERTORY

TO THE

HOMŒOPATHIC

MATERIA MEDICA.

LONDON:

W. DEWICK AND SONS, STEAM PRINTERS, 46, BARBICAN, CITY.

COMPLETE REPERTORY

TO THE

HOMŒOPATHIC

MATERIA MEDICA.

—o—

Second Edition.

—o—

REVISED, RE-ARRANGED, AND VERY MUCH ENLARGED.

DISEASES OF THE EYES.

BY E. W. BERRIDGE, M.D.,

Bachelor of Medicine and Bachelor of Surgery of the University of London; Doctor of Medicine (by Examination) of the Homœopathic College of Pensylvania; Formerly Resident Medical Officer to the Liverpool Homœopathic Dispensary.

Author of "Index to Cases of Poisoning in the Allopathic Journals;" "Pathogenetic Record," Contributions to the "American Journal of Homœopathic Materia Medica," "North American Journal of Homœopathy," "Hahnemannian Monthly," "Hering's Complete Materia Medica," "Monthly Homœopathic Review," "Gregg's Homœopathic Quarterly," "British Journal of Homœopathy," &c. &c.

—oo—

ἡ δέ Κρίσις χαλεπή.

—oo—

LONDON:

ALFRED HEATH, 114, EBURY STREET.

PREFACE.

A PERFECT Repertory should contain a reference to *every* symptom of the Materia Medica under *every* rubric where it can possibly be looked for. To effect this, I have divided each chapter of this Repertory into two Sections: I.—The *Symptoms* themselves; and II.—Their *Conditions*, (including *Concomitants*).* Section I. is further divided into five sub-sections: A. Functional Symptoms; B. Anatomical Regions; C. General Character, Sequence, and Direction; D. Right Side; and E. Left Side: and Section II. into two subsections; A. Aggravations; and B. Ameliorations. All the symptoms in these sub-sections are arranged *alphabetically*, excepting the *peculiar symptoms*, which, not falling under any general heading, are placed last. All symptoms of a nearly identical

* Here we discover the great value of *Clinical Cases.* It is often difficult or impossible to decide from the provings *alone* what symptoms are really connected with each other; because, if the prover has repeated the dose after the medicine has begun to act on him, the symptoms produced by the different doses are mixed up together—a *rudis indigestaque moles:* whereas, if a group of symptoms is cured homœopathically, there can be no doubt of the necessary connection of its constituent elements. (Hence in a Materia Medica, such clinical symptoms should always be given in their integrity *as a group*, and not be merely scattered throughout the Schema under the various rubrics to which their constituent elements respectively belong.) In making use of such a clinical confirmation, however, we must not only be sure that it is a *cure* and not a *recovery;* but that the case has been cured by the *Homœopathic* and not by the *Allopathic* or *Antipathic* action of the medicine. For this reason, cases cured rapidly, permanently, and without perturbative action, by single doses of high potencies, without the use of auxiliaries of any kind, are the *most*, if not the *only*, reliable ones.

meaning are placed under the same rubric, according to the Table of Synonyms.

The *Conditions* including the *Concomitants*, are arranged in 23 groups as follows:—(1) Time, (2) Situation and External Influences, (3) Posture, (4) Touch, (5) Motion, (6) Head (including Mental Symptoms), (7) Eyes, (8) Ears, (9) Nose, (10) Face and Front of Neck, (11) Teeth, (12) Mouth, and Throat, (13) Abdomen (including Stomach, Anus, and all Functional Symptoms thereof, (14) Urinary Organs, (15) Sexual Organs, (16) Chest and Larynx, (17) Back and Nape of Neck, (18) Arms, (19) Legs, (20) Sleep, (21) Fever, (Chills, Heat, and Sweat), (22) Generalities (including Skin, Bones, Convulsions, Other Drugs, &c.)

The arrangement of the symptoms in Section II is in every respect exactly the same as that of Section I.

In the sub-section I. C. *Direction*, the symptoms are given in the chapter belonging to the organ in which they *commence*, thus "Shooting from Eyeball to Head" is given in the subsection I. C. of the chapter on "Eyes," but not in that on "Head."

Sometimes in a complex group of symptoms one symptom *follows* another; in this case if they are both in the *same* organ they are given in Section I., sub-section C.; if in *different* organs, in Section II. Thus "Blindness followed by Heat in Eyes" would be given in I. C. under the rubric "*Symptoms Changing Character;*" but "Blindness followed by Heat in Head," would be given in II under rubric "*Before Head Symptoms*," and also in the Head Chapter under "*After Eye Symptoms.*"

As our Materia Medica is still incomplete, we are often obliged to select the remedy to a certain extent *by Analogy*;

hence we require a Collective view of the medicines acting on any organ which agree as to *Specific Character*, *Anatomical Regions*, *General Character*, *Sequence*, *Direction*, *Sides*, and *Conditions* (including *Concomitants*).

In order to give Collectives according to *Specific Character*, the following plan has been adopted:—Under every rubric in I. A., and in the *principal* subdivision of I. B., are placed all the medicines from all the other subdivisions which agree in that particular point; and also all the varieties of that symptom which are given separately; *enclosed in brackets*. Thus under "Shooting in Eyeball" are placed *bracketed* the medicines possessing any *variety* of Shooting which may be given separately, or Shooting in *right* or *left* eye separately, or Shooting in any *subregion* of eye (*e.g.* Orbit), or Shooting in any *direction* in eye, or Shooting *to or from eye from or to any other organ*. When a symptom refers necessarily to one subregion *only* (*e.g.* Closing of Eyelids), this collective is given there. In I. A. and I. B., the medicines not bracketed affect both sides *simultaneously*; if either is affected separately, it is given in I. D. or I. E.

Collectives of medicines agreeing with regard to *Anatomical Regions*, the chief divisions of the *Functional Symptoms*, *General Character*, *Sequence*, *Direction*, and *Sides*, are given under their respective rubrics, and in *these* collectives doubtful symptoms *only* are bracketed. In these collectives also, the principal one contains the less; thus under the general rubric "Eye to Face" are given all the medicines which have any variety of the above, *e.g.* "Eye to Lower Jaw," to make the collective complete; but, "Shooting from Eyeball to Lower Jaw" is given under the latter rubric only, and not under both. In the rubrics "Changing or Alternating in Character or Place in Eye," collectives as to the *varieties* of change of character or place are also given; thus we have collectives of "Eyeball then Orbit," "Heat then Shooting," &c., &c.

In the Rubrics "Right then Left," "Above then Below," and the reverse, Clinical symptoms are marked with an *asterisk*, to facilitate the application of Hering's Law of *Inverse Directions.*

To make the *Conditions* as useful as possible, we require to show (1) the conditions belonging to any symptom in the *whole body*; (2) those belonging to the *organ generally*; (3) those belonging to each *Anatomical Region*; (4) those belonging to each *variety of symptom* in the organ irrespective of the subregion to which it belongs; and (5) those belonging to *each symptom* separately. Thus, under the Rubric "By Reading" we have (1) the medicines found under this condition which have reference to *any* part of the body (this will be given in the General Chapter which will resemble Bœnninghausen's *Taschenbuch*); (2) those belonging to the *entire organ* which is the subject of each chapter; (3) those belonging to each *Anatomical Region*, *e.g.* Orbit; (4) those belonging to each *variety of symptom* in whatever subregion of the organ it may be; and (5) those belonging to *each individual symptom.* I have accordingly divided this Repertory into 17 chapters; the list of which will be found above where the groups of the Conditions are referred to.

In the last—the General—Chapter, the arrangement is similar to that of the preceding ones. First is the arrangement according to *Specific Character*, the medicines to which belong any *variety of symptom*, (*e.g.* Shooting) in *any* part of the body being arranged under their respective rubrics (as in Bœnninghausen's *Taschenbuch*); next comes the arrangement according to *Tissues* (*e.g.* Glands, Skin, Bones, Entire Body, &c). which corresponds to the Anatomical Regions of the preceding chapters; followed by *General Character Sequence* and *Direction*, *Right Side*, and *Left Side*, just as before. In the *Conditions* of this chapter the same rule is observed; thus, under aggravation "By Warmth" we have (1) a collective of all the medicines having aggravation of *any symptom* by warmth; (2) those having aggravation of any particular *variety of symptom* (*e.g.* Shooting) in *any* part of the body; (3) those having aggravation of any *Tissue* (*e.g.* Bones); and (4) those having aggravation of *any variety of symptoms in each of these tissues*. In this chapter *only* doubtful symptoms are bracketed.

With regard to the abbreviations of the names of the medicines, I have adopted an uniform and scientific method of cyphering, as it is quite time that such absurd names as Hepar Sulphuris, Alcohol Sulphuris, &c., be discarded for a more scientific nomenclature. The cyphers of the *elements* and *simple haloid salts* are the same as their *chemical symbols;* the *—ate* salts are cyphered by adding *—a*, and the *—ite* salts by adding *—i*, to the cyphers of the corresponding haloid salt. The *—ic* acids are cyphered by adding *—x*, the *—ous* acids adding *—ix*, and the *hydracids* by adding *—hx* to the cypher of the element or compound radical from which they are formed. Thus:

Na. = Sodium.	S. = Sulphur.
Na-s. = Sulphide of Sodium.	S-x. = Sulphuric acid.
Na-sa. = Sulphate of Sodium.	S-ix. = Sulphurous acid.
Na-si. = Sulphite of Sodium.	S-hx. = Sulphydric acid.

In the medicines derived from the Animal and Vegetable kingdoms, each genus is invariably expressed by a different cypher and by that only.

Hahnemann and Bœnninghausen insisted upon the necessity of having the medicines in a Repertory distinguished by *different types* to show their relative value, but hitherto such classification has been entirely arbitrary. The plan I propose is based entirely on the *provings*, not on the clinical experience of any one individual, and shows the relative frequency with which any symptom has been produced, compared with every other symptom of the Materia Medica.

This plan, however, cannot be satisfactorily carried out till we have a complete Materia Medica arranged like that of C. Hering, but I give it here for future adoption if thought useful. It is this—count the number of distinct *Pathogenetic* symptoms of each medicine obtained from *different* provers irrespective of their conditions or concomitants; those symptoms being considered distinct which are given as such in this Repertory. Thus if "Dilated Pupils" has been produced by a medicine on 20 *different* provers, it is counted as *twenty* symptoms; but if 20 times in the *same* prover, only as *one*, even though the conditions and concomitants should vary each time. Then if the total number of *provers* upon whom a symptom of any medicine has occured amounts to 1-25th of the total number of symptoms of the medicine obtained as stated above, the medicine producing that symptom is placed in the first rank, *Italic Capitals*; if from 1-50th to 1-25th, in the second rank, *Plain Capitals;* if from 1-75th to 1-50, in the third rank, *Italics;* if below 1-75rd in the fourth rank, *Roman Letters.* Clinical symptoms never rise above the fourth rank, and all *doubtful* symptoms are bracketed. The names of medicines enclosed in brackets for reference (as in the collectives of Specific Character) are invariably in *Roman letters.* In the *Conditions* the same rule is observed, as also in the Collectives of *Anatomical Regions*, *General Character*, *Sequence*, *Direction*, *Right Side*, and *Left Side;* the rank of the medicine being decided according to the number of *provers* whose symptoms refer to each respective rubric.

C. Hering's Materia Medica, which is the most complete in arrangement and execution of any yet published, has been used so far as it has extended (*i.e.* up to *Formica*) as the basis of this Repertory, but I have added some additional symptoms from later provings. I have also added many valuable symptoms from cases of poisoning, reported in the Allopathic Journals, which will in due time appear in the "Pathogenetic Record," now being published as an appendix to the British Journal of Homœopathy.

In order to illustrate the use of this Repertory, I give the two following cases from my own practice:*

CASE I.—Aug. 9, 1871. At 2 P.M., a child put its finger into its mother's left eye, scratching the upper part of eyeball; smarting in the eye followed, with heat, redness, and hot lachrymation; cannot open the eye from pain. Cold water applications relieve the pains and watering; the light of day increases the watering.

* As the selection of the remedy by means of the Repertory and Materia Medica is the *only* sure and scientific way of prescribing, it may not be inopportune to warn the public against the use of those very imperfect and deceptive works published under the names of "Domestic Homœopathy," &c. &c. In the first place, the plan of many of these works is entirely erroneous, the medicines being arranged *under the names of diseases*, and followed by their symptoms, instead of being arranged under *the symptoms*, as in the Repertory. Secondly, these works are often written by men possessed of very little knowledge of Homœopathy, who wish to gain notoriety by continually thrusting themselves upon the notice of the public by *popular* books, tracts, pamphlets, journals, &c.—a sort of "Homœopathy made Easy,"—the chief feature of which consists in the glorification of the author, and the vilification of Hahnemann and his *true* followers. Thirdly, they almost all encourage the public in that *curse* of homœopathy, the alternation of medicines; a method which is not only subversive of all *scientific* practice, but is, moreover, entirely opposed to the teachings of the inspired Hahnemann *from first to last*,—the apparent exceptions to this statement resting merely on perverted translations and mutilated quotations of his original works. To those who wish to practice Homœopathy scientifically, I can confidently recommend Simmons' Repertory on Cough, and Bell's Repertory on Diarrhœa and Dysentery, as most excellent. Fenton Cameron's pamphlet on "Imperfect Digestion, with an Appendix for those who desire to know the difference between True and Delusive Homœopathy," will best explain to the public the science of Homœopathy, and enable them to distinguish between its *true* practitioners and *pretenders*, of which latter class there are, unfortunately, many in the present day.

Diagnosis of the Remedy.

(As the symptoms arose from a mechanical cause, I did not consider the locality (*left* eye) as a characteristic of the case).

Page 290. **Relief from Cold.—Heat.** alo. amm-cl. (thu).
,, **Lachrymation.** al-o.
,, **Smarting.** al-o. n-x.

Page 293. **Relief from Washing.—Heat.** al-o. amm-cl. asr. k-na. (thu)
,, **Lachrymation.** al-o. asr. mg-ca.
,, **Smarting.** al-o. na-ca.

Page 175. **Worse from Natural Light.—Lachrymation.** al-o. bry. dig. dl-s. dt. eug. grp. k-bicra. kre. lyc. mg-cl. qu-sa. s-x. (str-i). vr-s. zn.

Thus *Alumina* alone corresponds to all these symptoms, and it will be found to have also Redness of eyes (page 16), Difficult opening of Eyelids (page 47) and Hot Lachrymation (page 24). Accordingly at 7 p.m., the symptoms having lasted five hours, I gave a single dose of *Alumina* C. M. (Fincke). In *fifteen minutes* all the symptoms were gone, except a little feeling of stiffness.

Case II.—November 6th. Three weeks ago, when blowing her nose, she felt as if something broke in the right eye, which watered much. Since then, at times, when blowing nose, has had a feeling as if a tight skin came half way down over right eye, preventing the sight of that eye; removed by rubbing. After it has gone, feeling as if something were pricking the eye; eye waters. On the last two occasions this sensation came on without blowing the nose.

Diagnosis of the Remedy.

Page 209. **By Blowing Nose. Sight Impaired.** k-o.
,, **Pellicle.** k-o.

As *Kali Oxidum (Causticum)* was the only medicine which possessed these most characteristic symptoms, and, moreover, corresponded to the remaining symptoms as a reference to the Repertory will show, I gave one dose of *Causticum* 6 m. (Jenichen).

Dec. 11. Reports that the symptoms ceased at once and did not return.

With these prefatory remarks, I give this work—the labour of many years—to the Homœopathic body, only asking that it may be *used*; and if others find it of as much service in the relief of suffering humanity as I have done, I shall feel amply repaid for all my trouble. Let me however, state here, that if we wish to obtain the *maximum* amount of benefit from Homœopathy, we can only do so by faithfully following the three great rules of the Master:—(1) The careful selection of the SIMILIMUM; not an *imperfectly homœopathic* remedy, or *allopathic palliative:* (2) the SINGLE REMEDY; all *mixing* of medicines, or *a priori alternation* or change of medicines *without* a corresponding alternation or change of the symptoms of the patient, being opposed to this law; and (3) the MINIMUM DOSE, which experience has shown to be a dose of one of the *highest potencies*, (repeated at such intervals as the case may require, till an improvement or medicinal aggravation sets in, and then allowed to act uninterruptedly so long as the patient improves, *without repetition of the dose or change of medicine*), PROVIDED ALWAYS *that the medicine be* PERFECTLY HOMŒOPATHIC *to the case.*

The volumes on the *Head* (including the Mental Group) and also on the *Ears* are being prepared, and will be published as soon as completed; whether I publish any more on the same plan, depends upon the encouragement I receive from the profession; I hope however, that others may be induced to take up the work, for to arrange the whole Materia Medica Repertorially, would alone occupy the lifetime of any one individual. I have spared no pains to make this work as accurate and complete as possible, both in execution and arrangement. To this end, I have examined all the English, French, and German Repertories which I could obtain, in order to combine all their excellences, at the same time excluding their defects. I have also endeavoured to extract the symptoms from the most reliable, and where possible the original, sources, thereby avoiding the many clerical and printer's errors which have crept into our Materia Medica. I cannot hope however to have avoided all these, and I shall feel grateful to any one who will point out any omission or error in this work, as it is my intention at the end of the third volume, (on the *Ears*) to print an Appendix, giving a list of the *errata* and *addenda* to all three volumes, thus bringing the entire work down to the date of the latest portion of it.

4, Highbury New Park,

London, N.

April, 1873.

SYNONYMS.

—o—

In this Table I have arranged under one rubric all the varieties of expression which *in practice* I have found to be synonymous. Hair-splitting distinction should be avoided in a Repertory, (though in the Materia Medica the *ipsissima verba* of the provers should be given), as different provers will often describe the same symptoms by different terms: conversely moreover, symptoms *verbally* the same may *actually* be different, according to their locality; thus *Pressing Out* in the *Head Generally* is equivalent to *Bursting;* in the *Forehead* to *Pressing Forwards;* in the *Occiput* to *Pressing Backwards;* in the *Vertex* to *Pressing Upwards,* &c.: all such symptoms I have arranged under their *real* not *verbal* rubrics.

Boring. Digging, Rooting.

Broken. Crushed, Demolished.

Bursting. Breaking, Expanding, Fulness, Pressing Asunder or Centrifugally, Torn Asunder, as if all would Come Out.

Coldness. Cool, Frozen, Icy, Subjective Coldness; (Objective Coldness is given separately as a variety.)

Contractive. Compressive, Constrictive, Grasping, Pinching, Pressing Centripetally, Screwed together, Squeezing.

Convulsions. Contortion, Distortion, Spasms, Twitches.

Crampy. Griping, Spasmodic.

Cutting. Acute, Sharp.

Drawing. Dragging, Pulling.

Heat. Burning, as if Burnt, Scalding, Warm, Subjective heat. (Objective Heat is given as a variety separately).

Itching. Irritation, Tickling.

Numbness. Deadness, Insensibility, Torpidity.

Paralysis. Weakness, Weariness.

Pressing. Aching, Forcing, Pushing.

Scraping. Grating, as if Rubbed.

Screwing. Twisting.

Shooting. Darting, Knife-thrusts, Lancinating, Penetrating, Piercing, Pricking, Sticking, Stitching, Stinging.

Smarting. Abscess-like, Biting, Corrosive, Eroding, Festering-like, Raw, Sore, Ulcerative.

Sprained. Dislocated.

Tensive. Stretching, Tight.

Throbbing. Beating, Blows, Hammering, Jerking, Pulsating, Shocks, Twitching.

Undefined. Dull, Congestive, Neuralgic, Rheumatic, and all other vaguely described pains.

LIST OF MEDICINES.

—o—

1 a. acetyl
2 a-x. aceticum acidum
3 ac-s. actæa spicata
4 aca. acacia catechu
5 acan. acanthus mollis
6 ach. achillea millefolium
7 acl. acalypha indica
8 aco. aconitinum
9 acon. aconitum napellus
10 acon-c. ,, cammarum
11 acon-f. ,, ferox
12 acon-l. ,, lycoctonum
13 ada adamas
14 adi. adianthum aureum
15 ægl. ægle marmelos
16 ægo. ægopodium podagraria
17 æsc. æsculus hippocastanum
18 æsc-g. ,, glabra
19 æth. æthusa cynapium
20 ag. argentum metallicum
21 ag-cl. ,, chloridum
22 ag-cy. ,, cyanidum
23 ag-i. ,, iodidum
24 ag-na. ,, nitricum
25 ag-o. ,, oxidum
26 ag-pa. ,, phosphoricum
27 aga. agaricus muscarius
28 aga-b. ,, bulbosus
29 aga-c. ,, campanulatus
30 aga-ca. ,, cacumenatus
31 aga-cm ,, campestris
32 aga-e. ,, emeticus
33 aga-g. ,, glutinosus
34 aga-p. ,, procerus
35 aga-pi. ,, piperitidis
36 aga-v. ,, verrucosus
37 agr. agrostema githago
38 agv. agave americana
39 ail. ailanthus glandulosa
40 aju. ajuga reptans
41 al. aluminium metallicum
42 al-cl. ,, chloridum
43 al-o. ,, oxidum(alumina)
44 ali. alisma plantago
45 all. allyl.
46 allyl. allylia
47 alli. allium cepa
48 alli-p. ,, porrum
49 alli-s. ,, sativum
50 alm. alumen. (potash-alum)
51 aln. alnus rubra
52 aln-s. ,, serratula
53 alo. aloes
54 alp. alpinia galanga
55 als. alstonia scholaris
56 alsi. alsine media
57 alt. aletris farinosa
58 alth. althæa
59 am. amyl
60 am-a. ,, aceticum
61 am-alc. ,, alcohol
62 am-gly. ,, glycol.
63 am-na-alc. ,, sodium alcohol
64 am-ni. ,, nitrosum
65 am-o. ,, ether
66 am-zn. ,, zinc
67 amar. amaranthus communis
68 amb. ambra grisea
69 amm-a. ammonium aceticum
70 amm-br. ,, bromidum
71 amm-bz. ,, benzoicum
72 amm-ca. ,, carbonicum
73 amm-cl. ,, chloridum
74 amm-ct. ,, citricum
75 amm-i. ,, iodidum
76 amm-pa. ,, phosphoricum
77 amm-s. ,, sulphuratum
78 amm-sc. ,, succinicum
79 amm-t. ,, tartaricum
80 ammon. ammonia
81 amn-c. anamirta citrina
82 amo. amomum cardamomum
83 amp. ampelopsis quinquefolium
84 amph. amphisbæna vermicularis
85 amy. amygdalæ amaræ
86 amyl. amylia
87 amyl-sa. ,, sulphurica
88 amylen. amylene
89 amyr. amyris gileadensis
90 ana. anagyris fætida

91 anac. anacardium occidentale
92 anacy. anacyclus officinarum
93 anacy-p. ,, pyrethrum
94 anag. anagellis arvensis
95 anan. anantherum muricatum
96 and. andira inermis
97 ane. anemone nemorose
98 anem. anemorrhena asphodeloides
99 aneth. anethum graveolens
100 ang. angelica archangelica
101 ani. anisodus luridus
102 ank. anthrokokali
103 anm. anamirta cocculus (cocculus indicus)
104 anth. anthemis nobilis
105 anthr. anthroxanthum odoratum
106 anthra. anthracite
107 antiar. antiaria toxicaria
108 ap. apium graveolens
109 aph. aphis chenopodium glaucum
110 apo. apocynum cannabinum
111 apo-a. ,, androsemifolium
112 aps. apis mellifica
113 aqui. aquilegia vulgaris
114 ara. aranea domestica
115 ara-d. ,, diadema
116 ara-s. ,, scinensia
117 arc. arctium lappa
118 arct. arctostophylos uva ursi
119 are. areca catechu
120 arch. archangelica officinalis
121 arg. argemone mexicana
122 argas. argas persicus
123 ari. aristolochia milhomens
124 ari-c. ,, clematitis
125 ari-s. ,, serpentaria
126 arl. aralia racemosa
127 arma. armadillo vulgaris
128 arn. arnica montana
129 art. artemisia vulgaris
130 art-a. ,, absinthium
131 art-v. ,, vahliana (cina)
132 artan. artanthe elongata
133 arum. arum maculatum
134 arum-t. ,, triphyllum
135 arun. arundo donax
136 arun-m. ,, mauritanica
137 as. arsenicum metallicum
138 as-h. arsenicum hydrogenisatum
139 as-i. ,, iodidum
140 as-o. ,, oxidum (album)
141 as-s. ,, sulphuratum
142 as-ters. ,, tersulphuratum
143 asag. asagræa officinalis
144 asc. asclepias tuberosa
145 asc-c. ,, currasavica
146 asc-g. asclepias gigantea
147 asc-i. ,, incarnata
148 asc-s. ,, syriaca
149 asc-v. ,, vincetoxicum
150 ask. askalabotes lævigatus
151 asp. asparagus officinalis
152 asper. asperula adorata
153 aspid. aspidium filix mas
154 asr. asarum europæum
155 asr-c. ,, canadense
156 ast. astacus fluviatilis
157 ath. athamanta oreoselinum
158 atp. atropa belladonna
159 atp-m. ,, mandragora
160 atr. atriplex
161 atrac. atractylis gummifera
162 atrop. atropinum
163 atrop-sa. ,, sulphuricum
164 au. aurum metallicum
165 au-cl. ,, chloridum
166 au-f. ,, fulminans
167 au-na-cl. ,, et natrum chloridum
168 au-o. ,, oxidum
169 aza. azalea procumbens
170 b. boron
171 b-x. boracicum acidum
172 ba-a. baryta acetica
173 ba-ca. ,, carbonica
174 ba-cl. ,, chlorida
175 ba-i. ,, iodida
176 bal. ballota lanata
177 bals. balsamodendron myrrha
178 bap. baptisia tinctoria
179 bar. baryosma tongo
180 be. beryllium
181 ber. berberis vulgaris
182 bgn. bignonia
183 bi. bismuthum metallicum
184 bi-cl. ,, chloridum
185 bi-na. ,, subnitricum
186 bi-v. ,, valerianicum
187 bid. bidens parviflora
188 bll. bellis perennis
189 blt. blatta americana
190 bnz. benzine
191 boa. boa crotaloides
192 bol. boletus suaveolens
193 bol-l. ,, laricis
194 bol-s. ,, satanas
195 bom. bombus
196 bothr. bothrops lanceolatus
197 br. brominum
198 br-x. bromicum acidum
199 bra. brayera anthelmintica
200 brf. bromoformum

201 brg. borago officinalis
202 brom. bromal
203 brs. brassica napus
204 bru. brucea antidysenterica
205 bruc. brucia
206 bruc-na. ,, nitrica
207 bry. bryonia alba
208 bry-d. ,, dioica
209 btl. betula alba
210 btn. betonia
211 bu. butyl (tetryl)
212 buf. bufo rana
213 buf-s. ,, sahytiensis
214 bung. bungarus lineatus
215 but. butea frondosa
216 bux. buxus sempervirens
217 bz. benzoyl
218 bz-x. benzoicum acidum
219 c-bicl. carbo bichloridum
220 c-bis. ,, bisulphuratum
221 c-h. ,, hydrogenisatum
222 c-o. ,, oxidum
223 c-tetracl. ,, tetrachloridum
224 c-x. ,, acidum
225 ca-a. ,, calcarea acetica
226 ca-asa. ,, arsenica
227 ca-ca. ,, carbonica
228 ca-cl. ,, chlorida
229 ca-f. ,, fluorida
230 ca-i. ,, iodida
231 ca-o. ,, oxida (caustica)
232 ca-pa. ,, phosphorica
233 ca-s. ,, sulphurata(hepar)
234 cac. cactus grandiflorus
235 cal. calla æthiopica
236 calth. caltha palustris
237 can. cannabis sativa
238 can-i. ,, indica
239 cap. capsicum annuum
240 cap-j. ,, jamaicum
241 car. carica alba
242 car-p. ,, papaya
243 carum. carum carui
244 cary. caryophyllus aromaticus
245 cast. castoreum
246 castor. castor equorum
247 cau. caullophyllum thalictroides
248 cb-a. carbo animalis
249 cb-v. ,, vegetabilis
250 cbz-x. carbazoticum acidum
251 cch. colchicum autumnale
252 ccn. coccionella septem-punctata
253 ccs. coccus cacti
254 cd. cadmium metallicum
255 cd-ca. ,, carbonicum
256 cd-cl. ,, chloridum
257 cd-i. cadmium iodidum
258 cd-sa. ,, sulphuricum
259 ce. cerium metallicum
260 ce-ox. ,, oxalicum
261 cer. cerastes
262 cetr. cetraria islandica
263 chæ. chærophyllum temulum
264 chd. chelidonium majus
265 che. chelone glabra
266 chi. china officinalis
267 chio. chiococca racemosa (cainca)
268 chlor. chloral
269 chm. chimaphila umbellata
270 chp. chenopodium vulvaria (atriplex olida)
271 chp-a. ,, anthelminticum
272 chp-am. ,, ambrosioides
273 chp-b. ,, botrys
274 chv. chavica roxburghii
275 chv-b. ,, betel
276 cic. cicuta virosa
277 cic-m. ,, maculata
278 cic-t. ,, tenuifolia
279 cich. cichorium intybus
280 cis. cistus canadensis
281 cit-c. citrullus colocynthis
282 citr. citrus limomum
283 cl. chlorinum
284 cl-hx. chlorhydricum (muriaticum) acidum
285 clb coluber berus
286 cld. caladium seguinum
287 cle. clematis erecta
288 clf. chloroformum
289 cll. collinsonia canadensis
290 clm. calamus aromaticus
291 clotho. clotho arietans
292 cln. calendula officinalis
293 clt. callotropis procera
294 clt-g. ,, gigantea
295 clv. claviceps purpurea(secale)
296 cmc. comocladia dentata
297 cmf. cimicifuga racemosa
298 cmx. cimex lectularius
299 cn. cinchoninum
300 cn-cl. ,, chloridum
301 cn-sa. ,, sulphuricum
302 cnm. cinnamonium zeylandicum
303 cnn. canna angustifolia
304 cnv. convolvulus arvensis
305 cnv-d. ,, duartinus
306 cnv-s. ,, scammoniæ
307 co. cobaltum metallicum
308 coc. cocculus palmatus
309 cochl. cochlearia armoracia
310 cod. codeinum

311 cof. coffea arabica
312 con. conium maculatum
313 conv. convallaria majalis
314 cop. copaifera multijuga
315 cor. corallia rubra
316 cori. coriaria myrtifolia
317 cori-r. „ ruscifolia
318 corian. coriandrum sativum
319 cory. corydalis formosa
320 cos. costus dulcis
321 cot. cotyledon umbilicus
322 cp. capryl.
323 cpo. caproyl
324 cph. cephaelis ipecacuanha
325 cr. chromicum metallicum
326 cr-o. „ oxidum
327 cr-x. „ acidum
328 cra. cratægus
329 crb-x. carbolicum acidum
330 crd. carduus benedictus
331 crd-m. „ marianus
332 crn. cornus cincinata
333 crn-f. „ florida
334 crn-s. „ sericea
335 cro. crocus sativus
336 crot. croton tiglium
337 crot-c. „ eluteria
338 crp. carapa touloucoma
339 crs. cerasus virginiana
340 crt. crotalus horridus
341 crt-c. „ cascavella
342 crt-co. „ confluentus
343 crt-d. „ durissus
344 crv. cervus braziliensis
345 cs. cæsium metallicum
346 csm. cissampelos pareira
347 css. cassia lanceolata
348 css-f. „ fistula
349 ct-x. citricum acidum
350 cth. cantharis vesicatoria
351 ctn. cetonia aurata
352 ctr. citrallus chinensis
353 cu. cuprum metallicum
354 cu-a. „ aceticum
355 cu-asi. „ arsenicum
356 cu-ca. „ carbonicum
357 cu-sa. „ sulphuricum
358 cub. cubebæ
359 cuc. cucurbita pepo
360 cum. cuminum cyminum
361 cund. cundurango
362 cup. cupressus sempervirens
363 cus. cuscuta europæa
364 cy. cyanogen
365 cy-hx. cyanhydricum acidum
366 cyc. cyclamen europæum
367 cyn. cynanchum argel
368 cynob. cynobatus
369 cynog. cynoglossum officinale
370 cyp. cypripedium pubescens
371 cyper. cyperus rotundus
372 cypr. cyprinus barbus
373 cyt. cytisus laburnum
374 cyt-s. „ scoparius
375 delph. delphinus amazonicus
376 di. didymium metallicum
377 dic. dictamnus albus
378 dichr. dichroa febrifuga
379 dig. digitalis purpurea
380 dig-l. „ lutea
381 dim. dimorephanthus edulis
382 dio. dioscorea villosa
383 dios. diosma fœtida
384 dios-c. „ crenata
385 dl-s. delphinium staphysagria
386 dlp. delphininum
387 dol. dolichos pruriens
388 dor. doryphora decemlineata
389 dph. daphne mezereum
390 dph-i. „ indica
391 dph-l. „ laureola
392 dps. dipsacus sylvestris
393 dpt. dipterix odorata
394 dra. dracontium fœtidum
395 dra-p. „ polyphyllum
396 drm. dorema ammoniacum
397 dro. drosera rotundifolia
398 dry. dryobalanops camphora
399 dt. datura stramonium
400 dt-a. „ alba
401 dt-ar. „ arborea
402 dt-f. „ ferox
403 dt-fa. „ fastuosa
404 dt-m. „ metel
405 dt-s. „ sanguinea
406 dt-t. „ tatula
407 eb. erbium metallicum
408 ecb. ecbalium officinarum
409 ech. echites suberecta
410 elæ. elæagnus angustifolia
411 elaps. elaps corallinus
412 ele. eleis guineensis
413 elet. elettaria cardamomum
414 elp. elaphrium elemiferum
415 elt. elater noctulicus
416 epg. epigæa repens
417 equi. equisetum arvense
418 erc. erica vulgaris
419 erech. erechthites hieracifolius
420 erig. erigonon canadense
421 ero. erodium cicutarium
422 eru. eruca
423 erv. ervum ervilia
424 ery. erythroxylon coca
425 eryn. eryngium aquaticum

426 erys. erysimum officinale
427 eryth. erythræa chilensis (canchalagua)
428 erythr. erythrophlæum judiciale
429 et-fr. ethyl formiatum (formic ether)
430 et-o. ethyl oxidum (ether)
431 eug. eugenia iambos
432 eug-p. ,, pimenta
433 eup. eupion
434 eupat. eupatorium perfoliatum
435 eupat-a. ,, aromaticum
436 eupat-c. ,, cannabinum
437 eupat-p. ,, purpureum
438 euph. euphorbia officinarum
439 euph-a. ,, amydaloides
440 euph-c. ,, corollata
441 euph-cy. ,, cyparissias
442 euph-e. ,, esula
443 euph-h. ,, helioscopia
444 euph-i. ,, ipecacuanha
445 euph-l. ,, lathyris
446 euph-p. ,, peplus
447 euph-s. ,, splendens
448 euph-v. ,, villosa
449 euphr. euphrasia officinalis
450 evo. evonymus europæus
451 evo-a. ,, atropurpureus
452 exo. exogonium purga (jalappa)
453 f-hx. fluorhydricum acidum
454 fag. fagus
455 fe. ferrum metallicum
456 fe-a. ,, aceticum
457 fe-asi. ,, arseniosum
458 fe-ca. ,, carbonicum
459 fe-cl. ,, chloridum
460 fe-cy. ,, cyanidum
461 fe-i. ,, iodidum
462 fe-l. ,, lacticum
463 fe mgs. ,, magneticum
464 fe-pa. ,, phosphoricum
465 fe-s. ,, sulphuratum
466 fe-sa. ,, sulphuricum
467 fe-t. ,, tartaricum
468 fel. fel tauri
469 fel-v. ,, vulpis
470 fer. ferula officinalis
471 fer-g. ,, glauca (bounafa)
472 flg. fuligo
473 fmr. fumaria officinalis
474 fœn. fœniculum vulgare
475 fœn-d. ,, dulce
476 fr-x. formicum acidum
477 frg. fragraria vesca
478 frm. formica rufa
479 frm-o. ,, omnivora
480 frm-s. ,, subsericea
481 frn. franciscea uniflora
482 frs. frasera carolinensis
483 frx. fraxinus
484 fu-v. fucus vesiculosus
485 ga-x. gallicum acidum
486 gad. gadus morrhuæ
487 gal. galium aparine
488 gale. galeopsis ochroleuca
489 gau. gaultheria procumbens
490 gel. gelseminum sempervirens
491 gettys. gettysburg
492 geum. geum rivale
493 geum-u. ,, urbane
494 gl. glucinum
495 glan. glanderinum
496 glb. galbanum officinale
497 glech. glechoma hederaceum
498 glo. glonoinum
499 glp. galipea cusparia. (augustura)
500 gn-c. gentiana cruciata
501 gn-l. ,, lutea
502 gna. gnaphalium polycephalum
503 gna-a. ,, arenarium
504 gna-m. ,, margaritaceum
505 gns. genista tinctoria
506 grc. garcinia morella (gamboge)
507 grc-c. ,, elliptica
508 gri. grindelia robusta
509 grn. geranium maculatum
510 grn-d. ,, dissectum
511 grn-o. ,, odoratum
512 grn-r. ,, robertianum
513 grp. graphites
514 grt. gratiola officinalis
515 grs. gossypium herbaceum
516 gua. guano
517 guar. guarea trichilioides
518 gui. guiacum officinale
519 gym. gymnocladus canadensis
520 gyn. gynocardia odorata
521 hæm. hæmatoxylon campechianum
522 ham. hamamelis virginica
523 hdm. hedeoma pulegioides
524 hed. hedysarum ildefonsianum
525 hel. helianthus
526 heli. helianthemum vulgare
527 helo. heloella esculenta
528 hem. hemisdesmus indicus
529 hg. mercurius (hydrargyrum) metallicus

530 hg-a. mercurius aceticus
531 hg-am-cl. „ ammonio-chloridus
532 hg-bibr. „ bibromidus
533 hg-bicl. „ bichloridus
534 hg-bini. „ biniodidus
535 hg-br. „ bromidus
536 hg-cla. „ chloratus
537 hg-cl. „ chloridus
538 hg-cy. „ cyanidus
539 hg-i. „ iodidus
540 hg-me. „ methidus (mercuric methide)
541 hy-o. „ oxidus
542 hg-pa. „ phosphoricus
543 hg-s. „ sulphuratus (cinnabar)
544 hg-sa. „ sulphuricus
545 hier. hieraceum pilosella
546 hier-u. „ umbellatum
547 hll. helleborus niger
548 hll-f. „ fœtidus
549 hlm. helminthocortos officinarum
550 hln. helonias dioica
551 hln-e. „ erythrosperma
552 hlt. heliotropum peruvianum
553 hlx. helix pomatia
554 hom. homeria collinea
555 hpm. hippomane mancinella
556 hpp. hippomanes
557 hpt. hepatica triloba
558 hrc. heracleum spondylium
559 hrn. herniaria glabra
560 hum. humulus lupulus
561 hur. hura braziliensis
562 hur-c. „ crepitans
563 hyd. hydrocotyle asiatica
564 hydr. hydrastis canadensis
565 hydro. hydrophobinum
566 hydrus. hydrus colubrinus
567 hyo. hyoscyamus niger
568 hyo-a. „ albus
569 hyo-s. „ scopolia
570 hyp. hypericum perfoliatum
571 hyp-p. „ pulcrum
572 hypoph. hypophyllum sanguineum
573 i. iodinum
574 if iodoform
575 ilex. ilex aquifolium
576 ilex-p. „ paraguaensis
577 ill. illicium anisatum
578 imp. imperatoria ostruthinum
579 in. indium metallicum
580 ind. indigo
581 inu. inula helenium
582 ipo. ipomæa jalappa
583 ir. iridium metallicum
584 irs. iris versicolor
585 irs-f. „ fœtidissimus
586 irs-g. „ germanicus
587 irs-ps. „ pseudacoras
588 irs-t. „ tricolor
589 itu. itu resina
590 jan. janipha manihot
591 jat. jatropha curcas
592 jat-m. „ multifida
593 jat-u. „ urens
594 jcr. jacaranda caroba
595 jnc. juncus effusus
596 jnc-p. „ pilosus
597 jnp. juniperus communis
598 jnp-s. „ sabina
599 jnp-v. „ virginiana
600 jug. juglans regia
601 jug-c. „ cinerea
602 jus. justicia adhatoda
603 k-a. kali aceticum
604 k-asa. „ arsenicum
605 k-asi. „ arseniosum
606 k-bica „ bicarbonicum
607 k-bicra. „ bichromicum
608 k-br. „ bromidum
609 k-ca. „ carbonicum
610 k-cl. „ chloridum
611 k cla. „ chloricum
612 k-cra. „ chromicum
613 k-cy. „ cyanidum
614 k-ct. „ citricum
615 k-fcy. „ ferrocyanidum
616 k-i. „ iodidum
617 k-mna. „ manganicum
618 k-na. „ nitricum
619 k-o. „ oxidum (causticum)
620 k-ox. „ oxalicum
621 k-permna. „ permanganicum
622 k-sa. „ sulphuricum
623 k-scy. „ sulphocyanidum
624 k-sia. „ silicatum
625 k-t. „ tartaricum
626 kao. kaolin
627 kd. kakodyl
628 kd-o. „ oxidum
629 kis. kissengen
630 klm. kalmia latifolia
631 kre. kreasotum
632 kreu. kreutznach
633 krm. krameria triandra (ratanhia)
634 l-x. lacticum acidum
635 la. lanthanium metallicum
636 lac. lac vaccinum
637 lac-b. „ „ butyrum
638 lac-bu. „ „ butyraceum
639 lac-c. „ caninnm

640 lac-cg. ,, vaccinum coagulum
641 lac-cs. ,, ,, caseum
642 lac-d. ,, ,, defloratum
643 lac-f. ,, felinum
644 lac-fl ,, vaccinum flos
645 lac-sr. ,, ,, serum
646 lam. lamium album
647 lap. lapathium acutum
648 lau-c. laurus camphora
649 lava. lava (Heckla)
650 lch. lachnanthes tinctoria
651 lcp. lycopus virginianus
652 lcp-e. ,, europæus
653 lcr. lacerta agilis
654 lct. lactuca virosa
655 led. ledum palustu
656 lgs. ligustrum vulgare
657 li-ca. lithium carbonicum
658 li-cl. ,, chloridum
659 lich. ,, vulgaris
660 lil. lilium candidum
661 lil-a. ,, album
662 lil-t. ,, tigrinum
663 lin. linum catharticum
664 lir. liriodendron tulipifera
665 lmx. limax ater
666 lnc. lonicera xylosteum
667 lnr. linaria vulgaris
668 lo-c. lobelia cardinalis
669 lo-cœ. ,, cœrulea
670 lo-i. ,, inflata
671 loa. loasa tricolor
672 lol. lolium temulentum
673 lpd. lepidium bonarense
674 lpt. leptandria virginica
675 lth. lathyrus sativus
676 lth-o. ,, odoratus
677 lvn. lavandula vera
678 lvs. levisticum officinale
679 ly-b. lycoperdon bovista
680 lyc. lycopodium clavatum
681 lyc-s. ,, selago
682 lyci. lycium berberis
683 lys. lysimachia nummularia
684 mam. mammæa americana
685 mar. marchantia polymorpha
686 me. methyl
687 med. medusa
688 meli. melilotus officinalis
689 meli-a. ,, albus
690 melia. melia azediracta
691 melis. melissa officinalis
692 melo. melolontha vulgaris
693 meloe. meloe majalis
694 men. menyanthes trifoliata
695 meni. menispermum canadanse
696 meni-c. ,, cordifolium
697 menth. mentha pulegium
698 menth-a. ,, aquatica
699 menth-p. ,, piperita
700 menth-v. ,, viridis
701 mg. magnesium metallicum
702 mg-ca. ,, carbonicum
703 mg-cl. ,, chloridum
704 mg-sa. ,, sulphuricum
705 mgs. magnes
706 mgs-ar. ,, arcticus
707 mgs-au. ,, australis
708 mgn. magnolia glauca
709 mik. mikania guaco
710 mim. mimosa humulis
711 mitch. mitchella repens
712 mll. melaleuca minor (cajeput)
713 mll-h. ,, hypericifolia
714 mls. melastoma ackermani
715 mn. manganum metallicum
716 mn-a. ,, aceticum
717 mn-ca. ,, carbonicum
718 mn-o. ,, oxidum
719 mn-sa. ,, sulphuricum
720 mnr. monarda didyma
721 mo. molybdenum metallicum
722 mo-s. ,, sulphuratum
723 mo-x. ,, acidum
724 mom. momordica balsamica
725 mon. monotropa uniflora
726 morph. morphium
727 morph-a. ,, aceticum
728 morph-cl ,, chloridum
729 morph-sa ,, sulphuricum
730 mph. mephites putorius
731 mrl. mercurialis perennis
732 mrr. marrhubium vulgare
733 mrx. murex purpurea
734 msc. moschus
735 msm. mesambryanthemum chrysanthemum
736 mth. methonica gloriosa
737 mtr. matricaria chamomilla
738 mur. murure leite
739 myg. mygale lasiodora cubana
740 myg-a. ,, avicularia
741 myo. myosurus minimus
742 myr. myrica cerifera
743 myro. myrospermum
744 myrox. myroxylon peruiferum
745 myrt. myrtus communis
746 myris. myristica officinalis (nux moschata)
747 myris-s. ,, sebifera
748 myris-t. ,, tomentosa
749 n-o. nitrogen oxidum
750 n-x. nitricum acidum

751 na-asa. natrum arsenicum
752 na-asi. ,, arseniosum
753 na-ba. ,, biboracicum (borax)
754 na-br. ,, bromidum
755 na-ca. ,, carbonicum
756 na-cl. ,, chloridum
757 na-hpa. ,, hypophosphoricum
758 na-i. ,, iodidum
759 na-na. ,, nitricum
760 na-o. ,, oxidum
761 na-pa. ,, phosphoricum
762 na-sa. ,, sulphuricum
763 na-sc. ,, succinicum
764 na-si. ,, sulphurosum
765 naj. naja tripudians
766 naph. napthalinum
767 narc. narcissus pseudo-narcissus
768 narth. narthex asafœtida
769 nb. niobium metallicum
770 nbl. nabulus serpentaria
771 nct. nectandra rodiæi
772 nct-p. ,, puchury major (pichurim)
773 ner. nerium oleander
774 ner-a. ,, antidysentericum
775 ngl. nigella sativa
776 ngl-d. ,, damascena
777 ni. niccolum metallicum
778 ni-ca. ,, carbonicum
779 nic. nicotiana tabacum
780 nitro-bnz. nitro-benzine
781 no. norium metallicum
782 nrc. narcotinum
783 nrc-a. ,, aceticum
784 nrc-cl. ,, chloridum
785 nst. nasturtium officinale
786 nst-a. ,, aquaticum
787 nuph. nuphar lutea
788 nym. nymphæa odorata
789 oci. ocimum canum
790 œn. œnanthyl
791 œna. œnantha crocata
792 œna-a. ,, apifolia
793 œno. œnothera biennis
794 oid. oidium
795 ol-a. oleum animale
796 ol-m. ,, morrhuæ
797 ol-t. ,, terebinthinæ
798 oni. oniscus asellus
799 ono. ononis arvensis
800 oph. ophelia chiretta
801 opo. opoponax chironicum
802 org. orgianum majorana
803 ori. origanum vulgare
804 oro. orobanche virginiana
805 os. osmium metallicum
806 os-bino. osmium binoxidum
807 os-x. ,, acidum
808 ost. ostrya virginica
809 ott. ottonia anisum
810 ox-x. oxalicum acidum
811 oxl. oxalis acitosella
812 ozæ. ozænin
813 p. phosphorus
814 p-h. ,, hydrogenisatus
815 p-x. phosphoricum acidum
816 pæo. pæonia officinalis
817 pan. panacea
818 pap. papaya vulgaris
819 par. paris quadrifolia
820 pass. passerina chamædaphne
821 pau. paullinia pinnata
822 pau-s. ,, sorbilis
823 pav. pavia ohio
824 pb. plumbum metallicum
825 pb-a. ,, aceticum
826 pb-bini. ,, biniodium
827 pb-ca. ,, carbonicum
828 pb-cra. ,, chromicum
829 pb-i. ,, iodidum
830 pb-na. ,, nitricum
831 pc-x. picricum acidum
832 pcr. picræna excelsa
833 pd. palladium metallicum
834 pe. pelopium metallicum
835 ped. pediculus capitis
336 pet. petroleum
837 peu. peucedaneum officinale
838 phen-h. phenyl hydride (benzol)
839 phenyl. phenylia (aniline)
840 phenyl-sa. phenylia sulphurica
841 phil. philadelphus coronarius
842 phl. phellandrium aquaticum
843 phlo. phlomis esculenta
844 phs. phaseolus angulatus
845 phy. phytolacca decandra
846 phys. physalis
847 physo. physostigma venenosum
848 picro. picrotoxin
849 pim. pimpernella saxifraga
850 pim-a. ,, anisum
851 pin. pinus sylvestris
852 pin-a. ,, abies
853 pip. piper niger
854 pip-m. ,, methysticum
855 pist. pistachia vera
856 plb. plumbago littoralis
857 plb-e. ,, europæa
858 plc. plectranthus fruticosus
859 plg. polygonum hydropiper
860 plg-a. ,, amphibium
861 plg-m. ,, maritimum

862 plm. polemonium cæruleum
863 pln. plantago major
864 pln-l. „ lanceolata
865 plp. polyporus officinalis
866 pnc. punica granatum
867 pnx. panex ginseng
868 pnx-q. „ quinquefolium
.869 pod. podophyllum peltatum
870 pog. pogostemon patchouli
871 pol. polygala senega
872 pol-a. „ amara
873 pop. populus tremuloides
874 ppv. papaver somniferum (opium)
875 ppv-d. „ dubium
876 ppv-r. „ rhœas
877 prd. pardanthus chinensis
878 prf. paraffin
879 prin. prinos verticillatus
880 prm. primula vera
881 prn. prenanthus
882 prs. persica vulgaris
883 prt. portulaca
884 pru. prunus domestica
885 pru-l. „ laurocerasus
886 pru-m. „ mahelep
887 pru-p. „ padus
888 pru-sp. „ spinosa
889 prun. prunella vulgaris
890 psboa. pseudoboa fasciata
891 psc. piscidia erythrina
892 pso. psoricum
893 psr. psoralea bituminosa
894 pst. pastinaca sativa
895 psy. psycotria emetica
896 pt. platinum metallicum
897 pt-cl. „ chloridum
898 pt-i. „ iodidum
899 pth. pothos fœtidus
900 ptl. ptelea trifoliata
901 ptm. potamageton natans
902 ptn. potentilla tormentilla
903 ptn-a. „ aurea
904 ptn-r. „ reptans
905 ptr. pterocarpus marsupium
906 pts. petroselinum sativum
907 ptv. petiveria tetrandra
908 pul. pulsatilla nigricans
909 pul-n. „ nuttaliana
910 pulm. pulmonaria vulgaris
911 pulmo. pulmo vulpis
912 pup. pupalia geniculata
913 qu. quinia
914 qu-asa. „ arsenica
915 qu-bicl. „ bichlorida
916 qu-cy. „ cyanida
917 qu-pa. „ phosphorica
918 qu-sa. „ sulphurica
919 quas. quassia amara
920 raph. raphanistrum arvense
921 rb. rubidium metallicum
922 rbn. robinia pseudo-acacia
923 rehm. rhemannia chinensis
924 rh. rhodium metallicum
925 rhe. rheum palmatum
926 rhm. rhamnus catharticus
927 rhm-f. „ frangula
928 rho. rhododendron chrysanthemum
929 ric. ricinus communis
930 rmx. rumex crispus
231 rmx-a. „ acetosella
932 rmx-p. „ patientia
933 rn-a. ranunculus acris
934 rn-b. „ bulbosus
935 rn-f. „ flammula
936 rn-fi. „ ficaria
937 rn-g. „ glacialis
938 rn-r. „ repens
939 rn-s. „ sceleratus
940 rosa. rosa canins
941 rosa-c. „ centifolia
942 rs. rhus toxicodendron
943 rs-g. „ glabrum
944 rs-l. „ laurina
945 rs-r. „ radicans
946 rs-v. „ veneneta
947 rs-vx. „ vernix
948 rsm. rosmarinus officinalis
949 rtt. rottleria tinctoria
950 ru. ruthenium metallicum
951 rubi. rubia officinarum
952 rud. rudbeckia hirta
953 rut. ruta graveolens
954 s. sulphur
955 s-h. „ hydrogenisatum
956 s-i. „ iodidum
957 s-o. „ oxidum
958 s-x. sulphuricum acidum
959 sa-a. seccharum album
960 sa-l. „ lactis
961 sa-mgs. „ „ odo-magneticum
962 sang. sanguinaria canadensis
963 sant. santalum album
964 sas. sassafras officinalis
965 sb. antimonium metallicum (stibium)
966 sb-asa. „ arsenicum
967 sb-asi. „ arseniosum
968 sb-cl. „ chloridum
969 sb-o. „ oxidum
970 sb-s. „ sesquisulphuratum (crudum)
971 sb-t. „ tartaricum (tartar emetic)

972 sbc-x. sebacicum acidum
973 scol. scolopendron heros
974 scor. scorpio europæus
975 scp. scoparia
976 scr. scrofularia nodosa
977 scr-m. „ marilandica
978 scu. scutellaria laterifolia
979 se. selenium metallicum
980 sed. sedinha
981 sedum. sedum acre
982 sedum-t. „ telephium
983 sep. sepia officinalis
984 si. silicium metallicum
985 si-cl. „ chloridum
986 si-x. „ acidum (silica)
987 silph. silphium laciniatum
988 sld. solidago virgaurea
989 slm. salamandra maculata
990 slv. salvia officinalis
991 slx. salix alba
992 slx-p. „ purpurea
993 smb. sambucus nigra
994 smb-e. „ ebulus
995 smc. semecarpus anacardium (anacardium orientale)
996 smi. smilax officinalis (sarsaparilla)
997 smi-a. „ aspera
998 smp. sempervivum tectorum
999 smr. simaruba cedron
1000 sn. stannum metallicum
1001 sn-cl. „ chloridum
1002 snc. senecio aureus
1003 snc-o. „ obovatus
1004 sng. sanguisorba officinalis
1005 snp. sinapis alba
1006 snp-n. „ nigra
1007 snt. santoninum.
1008 so-a. solanum arrabenta
1009 so-d. „ dulcamara
1010 so-l. „ lycopersicon
1011 so-m. „ mammosum
1012 so-n. „ nigrum.
1013 so-ps. „ pseudo-capsicum
1014 so-t. „ tuberosum
1015 so-t-æg „ „ ægrotans
1016 so-v. „ vesiculosum
1017 spar. spartium scoparium
1018 spg. spiggurus martini
1019 sph. sophora japonica
1020 spi. spigelia anthelmintica
1021 spi-m „ marilandica
1022 spil. spilanthes oleracea
1023 spir. spiranthes autumnalis
1024 spo. spongia tosta
1025 spo-f. „ fluviatilis (badiaga)
1026 spr. spiræa ulmaria
1027 sr. strontiana metallica
1028 sr-ca. „ carbonica
1029 sr-cl. „ chlorida
1030 srb. sorbus aucuparia
1031 srr. sarracenia purpurea
1032 stach. stachys betonica
1033 stach-r. „ recta
1034 stc. sticta pulmonaria
1035 ster. sterculia acuminata
1036 stl. stillingea sylvatica
1037 str. strychnos nux vomica
1038 str-i. „ ignatia
1039 str-t. „ tieute
1040 str-tx. „ toxifera.
1041 stry. strychnia
1042 stryph. stryphnodendron barbatinum
1043 styr. styrax officinale
1044 styr-b. „ benzoin
1045 sum. sumbulus moschatus
1046 sxf. saxifraga granulata
1047 syc. sycosin
1048 sym. symphytum officinale
1049 syph. syphilin
1050 syr. syringa vulgaris
1051 ta. tantalum metallicum
1052 tam. tamus communis
1053 tb. terbium metallicum
1054 tcn. ticunas
1055 te. tellurium metalicum
1056 te-o. „ oxidum
1057 te-x. „ acidum
1058 tep. teplitz
1059 tephr. tephrosia apollinea
1060 teu. teucrium marum verum
1061 teu-c. „ creticum
1062 teu-ch. „ chamædris
1063 teu-s. „ scorodonia
1064 th. thorium metallicum
1065 thasp thaspium aureum
1066 the. thea
1067 thl. thlapsi bursa pastoris
1068 thr. theridion curassivicum
1069 thu. thuya occidentalis
1070 thv. thevetia ruscifolia
1071 thv-n. „ nereifolia
1072 thy. thymus vulgaris
1073 thy-s. „ serpyllum
1074 ti. titanium metallicum
1075 til. tilia europæa
1076 tl. thallium metallicum
1077 tl-sa. „ sulphuricum
1078 tn-x. tannicum acidum
1079 tnc. tanacetum vulgare
1080 tnc-b. „ balsamita
1081 tng. tanghinia venenifera
1082 tourn. tournfortia argusina
1083 trach. trachinus vipera

1084 trd. tradescantia diuretica
1085 trf. trifolium arvense
1086 trf-p. „ pratense
1087 trf-r. „ repens
1088 trg. trigonocephalus lachesis
1089 trg-a. „ atrox
1090 trg-c. „ contortrix
1091 trg-j. „ jararaca
1092 trg-p. „ piscivorus
1093 tri. triosteum perfoliatum
1094 trich. trichosanthes dioica
1095 trl. trillium repens
1096 trl-p. „ pendulum
1097 trm. trombidium muscæ domesticæ
1098 trn. tarantula hispanica
1099 trx. taraxacum dens leonis
1100 tss. tussilago petasites
1101 tss-f. „ farfara
1102 tt-x. tartaricum acidum
1103 tub. tuber cibarium
1104 tx-b. taxus baccata
1105 tx-e. „ erecta
1106 tyl. tylophora asthmatica
1107 u. uranium metallicum
1108 u-cl. „ chloridum
1109 u-na. „ nitricum
1110 u-o. „ oxidum
1111 ulm. ulmus campestris
1112 unc. uncaria gambir
1113 upas. upas antiar
1114 ure. uredo caricis
1115 urea. urea
1116 urea-na „ nitrica
1117 urg. urginea scilla
1118 urt. urtica dioica
1119 urt-m. „ marina
1120 urt-u. „ urens
1121 ust. ustilago madis
1122 v. vanadium metallicum
1123 vac. vaccininum
1124 val. valeriana officinalis
1125 van. vanilla planifolia
1126 var. variolinum
1127 vbr. viburnum prunifolium
1128 vbr-o. viburnum odoratissimum
1129 vcc. vaccinium myrtillus
1130 verb. verbena officinalis
1131 verb-h. „ hastata
1132 verb-j „ jamaicensis
1133 verb-u. „ urticæfolia
1134 vi-o. viola odorata
1135 vi-t. „ tricolor
1136 vin. vinca minor
1137 vit. vitis vinifera
1138 vnc. vincetoxicum officinale
1139 vp-r. vipera redi
1140 vp-t. „ torva
1141 vr-a. veratrum album
1142 vr-s. „ sabadilla
1143 vr-v. „ viride
1144 vr-b. verbascum thapsus
1145 vrn. veronica officinalis
1146 vrn-b. „ beccabunga
1147 vrt. veratrinum
1148 vsc. viscum album
1149 vsp. vespa vulgaris
1150 vsp-c. „ crabro
1151 vtx. vitex agnus castus
1152 w. tungsten metallicum
1153 wis. wisbaden
1154 woo. woorari
1155 xan. xanthoxylon fraxineum
1156 xanth. xanthium spinosum
1157 xyp. xyphosura americana
1158 y. yttrium metallicum
1159 ziz. zizia aurea
1160 zn. zincum metallicum
1161 zn-a. „ aceticum
1162 zn-ca. „ carbonicum
1163 zn-cl. „ chloridum
1164 zn-cy. „ cyanidum
1165 zn-fcy. „ ferrocyanidum
1166 zn-i. „ iodidum
1167 zn-o. „ oxidum
1168 zn-sa „ sulphuricum
1169 zn-v. „ valerianicum
1170 zng. zingiber officinalis
1171 zr. zirconium metallicum

EYES.

SECTION I. SYMPTOMS. A. FUNCTIONS.

OBJECTS, FALSE APPEARANCE OF.

ac-s. acon. æth. ag-na. aga. al-o. alm. am-ni. amm-ca. amm-cl. anan. anm. arn. art-v. as-o. atp. au. ba-ca. ba-cl. bap. ber. bry. buf. c-bis. ca-ca. ca-o. ca-s. can. can-i. cap. cb-a. cb-v. chd. chi. chio. chlor. cic. cit-c. cl-hx. cle. clf. cmc. cmf. co. con. cop. cph. crb-x. cro. cth. cu. cy-hx. cyc. dig. dl-s. dph. dph-i. dro. dt. ele. ery. eug. euph. euph-c. euphr. f-hx. fe. fe-mgs. frm. frm-s. gel. grp. grt. gua. hæm. hg. hg-bicl. hpp. hyo. i. irs-f. jnc. jnp-s. k-bicr. k-ca. k-na. k-o. kre. lac-c. lac-d. lau-c. lct. led. li-ca. lo-i. lpd. ly-b. lyc. men. mg-ca. mg-cl. mgs. mgs-au. mn-ca. morph. mph. mrl. msc. mtr. myris. n-x. na-ba. na-ca. na-cl. ner. ni-ca. nic. os. ox-x. p. p-x. par. pb. pet. phy. physo. pnx. pod. pol. ppv. pru-l. pso. pt. ptv. pul. rho. rn-b. rs. rs-r. rut. s. s-x. sb-t. sep. si-x. smc. smi. sn. so-d. spi. spo. sr-ca. srr. str. str-i. tep. thr. thu. til. trg. val. vi-o. vin. vr-a. vr-s. vr-v. vrb. vtx. wis. woo. zn.

BLACK, (**dark**). acon. al-o. amm-ca. amm-cl. anan. anm. as-o. atp. au. ba-ca. ca-ca. ca-s. cap. cb-v. chi. cic. clv. dl-s. dt. euphr. hg. k-ca. k-o. lyc. mg-ca. mn-ca. msc. n-x. (na-cl). p. p-x. pet. physo. rut. s-x. sep. si-x. smc. str. thu. val. vr-a.

BLUE, (**lilac, purple, violet**). ac-s. acon. atp. cph. dt. hpp. i. kre. lyc. ni-ca. s. snt. sr-ca. trg. zn.

BRIGHT. al-o. amm-ca. anan. as-o. atp. au. ba-ca bry. ca-ca. can. cb-a. cb-v. chd. chlor. cic. cit-c. clv. con. cro. dig. dph. dro. euphr. grp. hyo. i. jnp-s. k-ca. k-o. lau-c. lyc. men. mgs. mn-ca. na-ba. na-cl. ner. p-x. pol. ppv. pt. pul. rs. sb-t. so-d. spi. sr-ca. str. str-i. trg. val. vi-o. vr-a. zn.

CLOSER **together.** myris.

CONFUSED (**indistinct**). ag-na. anan. anm. atp. au. bry. c-bis. ca-ca. can. chd. chi. chio. cic. cl-hx. cle. co. con. crb-x.

cund. dl-s. dro. dt. ele. ery. eug. euphr. f-hx. frm-s. gel. grp. hæm. hyo. i. irs-f. (k-bicr). k-ca. k-o. lct. led. lyc. mph. mrl. n-x. na-ca. na-cl. na-sa. os. p. phy. pnx. pod. pol. ppv. pt. rs-r. si-x. til. trg. vi-o. woo.

Outlines. chi. k-bicr. p. pod.

DISTORTED. atp. hyo.

FAR, **too.** (atp). can-i. cb-a. chlor. cic. dt. gel. hg-bicl. myris. na-cl. ox-x. p. s. smc. sn. srr. thr.

GREEN. art-v. chi. clf. dig. dt. hg. lac-c. mg-cl. nic. p. rut. s. sep. snt. sr-ca. tep. vr-v. zn.

GREY. anan. dt. n-x. p. sep. si-x. str.

INVERTED. atp. eug. gel. glo. gua. k-ca. ly-b.

LARGE, **too.** æth. anan. atp. ber. can-i. dig. dl-s. dt. euph. hyo. k-o. mll. myris. na-cl. ni-ca. os. ox-x. p. physo. ppv. pru-l. vrb.

LOW **down.** can-i. dl-s.

MOVING. acon. ag-na. aga. al-o. amm-ca. anan. anm. arn. atp. au. ba-ca. ba-cl. bap. ber. bi-na. bry. ca-ca. ca-o. ca-s. can. can-i. cb-a. chd. cic. cl-hx. con. crb-x. cy-hx. dl-s. dro. dt. ery. eug. euph. euph-c. euphr. fe. frm. grt. gua. hg. hll. hyo. i. jnc. jnp-s. k-bicr. k-ca. k-o. kre. lac-d. lct. lpd. ly-b. lyc. men. mg-ca. mgs. mrl. msc. myris. na-cl. ner. nic. p. p-x. par. pet. pnx. pol. ppv. pru-l. pso. pul. rho. rn-b. rs. rs-r. rut. s. s-x. se. sep. si-x. smc. spi. spo. str. str-i. tep. thu. til. urg. val. vin. vr-a. vr-s. vtx. wis. woo. zn.

Backwards. atp.

Backwards and Forwards. atp. cic. crb-x. frm. p. tep.

Circularly. acon. ag-na. al-o. amm-ca. anm. arn. atp. au. ba-ca. ba-cl. ber. bi-na. bry. ca-ca. ca-o. ca-s. can. can-i. cb-a. chd. cic. cl-hx. con. cy-hx. dl-s. dro. ery. euph. euph-c. fe. grt. gua. hg. hll. jnc. k-bicr. k-ca. k-o. kre. lct. lpd. ly-b. lyc. mg-ca. mrl. msc. na-cl. ner. nic. p. p-x. par. ppv. pru-l. pso. pul. rho. rn-b. rs. rs-r. rut. s. s-x. se. sep. si-x. smc. spi. str. tep. thu. urg. val. vin. vr-a. vr-s. vtx. zn.

Slowly. cy-hx.

Slowly, then Quickly. msc.

Semicircle, in a. dl-s.

From Below Upwards. gua.

Jumping. men.

Sideways. cic. grt. lac-d.

To Right. lac-d.

To Left. grt.

Swaying. ner. str-i.

Undulating. atp.

Vertically. arn. con. dt. hyo. lpd. p-x. si-x. spo.
Downwards. arn. dt. lpd. p-x.
Up and Down. con. si-x. spo.
Vibrating. acon. atp. ca-ca. cic. dro. dt. eug. euphr. hg. hyo. i. jnp-s. k-o. lyc. men. msc. p. pet. pol. s-x. smc. str-i. tep. thu. til. wis. zn.
On the Surface. atp.
In all directions. lac-d.
MULTIPLIED. æth. aga. (alm). amm-ca. atp. au. ba-ca. bry. ca-ca. chd. cic. cle. clv. cmf. con. cy-hx. cyc. dig. dph. dt. ery. eug. euph. gel. grp. hg. hg-bicl. hyo. i. (k-bicr.) k-ca. k-i. kis. led. lyc. mgs-au. mtr. n-x. na-cl. ner. ni-ca. nic. pb. pet. physo. pnx. pol. pul. s. sb-t. spo. srr. thr. vr-a. vr-v.
Antero-Posteriorly. euph.
Horizontally. dt. n-x. ner. pol. sbt.
Vertically. atp. dt. (k-bicr). pol.
The Left image Highest. dt.
The Right image Highest. pol.
The two images alternately Approach and Recede from each other. con.
The Left image seen with Right eye. na-cl.
NEAR, **too.** (atp). cic. dt. (k-ca). ly-b. morph. physo. (pol). srr.
OBLIQUE. atp. buf. dt. myris.
PART VISIBLE. au. ca-ca. can. chio. cl-hx. cro. dl-s. dt. i. k-ca. k-o. lac-c. li-ca. lo-i. lyc. mtr. na-cl. p. pb. rs-r. sep. spi. ti. vr-v.
Centre Visible. pb. dt. mtr.
Circumference Visible. cro.
Horizontal. au. chio.
Lower part Visible. au.
Upper part Visible. au. chio.
Vertical. au. ca-ca. cl-hx. i. k-o. li-ca. lyc. na-cl. pb.
Left side Visible. i. li-ca. lyc.
Right side Visible. ca-ca.
Beginning and End Visible. k-o. pb.
RED. anan. atp. ca-s. can. chlor. cmc. con. cph. cro. dig. dt. hyo. lac-c. mg-cl. myris. rut. s. smi. smr. snt. spi. sr-ca. trg. vr-s. vr-v.
SMALL. cb-v. (chd). chlor. dt. glo. hg-bicl. hyo. pet. ppv. pt. thu.
STRANGE. ba-cl. ca-a. can-i. cic. cro. dl-s. dt. glo. hyo. na-cl. ppv. pt. rs-r. vr-a.

STRIPED. amm-ca. amm-cl. atp. con. i. k-ca. mgs. mtr. na-cl. p. pul. sep.

VARIEGATED. ag-na. atp. ba-ca. cic. con. dig. dt. euph. fe-mgs. k-ca. k-na. k-o. lac-c. ni-ca. p. p-x. s. sn.

WHITE, (**pale**). aga. al-o. amm-ca. atp. can. chd. chi. (cop). cro. dig. dl-s. dro. ery. grt. k-ca. k-o. p-x. pb. pet. pul. (rn-b). rs. rut. s. si-x. srr.

WIDE **apart.** cb-a.

YELLOW (**orange**). al-o. am-ni. amm-cl. art-v. as-o. atp. clf. cth. dig hyo. k-bicr. k-ca. lac-c. mn-ca. nic. p-x. ptv. s. sep. si-x. snt. sr-ca. tep. zn.

OBJECTS, IMAGINARY.

ac-s. ach. acon. æsc. ag. ag-na. aga. al-o. alo. am-ni. amm-ca. amm-cl. amb. anan. anm. aps. art-v. arum-t. as-o. asc. atp. au. ba-ca. ber. bi-na. br. bry. buf. c-bis. ca-ca. ca-pa. ca-s. cac. can. can-i. cast. cb-a. cb-v. chd. chi. chio. cit-c. cl-hx. cle. clv. cmc. cmf. co. cof. con. cop. cph. crd. cro. crot. crt-c. cth. cu. cu-asi. cund. cy-hx. cyc. dig. dl-s. dph. drm. dro. dt. elaps. ery. evo. eug. eupat-p. euph. euphr. f-hx. frm. frm-s. gel. glo. glp. gn-c. grp. hæm. hg. hg-i. hur. hydr. hyo. i. itu. jat. jnp-s. k-ca. k-cla. k-na. k-o. klm. kre. krm. lac-c. lau-c. lch. lct. led. lpd. ly-b. lyc. men. mg-ca. mg-cl. mgs. mgs-ar. mgs-au. mim. mn-ca. morph. msc. mtr. myris. n-x. na-ba. na-ca. na-cl. na-sa. narth. ner. nic. ol-a. ol-t. p. p-x. par. pb. pet. phy. physo. pim. pnx. pol. ppv. pru-l. pso. pt. ptv. pul. qu-sa. rho. rmx. rn-b. rs. rs-r. rut. s. s-x. sang. sb-t. scr-m. sep. si-x. smb. smc. smi. so-d. so-n. spi. spo. sr-ca. srr. str. str-i. sum. tep. thr. thu. til. trg. trn. tx-b. urg. val. vi-o. vi-t. vin. vr-a. vr-s. vr-v. vrb. woo. zn. zng.

BLACK. ac-s. acon. ag-na. aga. al-o. amm-ca. amm-cl. anan. anm. asc. atp. au. ba-ca. buf. ca-ca. ca-pa. ca-s. can. cb-a. cb-v. chd. chi. clv. cmf. co. cof. con. cop. cu-asi. (cund). dig. dl-s. dt. elaps. ery. evo. glo. hg. hg-i. hyo. itu. jat. k-ca. k-o. klm. lau-c. lct. lyc. mg-ca. mn-ca. msc. (myris). n-x. na-ca. na-cl. narth. nic. ol-a. ol-t. p. p-x. pb. pet. pnx. ppv. pso. pul. qu-sa. rs. rut. s. sb-t. scr-m. sep. si-x. so-d. spi. sr-ca. str. tep. thr. thu. trg. val. vr-a. woo. zn.

Centre. atp. thu.

BLUE. as-o. can-i. clv. (cph). crt-c. (cund). dt. elaps. fe-mgs. k-ca. pso. sr-ca. trg. zn.

BRIGHT (**fiery**). acon. æsc. ag-na. al-o. alo. amm-ca. anan. as-o. atp. atrop. au. ba-ca. br. bry. ca-ca. ca-pa. ca-s.

can. cast. cb-v. chd. chi. cit-c. cl-hx. cle. clf. clv. co. con. cph. cro. cu. cu-asi. cyc. dig. dl-s. dph. dro. dt. elaps. ery. eug. euphr. f-hx. fe-mgs. gel. glo. grp. hg. hur. hydr. hyo. i. jat. k-ca. k-cla. k-o. klm. lau-c. led. lyc. men. mgs. mgs-ar. mn-ca. mtr. n-x. na-ba. na-ca. na-cl. na-sa. narth. ner. nic. ol-a. p. p-x. par. pet. pol. ppv. pru-l. pt. pul. qu-sa. s. sang. sb-t. sep. si-x. smc. smi. so-d. spi. spo. sr-ca. str. str-i. thr. thu. til. trg. tx-b. val. vi-o. vin. vr-a. woo. zn. zng.

Border. atp. thu.

BROWN. (aga). na-cl.

BUBBLE **Bursting.** pul.

CIRCLES. am-ni. anan. bry. ca-pa. cac. can. cb-v. cit-c. cph. dig. elaps. f-hx. fe-mgs. i. k-ca. k-na. lch. mn-ca. na-ca. p. pso. pul. (s). sep. str-i. thu. tx-b. woo. zn.

Black. elaps. mn-ca. (s).

Blue. fe-mgs. zn.

Bright. anan. bry. ca-ca. can. cit-c. (cph). fe-mgs. pul. thu. tx-b. woo.

On Inner Edge. cb-v. k-ca.

At Side of Visual Ray. can.

Green. zn.

Grey. lch.

Increasing in Size. k-ca.

Moving Circularly. k-ca. tx-b.

Rays with. (cit-c). k-ca.

Red. cac. elaps. fe-mgs.

Side of Visual Ray at. can.

Sparks. mn-ca.

Variegated. (cph). k-na. p. sep. zn.

Vibrations Bright. dig.

White. can. k-ca.

Yellow. am-ni. k-ca. mn-ca. zn.

Zigzags. fe-mgs. sep. str-i.

COBWEB. aga. k-ca. k-o. mgs-ar. mrl. n-x. trn.

CORPSES. (**Skeletons**). as-o. atp. ca-s. can-i. crt-c. cth. hur. na-ca. ppv. smc. str.

CROSS **Bright**. dt.

High up. dt.

CRYSTALS **with Black tips.** (cund).

CURLS. (cund). i. k-ca.

CYPHERS. p. p-x. s.

Increasing in Size. p. s.

ELLIPSE, **Bright with Dark Centre.** thu.

FAR **off.** dt.

FEATHERS. (al-o). ca-ca. kre. lyc. mg-ca. na-ca. na-cl. phy. pol. spi.

FIGURES **of Living Objects.** æth. ag-na. aga. amb. anm. as-o. atp. br. bry. ca-ca. ca-pa. ca-s. can-i. cch. chi. clv. cmf. cof. con. (cu). dig. drm. dt. hg. hyo. k-o. lac-c. lau-c. mg-ca. mg-cl. mg-sa. mgs-au. myris. na-ca. nic. p. p-x. ppv. pru-l. ptv. pul. rhe. rs. s. sep. si-x. smb. str. trn. vr-a. zn.

Black. anm.

Moving with the Eye. anm.

High up. dt.

Moving. dt.

Moving from Right to Left. ca-pa.

Moving Downwards. dt.

Moving Upwards. dt.

Moving from Sides. dt.

Moving with the Eye. anm.

Side of Visual Ray at. dt. lac-c. myris.

FLAMES. atp. ba-ca. bry. ca-ca. ca-s. can. cph. dig. dt. ery. f-hx. hyo. k-ca. k-o. na-cl. p-x. ppv. pul. s. so-d. spi. spo. str. vi-o. vin. vr-a.

Moving. f-hx.

Red. f-hx. spi.

White Circle. can.

FLASHES **Bright.** ag-na. as-o. atp. atrop. br. clf. clv. cro. dl-s. dt. elaps. ery. f-hx. glo. i. k-ca. mgs. mgs-ar. mtr. na-ca. na-cl. ner. pul. sb-t. sep. si-x. spi. str. thr. thu trn. zn.

Moving Downwards. i.

Moving from Left to Right. elaps.

Side of Visual Ray at. thu.

GREEN. can-i. chi. dt. k-ca. k-o. lac-c. mg-cl. n-x. (na-sa). nic. p. rut. sep. sr-ca. vr-v. zn.

GREY. ag-na. ca-pa. chd. dt. elaps. lch. n-x. p. pnx. sep. si-x. str.

HALO. al-o. atp. ba-ca. ca-ca. chi. cic. cmc. con. cph. dig. dl-s. dt. euph. hyo. k-ca. k-na. k-o. mg-cl. mim. n-x. p. p-x. ptv. pul. rut. s. sep. smc. smi. sn. sr-ca. trg. vr-v. zn.

Black. k-o. p.

Blue. cph. sr-ca. trg.

Bright. ca-ca. trg.

Green. k-o. mg-cl. p. rut. sep. vr-v. zn.

Grey. dt. p. sep.

Red. atp. (cmc). cph. dt. ptv. rut. s. sr-ca. trg. vr-v.

Starlike. pul.

Variegated. atp. ba-ca. cic. con. hyo. k-na. k-o.
White. chi.
Yellow. hyo.
HIGH **up**. atp. dt. hg. mg-cl. rn-b.
HORNS **Black**. (cund).
INCREASING **in Size**. k-ca. p. s. so-d.
INCREASING **and** DECREASING **in Size**. lau-c.
LEAF. hg. (na-sa).
White. (na-sa).
LIGHT. al-o. chi. eug. k-cla. lau-c. p. qu-sa. val.
Red. chi.
Yellow. chi.
LOW **down**. cit-c. dt. hg. rs-r.
MIST **(clouds)**. ach. acon. ag. ag-na. aga. al-o. amb. amm-cl. anan. arum-t. atp. (au). bi-na. bry. c-bis. ca-ca. ca-pa. cac. can. cast. cb-a. chd. chio. (cit-c). clv. con. cro. crot. cth. cund. cy-hx. cyc. dig. dl-s. dt. (ery). frm-s. gel. glo. glp. grp. grt. hæm. hg. hg-i. jnp-s. k-ca. k-o. klm. lac-d. ly-b. (lyc). mg-ca. mg-cl. mrl. msc. myris. n-x. na-cl. (na-sa). narth. ni-ca. ol-a. p. p-x. par. pb. pim. pln. pnx. pod. pru-l. pt. pul. qu-sa. rmx. rn-b. rs-r. rut. s. sep. smi. so-n. spi. srr. trg. trn. vi-t. vin. zn.
Black. (ery). hg-i. ol-a. p.
Moving. hg-i.
Bright. k-ca. lyc.
Grey. anan.
High up. atp. mg-cl.
Moving. atp. con. evo. hg-i. pod.
Moving Upwards. jnp-s.
Moving from Left to Right. atp.
Red. (ery).
White. atp. con.
High up. atp.
Moving. atp. con.
Moving from Left to Right. atp.
Yellow. k-ca.
MOVING. aga. amm-cl. anm. atp. au. buf. ca-ca. ca-s. can. cb-v. chi. clv. co. cof. con. cop. (cund). dig. dl-s. dt. ery. evo. f-hx. hg. hg-i. hyo. itu. k-ca. k-o. klm. lch. lct. lyc. mg-ca. n-x. na-ca. na-cl. narth. ol-a. p. pb. pod. ppv. pul. rs. rut. s. sb-t. sep. si-x. so-d. spi. thu. trg. zn.
MOVING **with** EYE. anm. ca-ca. dt. n-x. na-cl. (qu-sa). s. thu.
MOVING CIRCULARLY. aps. ba-cl. k-ca. msc. tx-b. urg. zn.

MOVING DOWNWARDS. dt. ery. i. k-ca. na-ba. p-x. thu.
MOVING UPWARDS. dt. jnp-s.
MOVING UP **and** DOWN. (ery). msc.
MOVING **towards** EACH OTHER. dig.
MOVING **from** SIDES. dt.
MOVING **from** RIGHT **to** LEFT. ca-pa. na-ba.
MOVING **from** LEFT **to** RIGHT. atp. elaps.
NEAR EYES. lyc. na-sa. s.
OBJECTS **Previously Seen, (images retained long on retina)**. lac-c. nic.
PYRIFORM **body**. (cund).
Blue. (cund).
Red. (cund).
RAIN. au. k-ca. na-ca. na-cl. thu.
RAYS. atp. cit-c. i. k-ca. mtr. srr. trg.
RED. atp. cac. chi. (cmc). cot. (cph). (cund). dt. elaps. (ery). f-hx. fe-mgs. lac-c. ptv. rut. s. spi. sr-ca. trg. vr-v.
ROCKS. **High up**. mg-cl.
ROPE **Across Sky**. rn-b.
SEMICIRCLE. con. dt. vi-o.
Bright. dt. vi-o.
High up. dt.
High up. dt.
SERPENTINE **bodies**. ag-na. (cund). ery. str-i.
Black. (cund).
Moving. (cund).
Bright. ery.
Moving. (cund).
SHADOWS. ca-ca. pol. rut.
SIDE **of** VISUAL RAY **at**. can. cit-c. dt. grp. lac-c. mgs. myris. str. str-i. thu.
SPIRITS. as-o. atp. ca-s. can-i. cb-v. (cu). dt. hur. hyo. na-cl. ppv. pt. pul. s. sep. si-x. so-d. trg. trn.
Increasing in Size. so-d.
SPOTS (**balls, points**). ac-s. acon. ag-na. aga. al-o. amm-ca. amm-cl. anan. anm. as-o. asc. atp. au. ba-ca. bry. buf. ca-ca. ca-pa. ca-s. can. cb-a. cb-v. chd. chi. cit-c. clv. cmf. co. cof. con. cop. cot. cro. cu. cu-asi. cyc. dig. dl-s. dph. dt. elaps. ery. evo. glo. hg. hur. hyo. i. itu. jat. k-ca. k-o. klm. krm. lac-c. lau-c. lch. lct. lyc. mg-ca. mgs. mn-ca. msc. (myris). n-x. na-ca. na-cl. na-sa. narth. ner. nic. ol-a. ol-t. p. p-x. par. pb. pet. pnx. pol. ppv. pru-l. pso. pul. (qu-sa). rs. rut. s. sb-t. scr-m. sep. si-x. so-d. spi. sr-ca. srr. str.. tep. thu. trg. val. vr-a. woo. zn.
Black. ac-s. acon. ag-na. aga. al-o. amm-ca. amm-cl.

anan. anm. asc. atp. au. ba-ca. buf. ca-ca. ca-pa. ca-s. can. cb-v. chd. chi. clv. cmf. co. cof. cop. cu-asi. dig. dl-s. dt. elaps. ery. evo. glo. hg. hyo. itu. jat. k-ca. k-o. klm. lau-c. lct. lyc. mg-ca. mn-ca. msc. (myris). n-x. na-ca. na-cl. narth. nic. ol-t. p. pb. pet. pnx. ppv. pso. pul. (qu-sa). rs. rut. s. sb-t. scr-m. sep. si-x. so-d. spi. sr-ca. str. tep. thu. val. vr-a. woo. zn.

Bright. dl-s. thu.

With Bright Border. atp.

Low down. (cit-c). dt. hg.

Moving. aga. amm-cl. anm. atp. au. buf. ca-ca. ca-s. can. cb-v. chi. clf. co. cof. con. cop. dig. dl-s. ery. hg. hyo. itu. k-ca. k-o. klm. lct. lyc. mg-ca. n-x. na-ca. na-cl. narth. ol-a. p. pb. ppv. pul. rs. rut. s. sb-t. sep. si-x. so-d. spi. thu. zn.

Moving with Eye. ca-ca. dt. (qu-sa). (si-x).

Moving Downwards. thu.

Near Eyes. lyc. s.

Side of Visual Ray at. thu.

Symmetrical Lines in. cb-a.

Blue. as-o. clv. crt-c. dt. k-ca.

Moving. clv.

Bright (sparks). acon. ag-na. amm-ca. anan. as-o. atp. au. ba-ca. bry. ca-ca. chd. cit-c. clv. con. cro. crt-c. cu. cu-asi. cyc. dig. dph. dt. elaps. ery. glo. hg. hur. hyo. i. jat. k-ca. k-o. lau-c. lyc. mgs. mn-ca. n-x. na-cl. na-sa. narth. ner. nic. ol-a. p-x. par. pet. pol. ppv. pru-l. s. sb-t. sep. (si-x) so-d. spi. sr-ca. srr. str. tep. thu. val. vr-a. zn.

Far off. dt.

High up. dt. hg.

Low down. (cit-c).

Moving. clv. con. ery.

Moving with Eye. na-cl. thu.

Moving Circularly. zn.

Moving Downwards. ery. p-x. thu.

Side of Visual Ray at. (cit-c). dt. thu.

Brown. (aga). na-cl.

Far off. dt.

Green. dt. k-ca. lac-c. n-x. sr-ca.

Low down. dt.

Moving. dt.

Moving with Eye. n-x.

Grey. ag-na. ca-pa. chd. lch. n-x. p. pnx. si-x str.

Moving. lch.

High up. dt. hg.

Low down. (cit-c). dt. hg.

Moving. aga. amm-cl. anm. atp. au. buf. ca-ca. ca-s. can. cb-v. chi. clv. co. cof. con. cop. dig. dl-s. dt. ery. hg. hyo. itu. k-ca. k-o. klm. lch. lct. lyc. mg-ca. n-x. na-ca. na-cl. narth. ol-a. p. pb. ppv. pul. rs. rut. s. sb-t. sep. si-x. so-d. spi. thu. trg. zn.

Moving with Eye. ca-ca. dt. n-x. na-cl. (qu-sa). (s). thu.

Moving Circularly. zn.

Moving Downwards. ery. k-ca. thu.

Near Eyes. lyc. s.

Red. atp. cot. elaps. lac-c.

Side of Visual Ray at. (cit-c). dt. thu.

Symmetrical Lines in. cb-a.

White. al-o. amm-ca as-o. elaps. ery. k-ca. krm. p-x. pnx. s. sr-ca. thu. trg.

Moving. thu. trg.

Moving Downwards. k-ca. p-x.

Yellow. aga. amm-cl. cb-a. cot. lac-c. lch. na-sa.

Symmetrical Lines in. cb-a.

SQUARES. elaps. hydr.

Red. elaps.

White. elaps.

STARS. al-o. amm-ca. atp. (ca-ca). cast. cro. hyo. k-ca. k-o. mgs. mgs-ar. na-ca. (na-sa). p. physo. pso. pul. trn.

Blue. pso.

Bright. al-o. amm-ca. atp. (ca-ca). cast. cro. k-ca. (na-sa). p.

Moving with Eye. ca-ca.

Near Eye. (na-sa).

Green. (na-sa).

Near Eye. (na-sa).

Halo. pul.

High up. atp.

Moving with Eye. ca-ca.

Near Eye. (na-sa).

Shooting. mgs. mgs-ar.

Variegated. physo.

White. al-o. amm-ca: atp. k-ca. k-o. na-ca.

High up. atp.

Yellow. (na-sa).

Near Eye. (na-sa).

STRIPES, (**bars, columns**). con. crd. dig. dl-s. dt. elaps. hydr. i. na-ca. na-cl. nic. p-x. s. thu. zn.

Black. p-x. s. zn.
Moving. s.
Upwards to Left. zn.
Blue. dt.
Moving with Eye. dt.
Vertical. dt.
Bright. dig. dl-s. dt. na-ca. na-cl. nic.
High up. dt.
Moving towards Each Other. dig.
Upwards to Right. dt.
Vertical. dl-s. dt.
Green. dt.
Moving with Eye. dt.
Vertical. dt.
High up. dt.
Moving. s.
Moving with Eye. dt.
Moving towards Each Other. dig.
Red. elaps.
Transverse. elaps.
Transverse. elaps.
Upwards to Left. zn.
Upwards to Right. dt.
Variegated. con.
Vertical. dl-s. dt.
SYMMETRICAL LINES **in.** cb-a.
THREADS (**hairs**). al-o. cb-a. con. (cund). elaps. (ery). k-ca. pln. pol. spi. trg.
Moving. con. (ery). trg.
Moving Up and Down. (ery).
White. elaps.
TRANSVERSE. elaps. rn-b.
UPWARDS **to** LEFT. zn.
UPWARDS **to** RIGHT. dt.
VARIEGATED. atp. au. ba-ca. cic. con. (cph). cund. dig. ery. k-ca. k-na. k-o. p. physo. sep. zn.
VEIL. (**net**). ach. acon. ag. aga. al-o. amb. amm-cl. arn. art-v. arum-t. as-o. atp. au. ba-ca. ber. bi-na. bry. buf. c-bis. ca-ca. ca-pa. ca-s. can. cast. cb-a. chd. chi. chio. clv. con. cro. crot. cth. cu. cy-hx. cyc. dig. dl-s. dro. dt. elaps. euph. euphr. gel. glp. gn-c. grp. hæm. hg. hg-i. hyo. i. jnp-s. k-bicr. k-ca. k-o. klm. kre. krm. lct. lpd. ly-b. lyc. mg-ca. mg-cl. mgs-ar. mgs-au. morph. mrl. msc. n-x. na-ba. na-ca. na-cl. narth. ni-ca. nic. ol-a. p. p-x.

par. pb. pet. pim. pln. pnx. pol. ppv. pru-l. pt. pul. qu-sa. rho. rn-b. rs. rs-r. rut. s. sb-t. scr-m. sep. si-x. smc. smi. so-d. spi. srr. thr. thu. til. trg. trn. vi-t. vin. vrb. woo. zn.

Black. (p). s.

Blue. (elaps).

Crooked. (na-cl).

Grey. elaps. p. si-x.

Watery. cb-a.

White. dl-s. elaps. lpd. srr.

Yellow. k-bicr.

VERTICAL. dl-s. dt.

VIBRATIONS, (**flickering**). acon. æsc. aga. al-o. alo. amm-ca. aps. as-o. atp. ca-ca. ca-s. cb-v. chd. chi. cic. cit-c. cl-hx. cle. clv. co. con. cro. cu. dig. dl-s. dph. dro. dt. ery. euphr. f-hx. frm. gel. grp. hg. hur. hydr. hyo. i. jnp-s. k-ca. k-o. klm. led. lyc. men. mgs. mtr. na-ba. na-cl. ner. nic. p. p-x. par. pet. pol. pru-l. pt. pul. rs-r. s. s-x. sang. sb-t. sep. si-x. smc. smi. sr-ca. str. str-i. sum. thr. thu. til. trg. vi-o. vin. vr-a. vr-s. zn. zng.

Black. dl-s. thr. trg.

Bright. acon. æsc. al-o. alo. amm-ca. as-o. atp. ca-ca. ca-s. cb-v. chd. chi. cit-c. cl-hx. cle. clv. co. con. cro. dig. dl-s. dph. dro. (dt). euphr. f-hx. gel. grp. hg. hur. hydr. hyo. i. k-ca. k-o. klm. led. lyc. men. mgs. mtr. na-ba. na-cl. ner. nic. p. p-x. pet. pol. pt. pul. s. sang. sb-t. sep. smc. sr-ca. str. str-i. thr. thu. til. trg. vin. vr-a. zng.

Circle of. dig.

Red. f-hx.

Side of Visual Ray at. grp. mgs. str.

Variegated. dig. k-ca.

White. sep.

Yellow. hydr.

VISIONS. acon. al-o. art-v. atp. ca-ca. can. can-i. cb-a. cb-v. dt. hg. k-o. led. na-ca. p. p-x. ppv. pul. rs. smb. str. thu. trn.

Beautiful. can. can-i. ppv.

Horrible. atp. ca-ca. cb-a. cb-v. dt. k-o. p. ppv. pul. smb. trn.

Ludicrous. atp. can-i.

WATER. ca-s. hg. sb-t.

WAVES. ca-ca. hur. k-o. na-ba. (p). rs-v. sr-ca.

Concentric. (p).

Green. sr-ca.

Irregular Lines. rs-r.

Light of. ca-ca. hur. k-o. na-ba.
Moving Downwards. na-ba.
Moving from Right to Left. na-ba.
WHITE. al-o. amm-ca. as-o. atp. can. chi. con. dl-s. elaps. ery. k-ca. k-o. krm. lpd. na-ca. (na-sa). p-x. pnx. rn-b. s. sep. sr-ca. srr. str-i. thu. trg.
YELLOW. aga. amm-cl. cb-a. chi. cot. hydr. k-ca. lac-c. lch. mn-ca. na-sa. nic. zn.
ZIGZAGS. can. con. f-hx. fe-mgs. grp. hur. na-cl. p. rs-r. sep. str-i. trg. vi-o.
Bright. f-hx. na-cl. p. str-i.
Circle of. fe-mgs. sep. str-i.
Low down. rs-r.
Red. f-hx.
Side of Visual Ray at. str-i.
Variegated. sep.
White. str-i.
Side of Visual Ray at. str-i.

PHOTOMANIA (DESIRE FOR LIGHT).

acon. amm-cl. atp. ca-a. ca-ca. dt. gel. rut.
ARTIFICIAL **Light.** dt.
NATURAL **Light.** dt.

PHOTOPHOBIA (AVERSION TO LIGHT), SEE CONDITIONS—LIGHT.

SIGHT DAZZLED.

acon. as-o. ba-ca. buf. ca-ca. cb-a. chd. cic. con. crt-c. dig. dro. dt. euph. euphr. grp. hg. hyo. k-ca. k-o. lau-c. lyc. mn-ca. mrl. n-x. na-ca. na-cl. ner. p. p-x. pol. s. sa-l. sep. si-x. str. str-i. val.

SIGHT IMPAIRED. (DIMNESS. BLINDNESS).

ach. acon. æsc-g. ag. ag-na. aga. aga-c. al-o. alm. alo. amb. amm-ca. amm-cl. anan. anm. aps. arn. art-v. arum-t. as-o. asc. asr. ast. atp. au. ba-ca. bi-na. br. bru. bry. buf. c-bis. ca-a. ca-ca. ca-pa. ca-s. cac. can. cap. cast. cau. cb-a. cb-v. ccs. cd-sa. chd. chi. chio. cic. cit-c. cl hx. cle. clv. cmf. co. cochl. cof. con. cop. cot. cph. crb-x. crd. cro. crot.

crt. cth. cu. cund. cy-hx. cyc. dig. dl-s. dol. dph. drm. dro. dt. elaps. ery. eug. eupat. eupat-p. euph. euph-c. euphr. evo. f-hx. fe. fe-mgs. frm. frm-s. gel. glo. glp. gn-c. gn-l. grp. grt. gui. hæm. hdm. hg. hg-bi. hg-i. hg-s. hur. hyo. i. jnp-s. k-bicr. k-ca. k-i. k-na. k-o. klm. kre. krm. lac-d. lac-f. lam. lau-c. lch. lct. led. lol. lpd. ly-b. lyc. men. mg-ca. mg-cl. mgs. mgs-ar. mgs-au. mim. mll. mn-ca. morph-a. mrl. msc. mtr. myris. n-x. na-ba. na-ca. na-cl. na-sa. narth. ner. ni-ca. nic. ol-a. ol-t. os. p. p-x. par. pb. pet. phl. phy. physo. pim. pln. pnc. pnx. pol. ppv. pru-l. pso. pt. ptv. pul. qu-sa. rhe. rho. rmx. rn-b. rs. rs-r. rs-v. rut. s. s-x. sa-a. sang. sb-s. sb-t. scr-m. se. sep. si-x. smc. smi. smr. sn. so-d. so-n. spi. spo. sr-ca. srr. str. str-i. stry. sum. thr. thu. til. trg. trn. trx. urg. val. vi-o. vi-t. vin. vp-r. vr-a. vr-s. vr-v. vrb. woo. zn. zng.

TRANSIENT. acon. ag. ag-na. aga. al-o. amb. arn. art-v. as-o. asr. atp. au. br. bry. ca-ca. ca-s. cac. can. cap. cb-a. chd. chi. cic. cl-hx. cle. cochl. con. cop. cro. crt. cyc. dig. dl-s. dph. dro. ery. euphr. fe. gn-l. grp. grt. gui. hg. hyo. i. jnp-s. k-ca. k-na. k-o. lau-c. led. lyc. men. mg-ca. mg-cl. mgs-au. mn-ca. msc. mtr. myris. n-x. na-ba. na-cl. narth. ner. nic. p. pb. pet. pol. ppv. pru-l. pt. pul. qu-sa. rn-b. rut. s. sang. sb-t. sep. si-x. smc. so-d. spi. str. sum. thu. til. trg. urg. vi-t. vp-r. vr-a. vr-s. zn.

MYOPIA AND PRESBYOPIA.

SEE CONDITIONS—LOOKING AT DISTANT & NEAR OBJECTS.

B. ANATOMICAL REGIONS.

EYEBALL (INCLUDING CONJUNCTIVA BULBI).

ach. acon. æsc. æth. ag. ag-na. aga. al-o alli. alm. alo. amb. amm-ca. amm-cl. anag. anan. anth. aph. apo. aps. ara. arn. art-v. arum. arum-t. as. as-h. as-i. as-o. asc. asp. asr. ast. atp. au. ba-a. ba-ca. ba-cl. bap. bar. ber. bi-na. blt. br. bru. bry. buf. buf-s. bz-x. c-bis. ca-a. ca-ca. ca-i. ca-o. ca-pa. ca-s. cac. can. can-i. cap. cast. cau. cb-a. cb-v. cbz-x. cch. ccs. cd-sa. chd. chi. chio. chlor. clv. cmf. cop. cori. cot. cr-o. crot. cu. cu-a. cu-ca. cu-sa. cund. cy. cy-hx. cyc. dig. dl-s. dph. dph-i. drm. dro. dt. elaps. erig. ery. eryn. et-fr. eug. eupat. eupat-p. euph. euphr. evo. f-hx. fe. fe-mgs. frm. frm-o. frm-s. gel. glo. glp. gn-c. gn-l. grn. grc. grp. grt. gui. gym. hæm. hed. hg. hg-bi. hg-bicl. hg-cl.

hg-cy. hg-s. hll. hpm. hrc. hum. hur. hydr. hyo. hyp. i. ind. irs. jat. jnp-s. jug. k-bicr. k-ca. k-cla. k-i. k-na. k-o. klm. kre. krm. lac-ac. lac-c. lac-d. lac-f. lam. lau-c. lch. lct. led. li-ca. lo-c. lo-cœ. lo-i. lpd. lpt. ly-b. lyc. men. menth. mg-ca. mg-cl. mg-sa. mgs. mgs-ar. mgs-au. mitch. mn-ca. morph-a. mph. mrl. msc. mtr. mur. myr. myris. n-x. na-ca. na-cl. na-sa. narth. ner. ni-ca. nic. ol-a. os. ox-x. p. p-x. pæo. pan. par. pau. pb. pb-a. pd. ped. pet. phl. phy. physo. pim. plb. pnc. pnx. pol. ppv. pru-l. pso. pt. ptv. pul. pul-n. qu-cy. qu-sa. rhe. rho. rmx. rn-b. rn-s. rph. rs. rs-r. rs-v. rut. s. s-x. sa-a. sa-l. sang. sb-s. sb-t. scr-m. sep. si-x. smb. smc. smi. sn. snp-n. so-d. so-n. so-o. so-t. spi. spi-m. spo. spo-f. sr-ca. srr. stach. stc. str. str-i. sum. teu. thr. thu. til. trg. tri. trn. trx. urg. urt. urt-m. val. vi-o. vi-t. vp-t. vr-a. vr-s. vrb. vsp. vtx. woo. xan. ziz. zn. zn-s. zng.

APPEARANCE, EXPRESSION, **Anxious.** acon. alo. arn. as-o.

Astonished. glo. lau-c.

Bright, &c. ach. acon. æth. ag-na. (alm). alo. arn. as-o. atp. bap. bry. clv. cmf. (con). cori. crot. cth. cu. cy-hx. dt. eupat. hg-bicl. hyo. jat. jnp-s. k-ca. k-o. lch. (lyc). mgs. morph-a. msc. mtr. na-cl. pb. pet. ppv. pul. sep. so-n. spi. str. trg. trn. val. vp-t. vr-a.

Dim, &c. acon. æth. (alm). anan. arn. as-o. asc. asr. ast. atp. ber. br. bru. bry. buf. c-bis. ca-s. cb-a. (cch). chd. chi. cle. clv. cmc. cmf. con. (cph). crn. crt-c. cu. cu-asi. cyc. dig. dph-i. dt. elaps. ery. eryn. eug. fe. gel. glo. gym. hg. hg-bicl. hg-s. hyo. jnp-s. (k-bicr). k-ca. k-i. kre. lau-c. lch. ly-b. lyc. mn-ca. mrl. msc. mtr. n-x. narth. p. p-x. pb. phy. pol. ppv. qu-sa. rs-v. s. sang. sb-t. sep. sn. spi. spo. trg. urg. val. vr-a. zn. zn-s.

Glassy. anm. atp. bry. cmc. (con). cro. dt. elaps. glo. p-x. ppv. s. sep. sn. spi.

Impudent. (dt).

Spiteful. (dt).

Staring. ach. acon. æth. al-o. amm-ca. amy. anm. arn. art-v. as-o. asr. atp. ba-cl. bru. bry. c-bis. ca-s. can. cast. chi. cic. cl-hx. cle. clv. con. cro. crot. crt-c. cth. cu. cu-a. cu-sa. cy. cy-hx. dig. dol. dph. dt. ery. eupat-p. glo. glp. gui. hg. hg-bicl. hll. hyo. k-ca. lau-c. lch. lyc. mgs. mgs-ar. mrl. msc. mtr. myris. nic. p-x. pb. pol. ppv. pru-l. rs. rut. s. sb-t. sep. spi. spi-m. (spo). str. str-i. urg. vr-a. zn.

Downwards. dt. ery.
Sideways. (dt).
Strange. æth.
Suspicious. dt.
Transparent. (acon).
Upward-looking. jat.
Velvety. (con).
Wild. (alm). as-o. atp. clv. cu. cu-ca. dt. glo. hyo. lau-c. pb. ppv. spi-m. vp-t.

BORING. alli. aps. ber. bi-na. (br). (ca-a). ca-ca. (ca-o). (ca-s). cch. (cis). (cof). (con). (cu-asi). (elaps). (euph-a). (frm). hg. (i). k-ca. (lo-cœ). (myris). na-cl. nic. (ol-a). p. (ptv). pul. s. spi. (srr). thu. woo.

BROKEN **as if.** (lch). si-x.

BRUISED. acon. (alm). anm. (as-o). ca-pa. ca-s. (chlor). (cu). gel. (glo). (lch). (ly-b). lyc. (mg-cl). (na-cl). (pln). (pol). (pt). (ptv). (rs). s. sb-t. (smi). (str). urt. vr-a. vtx.

BURSTING. acon. al-o. aps. asr. (au). bap. bi-na. (buf-s). ca-s. can-i. (ccs). cot. dl-s. frm-s. (gel). grn. grp. gui. hyo. k-o. lac-ac. (lau-c). (mg-ca). (morph). (morph-a). myris. n-x. na-ca. (na-cl). (na-sa). par. pb. pol. pru. sb-t. spi. stach. srr. thu. woo.

COLDNESS. acon. (æsc). ag-na. al-o. amm-ca. asr. ber. (br). buf. ca-ca. ca-pa. chd. (chlor). con. cro. (dt). et-fr. f-hx. grp. hg-s. (hur). k-ca. k-o. lch. (li-ca). lyc. mgs-ar. mgs-au. narth. (ni-ca). (nic). p-x. par. pim. pnx. pol. pt. rs-r. s. sa-l. (sep). spo. thu. (trn). urg.

Burning. et-fr.

COLOR **Dark. (blue, brown, &c.).** (acon). (aga). (anm). (aps). (arn). (art-v). (as-h). (as-o). atp. (au). (ba-ca). (ber). (bi-na). (buf). (c-bis). (ca-ca). (ca-s). (can). (cch). (chd). (chi). (clv). (cn-sa). (con). (cph). (crn). (cu). (cyc). (dig). (dl-s). (dph). (dro). (dt). (ery). euphr. (fe). (glo). (grp). (gui). (hæm). (hg). (hg-bicl). (hg-s). (hll). (hpm). (hur). (hyo). (irs). (jat). (jnp-s). k-bicr. (k-ca). (k-o). (lyc). (mg-ca). (mrl). (mtr). (myris). (n-x). (na-ca). (ner). (p). (p-x). pb. (pod). (ppv). (pul). (rs). (rs-v). rut. (s). (s-x). (sa-l). (sb-t). (sep). (si-x). (smc). (smi). sn. (so-d). (spi). (spo-f). (sr-ca). (str). (str-i). (trg). (trn). (trx). (tx-b). vr-a. (vr-s). (woo). (zn).

Green. (cch). (myris). (p). (pb). (rs). (vr-a).

Red. acon. æth. (ag). ag-na. aga. al-o alli. (alm). alo. amb. amm-ca. amm-cl. anan. apo. aps. arn (as). as-o. asr. ast. atp. atrop. au. ba-ca. (ba-cl). bap. ber. bi-na.

br. bru. bry. buf. (c-bis). (ca-a). ca-ca. (ca-o). ca-pa. ca-s. can. can-i. cap. (cb-a). (cb-v). (cch). ccs. chd. chi. (chio). chlor. cit-c. cl-hx. cld. cle. cln. cmc. cmf. (cnv-d). cof. con. cop. cor. (cot). cph. crot. cth. cu. cu-a. cu-asi. cu-ca. cy-hx. dig. dl-s. dph-i. dt. elaps. (ery). (eryn). (eug). (eupat). (eupat-p). euph. euphr. fe. frm. gel. glo. glp. gn-l. grc. grp. grt. hæm, hg. (hg-a). hg-bi. hg-bicl. hg-s. (hll). hur. (hydr). hyo. i. (ind). irs. k-bicr. (k-br). k-ca. k-cla. k-i. (k-na). k-o. klm. kre. krm. (lac-f). lau-c. (lch). lct. led. lpd. ly-b. lyc. mg-ca. mg-cl. (mgs). (mgs-ar). mim. morph-a. mph. (mrl). mtr. myr. myris. n-x. (na-ba). na-ca. na-cl. na-sa. ner. ni-ca. nic. ol-a. p. (p-x). (par). (pau). pb. (pb-a). ped. pet. (phy). (plb). pnc. (pod). pol. ppr. (pru-l.) pso. ptv. pul. qu-cy. qu-sa. rho. rn-b. rn-s. rph. rs. rs-r. rs-v. rut. s. s-x. sa-a. sb-s. sb-t. scr-m. sep. si-x. (smi). smr. sn. so-d. so-o. so-t. spi. spo. spo-f. sr-ca. srr. str. str-i. teu. thu. trg. trn. trx. (u-na). (val). vi-o. (vin). vp-t. vr-a. vr-s. woo. ziz. zn.

White. (acon). (ag-na). (atp). (buf). (ca-i). (cub). (frm). (hg-bicl). (k-bicr). (pb). (s).

Yellow. acon. æsc. aga. amb. (anan). anm. as-h. as-o. atp. (blt). bry. ca-s. cbz-x. chd. chi. cle. clv. con. crn. crt. (crt-c). cth. cu-sa. (dig). (eupat). (eupat-p). fe. gel. hg-cl. i. k-bicr. mg-cl. mtr. myr. (n-x). p. p-x. pb. (pnc). ppv. pul. rs. s. sb-s. sep. (spi). str. str-i. trg. vp-r. vr-a. woo.

CONGESTION **see** COLOR **Red.**

CONTRACTIVE. acon. ag. aga. (amph). (anan). (ber). bi-na. (bry). (chd). (chi). (crn). cro. (crot). crt-c. (dl-s). elaps. (eug). (euph). (euphr). evo. grt. hæm. (hll). jnp-s. k-ca. k-na. krm. lac-d. (lch). lpd. (lpt). ly-b. lyc. mgs-au. (myris). n-x. na-ba. na-ca. (ner). p-x. pb. physo. (ppv.) pru-l. (pt). (rho). rs. sep. (si-x). (sn). (so-d). (so-t). (spi). (str). (trg). (urg). vi-t. vr-a. (vrb). woo.

Band, like a. lac-d.

Cord, like a. (amph). pru-l.

Horizontally. lac-d.

Vertically. (lch).

CRACKING (**snapping**). con.

CRAMPY. (aga). amb. (arn). (au). buf. can. (chd). (cit-c). (crot). (eug). glp. (hll). (k-cla). (mn-ca). (msc). na-ca. (narth). (p-x). (pt.) (vi-o).

CREEPING. (ach). (aga). (art-v). (as-o). (asr). atp. (ber). chi. (cop). cro. crot. frm-o. (k-bicr). mgs-ar. na-sa. ol-a. (par). (phl). (pol). (pt). (rn-b). sep. spi. str.

CUTTING. (alli). amm-ca. aps. (atp). au. ca-ca. (ca-s). (chi). cit-c. (cl-hx). (cr-o). (crd). crt-c. cth. (cund). (dl-s). (dro). hg. (hg-s). (i). (k-i). (na-ba). ol-a. pet. pul. (pul-n). rs. s. sep. (spi). (srr). stry. (thu). trg. (vi-t). vr-a. (zn). (zng).

DISCHARGE. ach. (acon.) æth. ag-na. aga. al-o. (alm). amm-ca. amm-cl. anan. anm. aps. art-v. arum-t. as-o. as-ters. asc. atp. ba-ca. ba-cl. ber. bi-na. br. bry. buf. c-bis. ca-a. ca-ca. ca-s. cast. cb-a. cb-v. cch. ccs. chd. chi. cic. cl-hx. cn-sa. cof. con. cph. cro. dig. dl-s. dro. (dt). erig. ery. eryn. (eupat). euph. euphr. fe. glp. grc. grp. grt. gui. hg. hll. hydr. hyo. i. k-bicr. k-ca. k-i. k-na. k-o. kre. (lac-ac). lch. lct. led. lpt. ly-b. lyc. men. mg-ca. mg-cl. mgs. mgs-ar. mgs-au. mn-ca. mrl. mtr. n-x. na-ba. na-ca. na-cl. na-sa. ni-ca. ol-a. ox-x. p. p-x. par. pb. pet. phy. pol. pru-l. pt. pul. pul-n. rhe. rho. rs. rs-r. rut. s. s-x. sb-s. sep. si-x. smi. sn. spi. spo. str. str-i. thu. trx. vi-t. (u-na). vr-a. vr-s. ziz. zn.

Corrosive. lyc. na-cl. s. (u-na).

Fetid. led.

Foam. ber.

Hard (æth.) ag-na. aga. al-o. (as-ters). atp. ba-ca. (bi-na). ca-ca. ca-s. chd. chi. cn-sa. (cof). con. (cph). (dig.) (dl-s). dro. (euph.) (euphr). fe. grp. gui. (hll). k-ca. (k-na). k-o. (kre). led. lyc. mtr. n-x. na-ca. ox-x. p-x. par. (pol). rhe. rho. rs. s. (sb-s). si-x. spi. (str). thu. trx. (vr-s).

Mucus. ach. æth. ag-na. aga. al-o. amm-ca. amm-cl. anan. anm. aps. art-v. arum-t. as-o. asc. atp. ba-ca. ba-cl. bry. c-bis. ca-a. ca-ca. ca-s. cb-a. cb-v. ccs. chd. cic. cl-hx. cn-sa. con. cro. dig. dro. erig. ery. eryn. euph. euphr. fe. glp. grc. grp. grt. hg. hydr. i. k-bicr. k-ca. k-i. k-na. k-o. kre. lct. led. lpt. ly-b. lyc. men. mg-ca. mg-cl. mgs. mgs-ar. mgs-au. mn-ca. mrl. mtr. n-x. na-ba. na-ca. na-cl. ni-ca. ol-a. ox-x. p. p-x. par. phy. pol. pru-l. pt. pul. pul-n. rho. rs. rs-r. s. s-x. sb-s. sep. si-x. sn. spi. str. str-i. thu. trx. vr-a. ziz. zn.

Pus. ag-na. al-o. (alm). amm-ca. art-v. as-o. atp. br. bry. (buf). ca-ca. ca-s. cb-v. chd. cro. dl-s. (dt). (eryn). euph. euphr. glp. grp. grt. k-ca. k-i. k-o. led. lyc. mg-ca. mn-ca. (mrl). (mtr). n-x. na-cl. na-sa. p. par. pb. pru-l. pt. pul. rhe. rho. rs. rut. s. s-x. sep. si-x. sn. (spi). spo. str. str-i. thu. trx. (u-na). (zn).

Tenacious (glutinous). (eupat). (lac-c).

Thick. hydr.

Thin (watery). mrl. na-cl. (pet). s. str.

White. ber. hydr. lch. (rs.)

Yellow. aga. (ca-ca). hg. k-bicr. n-x. rs. str. ziz.

DRAWING. acon. aga. (alli). (alo). (arn.) art-v. as-o. asr. (ast). atp. (bar). (ber). buf. ca-s. can. (cb-v). cch. (ccs). chd. (chio). (cic). cit-c. (cl-hx). con. (cor). cro. (crt-c). (cth). (dph). (dro.) (f-hx). (grp). (grt). (hg-s). (hll). (jcr). (k-i). k-o. klm. kre. (li-ca). (lo-cœ). lo-i. (ly-b). mgs. (mgs-ar). (mn-ca). myris. n-x. (na-ba). (narth). (nic). ol-a. p. (p-x). (par). pb. (pod). pol. (pru-l). pt. pul. (rhe). rho. (rs). (rut). (s). se. (si-x). (sn). (spo). sr-ca. (str). thu. (trg). (trx). tx-b. (val). vr-s. zng.

DRYNESS. acon. ag-na. aga. al-o. (anm). (arn). art-v. as-o. asr. atp. atrop-sa. ba-ca. bar. ber. bry. ca-ca. (cb-v). chi. cit-c. cle. (cln). co. cor. (cph). (cr-o). cro. crt. (cyc). dl-s. dph. (dph-i). drm. elaps. euph. euphr. gel. (glp). grc. (grp). grt. hg-bicl. (hpm). k-bicr. k-ca. k-o. kre. lch. li-ca. lyc. mg-ca. mg-cl. (mgs). (mgs-ar). (mgs-au). mn-ca. mrl. mtr. myris. (n-x). na-ca. na-cl. na-sa. narth. ni-ca. ol-a. p. pæo. pol. (pet). phl. ppv. pru-l. pul. qu-sa. rho. rs. s. (sa-l). si-x. (smi). spi. srr. str. (str-i). thu. trg. vr-a. zn.

Appearance of. kre.

ERUPTIONS. ach. (æth). ag-na. (al-o). (alm). (alo). amb. amm-cl. (anan). (aps). arn. as-o. (asc). atp. (au). ba-ca. (br). (bry). (buf). (c-bis). (ca-a). ca-ca. (ca-i). ca-pa. (ca-s). can. cap. cb-a. (cch). chd. (chio). (chlor). chm. cit-c. (cle). (co). (con). (cro). crot. (cth). (cub). (dig). dl-s. (elaps). (ery). (eryn). (euph). euphr. f-hx. (fe). (fe-pa). (frm). grp. (gui). hg. (hg-bicl). (hg-s). (hll). hydr. (i). jug-c. k-bicr. (k-ca). k-i. (k-o). kre. krm. lau-c. (lch). (led). lyc. (men). (mgs-ar). (mgs-au). (mrl). (msc). mtr. (myris). (n-x). (na-ba). na-ca. (na-cl). (na-sa). (ner). p. (p-x). (par). pet. phy. (pol). pul. (rho). (rn-s). (rs). rut. s. sb-s. sb-t. (se). sep. si-x. (smi). sn. (so-o). (spi). (spo). (srr). (str). (str-i). (te). thu. trg. (trm). (trn). (trx). (tx-b). (u-na). (val). (vtx). woo. (ziz). zn.

Abscess. (ca-ca). (ca-s). (hg.) (na-ca). (pul). (si-x).

Blisters. (arn). (ca-s). euphr. (k-bicr). (na-sa). sb-t. (thu). woo.

Boils. (bry). (ca-pa). (i). (na-cl). (p).

Cancer. as-o. atp. ca-ca. cb-a. hydr. p. sep. si-x. thu. trg.

Dry. (kre). (tx-b).

Encysted Tumors. (ca-ca). (thu).

Erythema Circumscripta. (ery).

Fistula. (alm). ca-ca. chd. dl-s. f-hx. grp. pet. pul. rut. s. si-x. sn. trg.

Fungus. as-o. can. cb-a. p. sep. thu.
Hæmatodes. atp. ca-ca. lyc. sep. si-x.
Medullaris. atp.
Granulations (roughness). ag-na. (aps). (as-o). (eryn). (k-bicr.) phy. sb-t.
Hard. sb-t.
White. sb-t.
Feeling of. elaps. (k-bicr). myris. (trn).
Hard. (au). (bry). (ca-ca). (dl-s). (gui). (lch). (rn-s). sb-t. (thu).
Herpes. (bry). (ery). (kre). (rs). (sep). (trn). (tx-b). (woo).
Dry. (kre). (tx-b).
Red areola with. (tx-b).
Hot. (c-bis). (smi). (sn). (woo).
Itching. (c-bis) (ca-ca) (na-cl). (se). (smi).
Moist. (ca-ca). sb-s.
Pimples. ach. (al-o). (asc). (au). ba-ca. (bry). (ca-s). (dl-s). (gui). (hg-s). (hur). (k-ca). (lyc). (msc). (n-x). (na-cl). (pet). (rho). (rn-s). (rs). (s). (smi). (sn). (thu). (trg). (trn). (trx).
Hard. (gui). (rn-s).
Hot. (sn).
Pressing. (sn).
Smarting. (gui).
Undefined pain. (asc).
Pterygium. ag-na. as-o. can. chd. chm. euphr. (frm). krm. myris. pul. rut. spi. (trm). zn.
Pustules. (æth). (al-o). (alo). atp. (c-bis). (ca-s). (chd). (chio). (con). (cro). (cth). hg. jug-c. k-bicr. (lyc). (na-cl). (p). (pet). (pol). (rs). (s). (se). (sep). (thu).
Hot. (c-bis).
Itching. (c-bis).
Red areola with. k-bicr.
Soft. (bry).
White. (k-bicr).
Red areola. k-bicr. (tx-b).
Rhagades (cracks). (anan). (grp). (zn).
Scabs. (buf). (co). (con). (f-hx). (grp). (hg). (lyc). (sb-t). (sep). (spo). (srr). (te).
Undefined pain. (spo).
Yellow. (spo).
Scales, (scurf). (kre). (pul).
Shooting. (smi).

Smarting. (gui). (s).
Smooth. (au).
Soft. (bry).
Spongy. (alm).
Stye. (Al-o). (amb). (aps). (as-o). (au). (ca-ca). (ca-s). (cch). (cit-c). (con). (cth). (cub). (dig). (dl-s). (elaps). (fe). (fe-pa). (grp). (hg). (k-o). (lyc). (men). (mgs-au). (na-cl). (p). (p-x). (pol). (pul). (rs). (s). (sep). (sn). (so-o). (thu). (trg). (u-na). (val). (ziz).
Smarting. (s).
Tubercles (warts). (alm). (au). (bry). (ca-ca). (dl-s). (hg-s). (k-i). (k-o). (lch). (n-x). (rn-s). (sb-s). (sb-t). (srr). (thu).
Smooth. (au).
Spongy. (alm).
Undefined pain. (bry). (sb-s).
White. (sb-s).
Ulcers. amb. (anan). arn. (as-o). atp. (buf). (ca-a). ca-ca. (ca-i). ca-pa. (ca-s). cap. (cch). cit-c. (cle). (con). (cro). crot. dl-s. (euph). (euphr). (frm). (hg). (hg-bicl). (k-i). (led). (lyc). (mrl). mtr. (na-ba). na-ca. (na-cl). p. (pul). (rs). (rut). s. (sb-s). si-x. (spi). (str). (str-i). trg. (woo). (zn).
Undefined pain. (asc). (bry). (hg-s). (sb-s). (sn). (spo). (thu).
Urticaria. (chlor). (f-hx). (smi).
Hot. (smi).
Itching. (smi).
Shooting. (smi).
Vesicles. amm-cl. (arn). atp. ba-ca. (br). cth. euphr. (lch). (mgs-ar). (pol). (rs). s. (se). srr.
White. (k-bicr). (sb-s). sb-t.
Yellow. (spo).
FALSE SENSATIONS. ag-na. (aga). (al-o). alli. amb. (amm-cl). (amph). anm. apo. aps. arn. art-v. as-o. asc. atp. au. ba-ca. (bar). ber. bru. bry. buf. ca-ca. ca-o. ca-pa. ca-s. cap. (cau). (cb-a). cb-v. ccs. chd. chi. cis. (co). con. cor. cro. (crt-c). dig. (dl-s). drm. (dt). et-fr. euph. euphr. f-hx. fe. frm. frm-s. gel. (grp). grt. hæm. hg. hg-s. hur. hyo. i. k-bicr. k-ca. (k-i). k-na. k-o. kre. lac-d. lch. li-ca. (lo-cœ). ly-b. lyc. (men). mg-cl. (mg-sa). mgs. mgs-ar. mgs-au. mph. msc. n-x. na-ba. na-ca. na-cl. (na-sa). narth. ner. ni-ca. (nic). ol-a. ox-x. p. p-x. pb. ped. pet. phy. pol. ppv. pt. ptv. pul. rhe. rho. rn-b. rs. rs-r. s. (s-x). sang. sb-t.

(se). (sep). si-x. smc. smi. (sn). spi. sr-ca. srr. (str-i). (te). teu. thu. trg. trn. trx. urg. urt. vi-t. zn. (zng).

Cutting. hg. k-bicr.

Fixed. k-i.

Hair. ccs. (k-na). mgs-au. na-ca. (nic). pul. rn-b. sang. (te). (trn).

Hard. ner.

Lime. rs-r.

Mucus (grease). aps. ca-ca. (euph). pul.

Pellicle (film). cro. k-o. ol-a. (s). scr-m.

Sand (dust, foreign body). ag-na. (aga). (al-o). (alli). amb. (amm-cl). (amph). anm. apo. aps. arn. art-v. as-o. asc. atp. au. ba-ca. (bar). ber. bru. bry. buf. ca-ca. ca-o. ca-pa. ca-s. cap. (cau). (cb-a). cb-v. ccs. chd. chi. (co). con. cor. cro. (crt-c). dig. (dl-s). drm. (dt). euph. euphr. (f-hx). fe. frm. frm-s. gel. (grp). grt. hæm. hg. hg-s. hur. hyo. i. k-bicr. k-ca. k-i. k-na. k-o. kre. lch. li-ca. lo-cœ. ly-b. (lyc). (men). mg-cl. (mg-sa). (mgs). mgs-ar. (mgs-au). mph. msc. n-x. na-ba. (na-ca). na-cl. (na-sa). narth. ner. ni-ca. (nic). ol-a. ox-x. p. p-x. ped. pet. phy. plb. pol. ppv. pt. ptv. pul. rhe. rho. rn-b. rs. (rs-r). s. (s-x). (sang). sb-t. (se). (sep). si-x. smc. smi. (sn). spi. sr-ca. srr. (str-i). teu. thu. trg. trn. trx. urt. vi-t. zn. (zng).

Smoke. (alli). (chi). sang.

Snow-flakes. et-fr.

Splinter (thorn). ca-o. s. trn.

Stones, surrounded by. k-na. lac-d.

Water. ber. buf. (dt). (ni-ca). (trn). urg.

Wind. ag-na. (asr). cro. f-hx. hg-s. mgs-ar. narth. (sep). thu.

GNAWING. (hyo). (k-i). (kre). ox-x. (pt). rn-s. s. (str-i). vtx.

HÆMORRHAGE. arn. atp. ca-ca. cb-v. crt. elaps. (ery). euphr. (grp). mtr. (pb). rut. str.

HARD. (acon). (bry). (cit-c). (dl-s). (n-x). (rn-s). (rs). (spi). (spo-f).

HEAT, (**burning**). ach. acon. (æsc). æth. ag-na. aga. al-o. alli. (alm). amb. amm-ca. amm-cl. anan. aph. apo. aps. ara. arn. (art-v). as. as-i. as-o. asr. ast. atp. au. ba-ca. bap. bar. ber. bi-na. br. bru. bry. (buf). bz-x. c-bis. (ca-a). ca-ca. ca-o. (ca-pa). ca-s. can. can-i. cap. cast. cb-a. cb-v. (cch). (ccs). chd. chi. chio. (chlor). cic. cit-c. cl-hx. cld. cle. (cmf). co. con. cor. crb-x. cro. crot. crt. cth. cu. cy-hx. cyc. dig. dl-s. dph. drm. (dro). dt. elaps. ery. eryn. et-fr.

eug. euphr. f-hx. fe. frm-s. (gel). glo. glp. grc. grp. gym. hg. (hg-a). (hg-bi). hg-bicl. (hg-s). hll. hpm. (hur). hydr. (ind). (irs). (itu). jnp-s. jug. k-bicr. k-ca. k-i. k-na. k-o. (klm). kre. krm. lau-c. lch. lct. led. li-ca. lo-c. (lo-cœ). lo-i. lpd. ly-b. lyc. (men). mg-ca. mg-cl. mg-sa. mgs. mgs-ar. (mgs-au). mn-ca. mph. mrl. mtr. mur. myris. n-x. na-ba. na-ca. na-cl. na-sa. narth. (ner). ni-ca. nic. ol-a. os. p. p-x. pæo. par. pb. pb-a. pet. phl. phy. pim. plb. (pnc). (pnx). pol. ppv. pru-l. pso. pt. ptv. pul. (pul-n). (rhe). rho. (rn-b). (rn-s). rs. rs-r. rs-v. rut. s. s-x. (sang). sb-t. sep. si-x. (smi). sn. so-d. so-t. spi. spo. (spo-f). sr-ca. srr. (stc). str. str-i. stry. (te). (thr). thu. til. trg. trn. trx. (tx-b). (urg). val. vi-o. (vin). vp-t. vr-a. vr-s. vrb. vtx. woo. ziz. zn. zng.

Cold. et-fr.

HEAVINESS. (acon). æsc. al-o. anan. aps. arum-t. as. as-o. asc. ast. atp. (atrop). (ber). br. (c-bis). (ca-ca). (ca-o). (cac). cb-v. (chd). chi. (cit-c). (cl-hx). cmc. cmf. (con). cph. (cr-o). crb-x. crn. cro. crot (crt-c). (dig). (dl-s). (dph-i). ery. (euph). euphr. fe. (gel). glo. (glp). hæm. hg-s. hll. hpm. hur. itu. k-bicr. k-ca. k-o. (lac-c). (lac-f). lch. (lpd). lyc. mitch. mrl. (mtr). myr. na-ba. (na-ca). (na-sa). (nuph). (ol-m). p. (p-x). pan. pb. (pd). (physo). (pnx). pod. (ppv). (pru-l). ptv. (pul-n). (rs). rs-r. s. sep. (si-x). so-t. (spi). (spo). stach. (str). str-i. stry. (thr). thu. (trn). (vi-o). (vr-a). (vr-v).

INFLAMED. **See** COLOR **Red.**

ITCHING. ach. acon. (æth). (ag). (ag-na). aga. al-o. alli. (alm). amb. amm-ca. amm-cl. anan. (anm). aps. (arn). art-v. arum. as-o. asc. atp. (au). ba-ca. (bar). ber. (br). bru. (bry). buf. buf-s. (by-x). (c-bis). ca-a. ca-ca. (can-i). cb-a. cb-v. chd. (chi). (chio). (chlor). (cit-c). cl-hx. (cle). con. cot. (cr-o). crd. cro. (crot). (crt). (crt-c). cth. cu. cyc. (dl-s). dph. dro. (dt). (elaps). eug. (euph). (euphr). (f-hx). fe. (frm). frm-s. (glo). (glp). grc. grp. (grt). hg. (hg-a). hg-bicl. hg-s. (hll). (hur). (hyo). (i). (ind). (jat). (jnc). k-bicr. k-ca. (k-i). k-na. k-o. klm. kre. (krm). lam. (lau-c). (lch). (led). (lo-cœ). (lo-i). lpd. ly-b. lyc. mg-ca. mg-cl. mgs. mgs-ar. mgs-au. mim. mn-ca. mrl. msc. n-x. na-ba. na-ca. na-cl. (na-sa). narth. ner. ni-ca. (nic). (ol-a). p. p-x. pæo. (par). (pb). (pb-a). pd. (ped). pet. phl. (phy). (pnc). (pnx). (ppv). (pru). pru-l. pt. pul. rho. rn-b. (rs). rs-r. (rut). s. (s-x). sb-s. (sb-t). (se). sep. si-x. (smi). smr. (sn). (spi). (spo). (sr-ca). srr. str. str-i. stry. (te). (til). trg. trn. tx-b. urg. vi-t. (vin). (vsp). (vr-a). (vr-v.) vtx. zn.

Desire to rub the eyes. aga. con. cot. cro. gym. k-bicr. k-o. urg.

LACHRYMATION. ach. acon. ag-na. aga. al-o. alli. (alm). alo. amb. amm-ca. amm-cl. (amph). anan. anth. aps. arn. art-v. arum-t. as-i. as-o. asr. ast. atp. au. ba-ca. bap. bar. ber. blt. br. bru. bry. buf. c-bis. ca-ca. (ca-i). ca-o. ca-pa. ca-s. cap. cast. cau. cb-a. cb-v. cch. cd-sa. chd. chi. cit-c. cl-hx. cle. clv. cmc. cmf. co. cof. con. cor. cph. cr-o. (crb-x). cro. crot. crt. crt-c. cth. cu. cu-asi. dig. dl-s. dph. dph-i. dt. (ery). eug. eupat. eupat-p. euph. euphr. f-hx. fe. fe-mgs. frm. gel. glp. grc. grp. grt. gym. hg. hg-bi. hg-s. hll. hrc. hydr. (hyo). i. irs. jnp-s. k-bicr. k-ca. k-i. k-na. k-o. kre. lac-d. (lac-f). lau-c. lch. led. lo-c. (lo-cœ). lpd. lpt. ly-b. lyc. men. mg-ca. mg-cl. mg-sa. mgs. mgs-ar. mgs-au. mitch. mrl. msc. myris. n-x. na-ba. na-ca. na-cl. na-sa. ner. ni-ca nic. ol-a. os. p. p-x. par. pau. pb. pb-a. (ped). pet. phl. phy. physo. plb. pnx. pol. ppv. pru-l. pt. ptv. pul. pul-n. qu-cy. qu-sa. rhe. rho. rn-b. rn-s. rs. (rs-r). rs-v. (rut). s. s-x. (sa-l). (sang). sb-t. se. sep. si-x. smc. smi. sn. snc. (snp). so-n. so-t. spi. spo. sr-ca. srr. str. str-i. stry. te. teu. thu. trg. trn. trx. tx-b. (u-na). urg. val. vi-o. vr-a. vr-s. vr-v. vtx. woo. xan. ziz. zn.

Cold. (trg).

Excoriating. as-o. led. pul. (u-na).

Greasy. s.

Hot (acrid). acon. al-o. arn. as-o. atp. au. bry. (ca-ca). (ca-i). cb-v. cd-sa. cit-c. con. cph. dig. dl-s. eug. euphr. glp. (grc). grp. hg. jnp-s. (k-na). k-o. kre. led. lyc. mgs. n-x. na-cl. (na-sa). p. p-x. pb. pb-a. pul. rs. s. sep. spi. str. str-i. teu. zn.

Salt. atp. kre. rs.

Thick. trn.

Appearance of. ca-ca. cro. hyo. kre. na-cl. ppv. sa-l. sep. so-n. teu. trg. vr-a.

Feeling of. arum-t. as-i. ba-ca. chi. cor. cro. (hg-s). hyo. kre. mitch. mrl. myris. n-x. na-cl. ner. ped. pt. s. sep. si-x. smr. sn. spi. teu.

LOOSE, **feel**. alli. cb-a. spi.

MOTION **in**. acon. ber. cb-a. cis. (dt). eug. (ly-b). mgs. (pt). (rs).

Bubbling. ber.

Jumping like something. (dt).

Passing round, like something. cis. (rs).

Pendulum, like. mgs.

Rolling. eug.
Undulation. acon. (pt).
Whirling. (ly-b).

MOVEMENTS. ach. acon. æsc. æth. ag-na. aga. al-o. (alm). amb. amm-cl. amph. amy. anan. anm. aps. ara. arn. art-v. arum-t. as-o. asr. ast. atp. ba-ca. bar. ber. br. bry. buf. (c-bis). ca-ca. (ca-i). ca-pa. cb-a. cb-v. cbz-x. cch. ccs. chd. chi. cic. cit-c. cl-hx. clv. con. (cop). cori. cph. crd. cro. crot. crt. crt-c. cth. cu. cub. cy-hx. cyc. dig. dl-s. dph. dt. (ery). eryn. eug. f-hx. (frm). gel. glo. glp. grp. grt. hg. hg-bicl. hll. hur. hyo. (hyp). i. ind. jat. jnp-s. k-bicr. k-ca. k-cla. k-i. k-o. kre. krm. (lac-ac). (lac-d). (lac-f). lau-c. lch. lyc. men. mg-ca. mg-cl. mgs. mgs-ar. mn-ca. mrl. msc. mtr. n-x. na-ca. na-cl. narth. ni-ca. nic. ol-a. p. p-x. par. pb. pet. phl. phy. pnc. pnx. pol. ppv. pru-l. pt. pul. qu-sa. rhe. rho. rs. rs-r. rut. s. s-x. (sa-l). sb-s. se. sep. si-x. smc. (smi). sn. so-d. so-t. spi. (spi-m). (spo). sr-ca. str. str-i. thu. trg. trn. urg. vi-o. vr-a. vrb. woo. zn.

Convulsions (rolling, quivering, twitching). ach. acon. (æsc). æth. ag-na. aga. al-o. alo. (amb). amm-cl. (amph). amy. anan. anm. (aps). arn. (art-v). (arum-t). as-o. (asr). (ast). atp. au. (ba-ca). (bar). (ber). bry. buf. (c-bis). ca-ca. ca-pa. cb-a. (cb-v). cbz-x. (cch). (ccs). (chd). chi. cic. (cit-c). (cl-hx). clv. con. cori. (cph). (crd). (cro). crot. (crt). (crt-c). cth. cu. (cub). cy-hx. cyc. dig. dl-s. (dph). dt. eryn. eug. (f-hx). (frm). gel. glo. glp. (grp). (grt). hg. hg-bicl. hll. (hur). hyo. i. (ind). (jat). (jnp-s). (k-bicr). (k-ca). (k-cla). k-i. (k-o). (kre). (krm). (lac-ac). (lac-d). (lac-f). lau-c. (lch). (lyc). men. (mg-ca). (mg-cl). (mgs). mgs-ar. mn-ca. mrl. msc. mtr. (n-x). (na-ca). na-cl. (narth). ni-ca. (ol-a). (p). p-x. par. pb. pet. (phl). (phy). (pnc). pnx. (pol). ppv. pru-l. pt. pul. qu-sa (rhe). (rho). (rs). rs-r. (rut). s. (s-x). (sa-l). (sb-s). (se). (sep). si-x. smc. (smi). sn. (so-d). (so-t). spi. sr-ca. (str). str-i. (thu). trg. (trn). (urg). (vi-o). vr-a. vr-s. (vrb). (woo). (zn).

Feeling of. ara. ca-ca. (can). clv. (dt). glo. (lch). (ol-a). pet. rs-r. trn.

Squinting. acon. æth. al-o. (alm). aps. (art-v). as-o. atp. ca-ca. ca-pa. clv. cu. cub. cyc. dig. dt. eryn. gel. hll. hyo. k-i. men. pb. pul. rs. s. s-x. spi. (spi-m).

Feeling of. ca-ca. men. pod. pul.

Downwards. æth. (cb-a). (chd). (elaps). (grp). (ind). (k-o). (phy). (ppv). (sep). (spi). (urg).

Feeling of. (can). (ol-a).

Upwards. ach. acon. aga. amy. anan. arn. as-o. buf. cic. cu. cub. glo. hll. jat. lau-c. (lch). msc. (na-cl). nic. pb. ppv. spi. vr-a.

Inwards. (alm). (art-v). (ca-ca). (cyc). (hyo). pb.

Outwards. (cph). (cro). glo. lau-c. (mtr). (rhe). (rut). s-x. vr-a.

Feeling of. arn.

To the left. buf. dig.

From side to side. cu.

As if turned round. (chi).

As if taken out, squeezed, and put back. trg.

NUMB. (acon). (as-h). hg-s. (mrl). (naj). (narth). (pb). (ppv). pt. trg.

PARALYSIS. (acon). (ag-na). (aga). al-o. (amb). (amm-ca). amph. (anan). (anm). aps. arn. art-v. as-o. asr. ath. atp. atrop. au. ba-ca. ba-cl. (bap). (br). bru. bry. ca-ca. (ca-s). can. (cap). cb-a. (cb-v). (chd). chi. (chlor). cle. con. cro. (cu). cy-hx. cyc. (dro). (dt). (elaps). (eug). (euph). (fe). (gel). glp. grp. (hg). hg-bicl. (hll). hur. (hyo). i. ind. (k-ca). k-i. k-o. (li-ca). (lpd). ly-b. lyc. (men). (mg-ca). (mg-cl). mg-sa. mrl. (mtr). (myris). n-x. (na-ba). na-ca. (na-cl). (nic). (p). p-x. (pæo). pb. ped. (pet). (physo). (pnx). pol. ppv. pru-l. (ptv). (pul). rhe. (rs). (rs-v). (s-x). (sa-l). sb-t. (sep). (si-x). sn. (so-d). spi. srr. (str). stry. (thu). trg. (trn). urg. val. (vi-t). vr-a. vr-s. (zn).

PECKING. (pet).

PRESSING. ach. acon. æth. ag-na. aga. (al-o). (alo). amb. (amm-ca). (amm-cl). (amph). anag. anan. anm. aps. (arn). art-v. (arum-t). as-o. (asr). (ast). (ath). atp. atrop. atrop-sa. au. ba-a. ba-ca. bap. (ber). bi-na. br. bry. buf. c-bis. (ca-a). ca-ca. (ca-o). ca-s. (can). (can-i). cap. (cau). cb-a. (cb-v). (cch). (ccs). chd. chi. (chio). (cic). (cit-c). cl-hx. (cld). (cle). clv. cmc. cmf. cn-sa. co. cof. con. cop. (cor). cph. (crd). cro. crot. (crt). crt-c. cth. cu. cyc. dig. dl-s. dph. (drm). dro. dt. elaps. erig. ery. (eryn). evo. (euph.) euphr. (f-hx). fe. (fe-mgs). (frm-s). (gel). glo. glp. gn-c. gn-l. grp. grt. (gui). gym. hæm. hg. (hg-bi). hg-bicl. (hg-i). hg-s. (hll). hur. (hydr). (hyo). i. ind. itu. (jcr). (jnp-s). k-bicr. k-ca. k-cla. (k-i). k-na. k-o. (klm). kre. krm. lac-c. (lac-f). lam. lau-c. lch. lct. led. lo-i. lpt. (ly-b). lyc. men. menth. mg-ca. mg-cl. mg-sa. (mgs-ar). mgs-au. mn-ca. (morph-a). mph. mrl. (msc). mtr. myr. (myris). n-x. (na-ba). na-ca. na-cl. na-sa. narth. ner. ni-ca. nic. nuph. ol-a. (ox-x). p. p-x. (pan). par. pb. (pd). pet. (phl). phy. pnx. pol. (ppv). pru-l. pso.

pt. ptv. pul. pul-n. (qu-sa). rhe. rho. rn-b. rn-s. rs. (rs-r). rs-v. rut. s. s-x. sang. (sb-s). sb-t. (scu). se. sep. si-x. smb. smc. smi. sn. snp-n. so-d. (spi). spo. sr-ca. str. str-i. stry. sum. (te). (teu). (thr). thu. trg. (trx). (urt). val. vr-a. vr-s. (vr-v). xan. (zn). (zng).

Like a Plug, &c. (asr). chi. (hll). n-x. (na-sa). smc.

As if pressed about in all directions. atrop.

PROJECTING. acon. æth. (alm). alo. amy. anan. anm. (aps). arn. as-o. atp. au. br. bru. ca-pa. ca-s. cap. (cch.) chi. cic. cl. con. cth. cu. cy-hx. dl-s. dro. dt. glo. glp. gui. gym. hg. hg-bicl. hyo. (k-bicr). mgs-ar. morph-a. mrl. msc. myris. na-ba. pb. ppv. pru-l. rs. (s). (si-x). sn. spi. spo. str. urg. vp-r. vp-t. vr-a.

Feeling. atp. (cmc). glo. gui. rs. scu.

SCRAPING. (chd). (k-bicr). (p). (pb). (pru-l). pul. s. (si-x). sn.

SENSITIVE. **See** CONDITIONS—TOUCH, &c.

SHOOTING. ach. acon. (æsc). (æth). (ag). aga. al-o. alli. (alo). amm-ca. amph. (anag). anan. (anm). aps. arn. as-o. atp. (au). ba-ca. (bar). ber. (blt). (br). bry. buf. c-bis. ca-a. ca-ca. (ca-o). ca-s. cap. cb-a. cb-v. (chd). (chi). (chio). (cic). (cis). cit-c. cl-hx. (cld). (cle). clv. (cmc). co. con. (cot). cph. (crd). cro. crot. (crt). (cth). (cub). cyc. dl-s. (dph). drm. (dro). (dt). (ecb). elaps. (eug). euphr. (f-hx). fe. (frm-s). (gel). glo. (glp). (grp). (grt). (gym). hed. hg. (hg-bi). hg-bicl. hg-cy. (hg-s). hll. hpm. hur. (hyp). (i). (ind). (irs-f). (itu). (jnp-s). (k-bicr). k-ca. k-cla. (k-i). k-o. klm. (krm). (lac-f). lau-c. (li-ca). lpd. ly-b. lyc. men. mg-ca. mg-cl. (mgs). mgs-ar. mgs-au. (mn-ca). mph. mrl. mtr. (myris). (n-x). na-ba. na-ca. na-cl. na-sa. narth. (ner). (ni-ca). (nic). ol-a. p. p-x. (pæo). (pan). par. pau. pb. pet. phl. (phy). pnx. pru-l. (pso). (ptv). pul. (rho). (rn-s). rs. rs-v. s. (s-x). sa-l. (sang). sb-s. (sb-t). se. sep. si-x. smi. (sn). (snc). snp-n. so-t. (spi). spo. sr-ca. srr. str. (str-i). stry. thu. trg. trn. (trx). (tx-b). (u-na). (urg). (val). (vi-t). (vr-a). (vr-v). vtx. woo. (ziz). (zn). (zng).

Cold. s. sa-l.

Hot. aps. (as-o). (con). (rho). (trg).

SMALL (**contracted**). (can-i). (crot). hg-s. (na-ba). (pb). (rho). (woo).

Feeling. al-o. cro. grt. (gui). hg-bicl. (kre). (lac-d). mrl. (par). (trg).

SMARTING. acon. æsc. æth. ag-na. aga. al-o. alli. amb. amm-ca. anan. aps. arn. art-v. arum-t. as-o. (asc). asp. asr. atp. (au). (ba-ca). bap. (bar). ber. br. bry. buf-s. (c-bis). ca-ca.

ca-s. (cac). cap. cast. cb-a. cb-v. cch. ccs. (chd). chi. (cl-hx). cld. cle. (cln). cit-c. cmc. cmf. cmx. co. con. cor. cot. cr-o. crn. cro. crot. cth. (cu). (cu-asi). dig. dl-s. dph. dro. dt. erig. eryn. eug. eupat. euph. euphr. fe. fe-mgs. (frm). gel. glo. glp. (gn-l). grp. (grt). (gui). gym. hg. (hg-i). hg-s. hll. (hur). hydr. (hyo). i. (jat). k-bicr. k-ca. k-i. k-na. k-o. klm. kre. (krm). (ind). (lac-ac). (lac-f). lau-c. lct. (led). li-ca. lo-c. lo-cœ. (lo-i). lpt. lyc. mg-ca. mg-cl. mg-sa. mgs. (mgs-ar). mgs-au. mn-ca. mrl. msc. (mtr). n-x. (na-ba). na-ca. na-cl. ner. ni-ca. nic. ol-a. ox-x. p. p-x. pæo. par. (pb). ped. pet. phl. phy. (pim). (pln). (pnc). (pnx). pod. pol. pru-l. pso. (pt). (ptv). pul. (pul-n). rhe. (rho). rmx. rn-b. rn-s. rs. rs-r. rs-v. rut. s. s-x. sa-l. sang. (sb-s). (sb-t). se. sep. si-x. smc. smr. sn. snp-n. so-t. spi. sr-ca. srr. stc. str. (str-i). stry. (te). teu. thu. trg. trn. trx. (u-na). (urt). val. (vi-t). (vr-a). (vr-v). vtx. woo. ziz. (zn).

SOFTNESS. (rs). (thu).

Feeling of. (na-sa).

STICKY **feeling.** elaps.

STIFFNESS. acon. (al-o). anm. as-o. atp. ber. (ca-ca). ca-s. chi. (chlor). cic. clv. eryn. (hg-s). hyo. k-o. klm. (krm). (men). mgs. mgs-ar. mrl. mtr. p. p-x. pol. pru-l. (rs). s. (spi). str-i. stry. trg. vr-a.

STRAINED. dph. s.

SUNKEN. (æth). ag-na. amb. anan. anm. as-h. as-o. ber. buf. c-bis. ca-ca. chi. cic. cit-c. clv. cn-sa. crn. crt. cu. cu-a. cyc. dl-s. dro. dt. ery. fe. glo. hg. hg-cy. hyo. i. irs. k-bicr. k-ca. lau-c. lyc. mgs-ar. morph-a. n-x. ner. ox-x. p. p-x. pb. phy. pnc. pod. ppv. pru-l. pul. qu-sa. rph. rs. s. smc. sn. spi. spo. str. teu. til. trg. urg. vp-t. vr-a.

Feeling. amb. hg-s. lac-f. teu.

SWEAT. (ca-pa).

SWELLING. (acon). æth. (ag). ag-na. (aga). (al-o). alli. (alm). (amb). anan. anm. (aps). arn. (arum-t). (as). as-o. (asr). atp. au. ba-ca. (ba-cl). br. bru. bry. buf. (ca-ca). ca-pa. ca-s. (can-i). cap. (cb-v). (cch). (cd-cl). chd. (chio). (chlor). (cit-c). (cl-hx). (cln). (clv). (cmc). (cmf). cn-sa. cochl. (con). cro. (crot). (cu). (cyc). (dig). dt. (elaps). (ele). (ery). (eryn). (eupat-p). (euph). euphr. (fe). (fe-mgs). (gel). (glo). (grp). gui. (hg). hg-bi. hg-bicl. hg-s. (hll). hum. hur. (hyo). (i). k-bicr. (k-br). (k-ca). k-i. (k-o). (kre). (lch). (lct). led. (lyc). mg-ca. (mg-cl). (mgs-au). (mn-ca). (morph-a). (msc). mtr. myris. n-x. na-ca. (na-cl). (ner). ol-m. ni-ca. (p). (p-x). pb. (pet). (phy). (physo). (pln). (pol). ppv. (pru-l). (pso). ptv. pul. rhe.

(rho). (rn-b). (rph). rs. (rs-r). rs-v. (rut). s. (sa-a). sb-t. sep. si-x. (smi). (sn). (spi). (spi-m). (spo). (srr). str. (str-i). (te). (teu). (thu). til. (trg). (u-na). (urg). (urt). urt-m. (urt-u). (val). (vp-r). (vsp). woo. (zn).

Air-like. (p).

Bag-like. (k-ca).

Blue. (phy).

Chemosis. acon. aps. (atp). cd-cl. euphr. k-bicr. k-br. k-i. physo. (vsp).

Hard. (acon). (thu).

Œdematous. (aps). (arn). (as-o). (chio). (crot). (hur). (i). (k-bicr). (k-i). mg-ca. (pb). (phy). (rph). (rs). (rs-r). rs-v. (sa-a). (te). (u-na). (urt). urt-m. (urt-u).

Red. (acon). (aps). (ner). rs. (sep). (te). (thu). (vsp).

Watery. (pul).

Feeling of, (feel large). acon. (al-o). (aps). asr. bap. (ber). bi-na. (buf-s). ca-s. can-i. cch. (ccs). (chd). (cit-c). cld. (cmc). cmf. con. cph. crd. cro. (cyc). dph. (dt). gel. grp. gui. (hg-s). hyo. k-o. lch. men. mg-ca. (morph). (morph-a). mrl. myris. n-x. na-ca. na-cl. ni-ca. p-x. par. pb. phy. pol. ppv. pru-l. (rs). (rs-r). (sa-l). sb-t. sep. spi. srr. thu. trg. trx. (val). (vi-o). (vr-v).

Veins swelled. acon. (alm). amb. (atp). (ca-s). dt. (ery). (mg-ca). (pru-l). sa-a. spi.

TEARING. (acon). (ag-na). (aga). al-o. (alli). (amb). amm-cl. (anm). arn. as-o. asr. atp. (au). (au-cl). ba-ca. (bar). ber. (bi-na). bry. (ca-a). ca-ca. (ca-o). (can). (cast). (cb-v). cch. ccs. chd. (chi). cit-c. (cl-hx). (cle). (con). cph. cro. cth. (dl-s). dph. (dro). (euph). grt. (hg-bicl). (hyo). (hyp). (i). (jnp-s). (k-ca). (k-i). (k-na). k-o. (krm). led. ly-b. lyc. (men). mg-ca. (mg-cl). mg-sa. mgs. (mrl). na-ba. na-ca. na-sa. (ni-ca). (ol-a). p. (p-x). par. (pb). (phl). (pnc). (pru). (pru-l). pul. (rs). rut. s. (s-x). sb-t. sep. (si-x). smc. (spi). (spo). str. (str-i). (teu). (thu). (trg). urg. (val). vr-a. zn.

TENSIVE. (ach). (acon). æth. al-o. (amm-ca). aps. (as-o). au. ba-a. ba-ca. (bar). ca-ca. (con). cro. (cth). (dl-s). (dro). dt. glp. (grt). (hg-s). (hll). hyp. i. jnp-s. k-ca. (k-o). lau-c. lct. led. (ly-b). (lyc). (men). mrl. (myris). n-x. (na-ba). na-ca. na-cl. narth. (ner). ni-ca. (nic). ox-x. p. (par). (phl). pol. pt. pul. s. (s-x). (sb-t). sep. si-x. (sn). spi. (spo). stach. str. (thu). trg. vi-t. (zn).

Like a Thread Stretched. (par). (s). (trg).

Laterally. (s).

THROBBING. aga. (amm-cl). aps. arn. as-o. asr. (atp).

(ba-a). (ba-ca). ber. (br). bry. (buf). bz-x. (c-bis). ca-ca. (cch). (ccs). (chd). (chi). (cl-hx). (cph). (cr-o). (cro). crot. (cth). (dig). dl-s. (euphr). (glo). hur. hyo. (i). (k-ca). (k-o). klm. (lau-c). (li-ca). (men). (mg-ca). (mgs). mgs-ar. mgs-au. mn-ca. mtr. (myris). (n-x). na-cl. (na-sa). ni-ca. p. (par). (pb). (pet). pol. (pru-l). rhe. (rho). (rs). (rs-r). (s). (s-x). (sep). sn. (so-t). (sr-ca). srr. (stry). (thr). thu. (trg). trn. (woo). (zn).

Single Throbs. cr-o.

TINGLING. aga. (art-v). (cro). crot. (drm). (ly-b). (par). (pol). spi.

UNDEFINED **Pain.** acon. (æth). ag-na. aga. al-o. (alli). alo. (amm-ca). (amm-cl). amph. anan. (anm). aps. arn. art-v. (arum-t). as. as-o. asc. ast. atp. atrop. atrop-sa. au. ba-ca. bap. (ber). bry. buf. bz-x. ca-ca. (ca-o). ca-pa. ca-s. cap. (cast). cau. cb-a. cb-v. cch. (ccs). chd. chi. (chio). cic. cit-c. (cl-hx). cld. cle. cmc. cmf. cn-sa. co. (cof). con. cph. crb-x. crn. cro. crot. (crt-c). (crv). cth. (cu). (cu-asi). cund. (delph). dig. dl-s. dph. dph-i. (drm). (dro). dt. (elaps). erig. ery. eryn. (eupat). euphr. (f-hx). fe. (fe-mgs). frm. (gel). gn-l. (grc). grp. gui. (gym). hg. hg-bi. (hg-i). (hg-s). hll. hpm. (hur). (hydr). hyo. hyp. i. (irs). (irs-f). (jan). (jcr). jnp-s. jug. k-bicr. k-ca. (k-cla). k-i. (k-na). k-o. klm. kre. lac-ac. lac-c. lac-d. (lau-c). led. li-ca. (lo-c). lo-i. lpd. (lpt). (ly-b). lyc. (mg-ca). mg-cl. (mg-sa). mgs-ar. mll. mn-ca. mph. mrl. (msc). mtr. myr. n-x. na-ba. na-ca. na-cl. narth. ner. (ni-ca). nic. (nuph). (ol-a). (ox-x). p. p-x. (pau). pb. (pd). pet. (phy). (pnx). pod. pol. ppv. (pru-l). (pso). pt. pul. pul-n. (qu-sa). rho. rn-b. rn-s. rs. (rs-r). rut. s. (s-x). (sa-a). (sang). (sb-s). (sb-t). (scu). (se). sep. si-x. smc. smi. sn. snp-n. (so-o). spi. spo-f. srr. str. str-i. stry. thu. trg. tri. trn. (trx). (urt). val. vr-a. vr-s. (vsp). (vtx). (woo). (xan). (ziz). zn. (zng).

WRINKLED. ag-na. br. (chio). (dt). (zn).

Feeling. anan.

EYEBALL SUPERIORLY.

acon. aga. alli. amm-cl. anan. as-o. ast. br. ca-ca. ca-o. cac. cb-a. cb-v. ccs. chd. cmf. co. cot. crt-c. dl-s. drm. hg. hll. i. lo-cœ. lo-i. mrl. ox-x. p-x. phy. pim. pru-l. s. sep. si-x. sn. snc. spi. sr-ca. str-i. thu. vi-t.

BORING. s.

BRUISED. s.

BURSTING. acon.
COLOR **Red**. str-i.
CONTRACTIVE. chd.
CUTTING. hg.
DRAWING. pru-l.
DRYNESS. s.
FALSE SENSATIONS, **Hair**. ccs.
Sand. aga. anan. ca-ca. ca-o. ccs. co. sn. str-i. vi-t.
Smoke. alli.
HEAT. p-x. pim. spi.
ITCHING. aga.
PRESSING. aga. cb-a. cb-v. chd. drm. lo-i. mrl. ox-x. phy. sep. spi.
SHOOTING. cb-a. hll. p-x.
SMARTING. cac. spi.
TEARING. amm-cl.
TINGLING. aga. drm.
UNDEFINED. (acon). as-o. cmf. crt-c.

EYEBALL INFERIORLY.

aga. aps. chi. glp. jnp-s. men. p-x. pol. s. se. sep. spi. str. zn.
COLOR, **Yellow**. str.
DRYNESS. s.
FALSE SENSATIONS, **Sand**. se. smc. (spi.)
Smoke. chi.
HEAT. glp.
PRESSING. p-x. pol. spi.
SMARTING. spi.
TENSIVE. jnp-s.

EYEBALL EXTERNALLY.

ca-a. ca-pa. cyc. dt. i. k-bicr. p-x. ptv. pul. rn-b. rs. smi. sn. spi. spo. trx. vr-a. vtx. woo.
BRUISED. vtx.
COLOR, **Red**. ca-a. ca-pa. pul. smi.
ERUPTIONS, **Blisters**. woo.
HEAT. trx.
PRESSING. rn-b.
SHOOTING. cyc. trx.
SWELLING. ptv.

EYEBALL INTERNALLY.

acon. ag-na. art-v. ber. ca-ca. ca-pa. ery. eug. glp. hæm. jnp.-s. k-bicr. k-o. li-ca. mtr. p-x. pru-l. pul. rs. rs-v. rut. s. str-i. thr. thu. trm. trx. woo. zn.

BORING. s.
BRUISED. s.
COLOR, **Red**. acon. ag-na. ca-pa. eug. hæm. p-x. pru-l. pul. rs-r. rs-v. zn.
Yellow. p-x.
DRYNESS. art-v. ber.
ERUPTIONS, **Blisters**. woo.
Pterygium. trm. zn.
Pustules. k-bicr.
FALSE SENSATIONS, **Pellicle**. k-o.
HEAT. glp. thr.
ITCHING. str-i.
PRESSING. ber.
SWELLING. ag-na.
TENSIVE. jnp-s.

EYEBALL ANTERIORLY.

acon. s-x. sb-s.
HEAT. s-x.
PRESSING. acon. s-x.
SHOOTING. acon. sb-s.

EYEBALL POSTERIORLY.

anth. asc. atp. au. bi-na. ca-pa. can. cau. co. f-hx. glo. led. menth. mrl. p. p-x. pd. s. sep. spi. spo-f. srr. thr. thu. urg.

BORING. thu.
COLDNESS. ca-pa.
HEAVINESS. thr.
ITCHING. sep.
PRESSING. anth. au. can. cau. f-hx. led. menth. mrl p-x. s. thr.
SHOOTING. p.
SMARTING. srr.
TEARING. bi-na. urg.
UNDEFINED. atrop. co. sep. spi.

EYEBALL INTERIORLY.

acon. al-o. alli. anag. art-v. as-o. asr. atp. ba-a. ba-ca. cch. chd. cis. cmf. dt. glo. hg. k-ca. lac-ac. lac-f. li-ca. men. mrl. pol. rn-b. spi. trn. vr-s.
BORING. cch.
BURSTING. acon.
DRAWING. cch.
DRYNESS. asr.
HEAT. hg.
PRESSING. anag. art-v. atp. ba-a. ba-ca. cmf. dt. hg. men. mrl. rn-b.
SHOOTING. k-ca.
SMARTING. al-o. spi.
TEARING. asr.
THROBBING. asr. trn.
UNDEFINED. as-o. cmf. li-ca.

EYEBALL CIRCUMFERENCE.

æsc. crt-c. gel. spo.
CUTTING. crt-c.
PRESSING. spo.

EYEBALL ROUND CORNEA.

ag-na. as-o. ba-ca. ca-s. hg-s. k-bicr. na-ca. pul. s. thu.
COLOR **Red**. ag-na. as-o. (ca-s). hg-s. k-bicr. pul. s.
ERUPTIONS **Blisters**. (ca-s).
Pimples. ba-ca.
Ulcers. na-ca.
Vesicles. s.

EYEBALL, CENTRE OF.

k-bicr. krm. lac-ac. lac-f. rs.
FALSE SENSATIONS, **Pellicle**. krm.
HEAT. krm.
SMARTING. lac-ac.

SCLEROTIC.

acon. anan. aps. as-o. atp. blt. ca-s. clv. cmc. con. dt. elaps. eupat. hg. hur. i. k-bicr. led. pau. pnc. rs. so-t. srr. str.

COLOR **Dark.** pb.

Red. aps. as-o. atp. ca-s. cmc. dt. elaps. eupat. hg. hur. i. led. pau. rs. so-t. srr. str.

Yellow. acon. anan. as-o. blt. clv. con. eupat. i. k-bicr. pnc.

SWELLING. atp. k-bicr. led.

Veins of. atp.

CORNEA.

acon. æth. ag-na. (alm). amm-ca. amm-cl. aps. art-v. atp. au. ba-ca. bry. buf. ca-ca. (ca-i). ca-pa. ca-s. can. cap. cch. chd. chi. con. cph. crot. cu. dig. dt. euph. euphr. fe. (frm). glp. grp. hg. hg-bicl. hyo. k-bicr. k-i. k-o. kre. lac-ac. ly-b. lyc. mg-ca. n-x. na-ca. na-cl. nic. p. pb. pb-a. physo. pol. ppv. pul. rs. rut. s. sa-a. sb-t. sep. si-x. smi. sn. so-d. spi. spo. str. thu. trg. trx. urg. val. vr-a. zng.

APPEARANCE, **Bright.** con.

Glassy. con.

ARCUS SENILIS. ca-ca.

COLOR. **Dark.** aps. crot. euph. euphr. glp. k-bicr. n-x. spi.

Red. (alm). amm-ca. au. can. nic. pb. pb-a. s. thu.

White. ag-na. (ca-i). (frm). hg-bicl. (k-bicr). pb. s.

ERUPTIONS, **Abscess.** ca-ca. ca-s. hg. si-x.

Pimples. rs.

Pustules. æth. ca-s. hg. k-bicr. (p). sep.

Ulcers. (aps). as-o. atp. buf. ca-ca. (ca-i). ca-pa. ca-s. con. crot. euphr. (frm). hg. na-ca. rut. s. sa-a. si-x. trg.

Vesicles. rs.

OPACITY (**specks**). æth. ag-na. (alm). aps. art-v. as-o. atp. au. ca-ca. ca-s. can. cap. cch. chd. chi. con. crot. (cu). euphr. (frm). glp. (k-bicr). k-i. k-o. lyc. mg-ca. n-x. pb. physo. pol. pul. (rs). rut. s. sa-a. sep. si-x. str. trx. zng.

PROJECTING. (alm.) aps. cch. (k-bicr). k-i. s. si-x.

SMARTING. lac-ac.

SUNKEN. æth.

CHAMBERS OF EYE.

as-o. (atp). ca-s. crot. hg-bicl. pb. s.

DISCHARGE, **Pus.** as-o. (atp). ca-s. crot. hg-bicl. pb. s.

IRIS.

acon. æth. ag. ag-na. aga. aga-p. (alm). amy. anan. anm. aps. arn. art-v. as-o. ast. atp. au. ba-a. br. buf. c-bis. ca-a. ca-ca ca-s. can. cap. cb-a. cch. chd. chi. chlor. cic. cl-hx. cle. clf. cln. clv. con. cop. cph. cro. crt. cth. cu. cu-a. cub. cy. cy-hx. cyc. cyt. dig. dl-s. dph. dph-i. dt. ery. euph. fe. gel. glo. glp. grp. gui. hæm. hg. hg-bicl. hg-cy. hg-s. hll. hyo. hyp. i. jat. jnp-s. k-br. k-i. k-o. kre. lam. lau-c. lch. lct. led. lol. lyc. men. mgs. mgs-ar. mgs-au. mn-ca. morph. morph-a. mrl. msc. mtr. myris. n-x. na-ca. narth. ner. nic. ol-t. p. p-x. par. pb. ped. pet. phy. physo. pnc. pnx. pol. ppv. pru-l. qu-sa. rhe. rho. rn-b. rph. (rs). rut. s. sang. sb-t. scu. si-x. smb. smc. smi. smr. sn. so-d. so-n. spi. spi-m. sr-ca. srr. str. str-i. thu. trg. trx. tx-b. urg. val. vi-o. vi-t. vr-a. vrb. vtx. woo. zn.

APPEARANCE **Dim.** cch. cph. (k-bicr).

COLOR **Discolored.** as-o. atp. cle. hg. hg-bicl. na-cl. ol-t. rs. s. zn.

Green. rs.

Red. s.

ERUPTIONS, **Tubercles.** hg-s.

PROLAPSUS. (alm).

PUPILS **Contracted.** acon. ag. ag-na. aga. aga-p. amy. anan. anm. arn. art-v. as-o. ast. atp. au. c-bis. ca-a. ca-ca. can. cap. cch. chd. chi. chlor. cic. cl-hx. con. cop. cph. (crb-x). cro. crot. cth. cu. cu-a. cub. dig. dl-s. dph. dph-i. dro. dt. glo. glp. hæm. hg-bicl. hg-cy. hll. hyo. jat. jnp-s. k-o. lam. lau-c. led. men. mgs-ar. mn-ca. morph. morph-a. msc. mtr. myris. na-ca. ner. nic. p. p-x. pb. phy. physo. pnc. pnx. pol. ppv. pru-l. pul. qu-sa. rhe. (rho). rs. rut. s. sb-t. sep. si-x. smb. smc. sn. srr. str. str-i. thu. trx. urg. vi-o. vi-t. vr-a. woo. zn.

Dilated. acon. æth. ag-na. aga. aga-p. (alm). anan. anm. aps. arn. art-v. as-o. atp. au. br. buf. c-bis. ca-a. ca-ca. ca-s. can. cap. cb-a. chi. chlor. cic. cl-hx. cln. clv. con. cph. cro.

crt. cth. cu. cub. cy. cy-hx. cyc. cyt. dig. dl-s. dph. dro. dt ery. euph. gel. glo. glp. gui. hg. hg-bicl. hg-cy. hyo. hyp. i. jnp-s. k-bicr. k-br. k-i. k-o. kre. lam. lau-c. lch. lct. led. lol. lyc. men. mgs. mgs-ar. mgs-au. mn-ca. morph. morph-a. mrl. msc. mtr. myris. n-x. na-ca. narth. ner. nic. p. (p-x). par. pb. ped. physo. pnc. pnx. ppv. pru-l. pul. qu-sa. rhe. rho. rph. rs. sang. scu. smb. smc. smi. smr. sn. so-d. so-n. spi. spi-m. sr-ca. str. str-i. thu. trg. trx. tx-b. urg. val. vr-a. vrb. vtx. woo. zn.

Insensible. acon. æth. ag-na. amy. arn. atp. ba-ca. buf. chi. chlor. cph. (crb-x). cu. cy-hx. dig. dt. fe. hg-bicl. hyo. k-bicr. lyc. mgs-ar. mtr. myris. n-x. pb. pnc. pol. ppv. pru-l. rn-b. (rs). spi. trg.

Irregular. ba-a. ca-ca. grp. hg-bicl. n-x. (nic). (rs). s. si-x. trg.

Mobile. anan. atp. buf. cph. mtr. pb. ppv. s. str-i.

LENS.

acon. aga. alli. amm-ca. amm-cl. anm. arn. art-v. as-o. atp. au. ba-ca. bry. buf. ca-ca. ca-pa. ca-s. can. cap. cch. chd. chi. clv. con. cro. cub. dig. dl-s. dt. euph. euphr. glp. gui. hg. hyo. k-o. kre. ly-b. lyc. men. mg-ca. mn-ca. n-x. na-ca. na-cl. p. pb. pol. ppv. pul. rs. rut. s. sa-a. sang. sb-t. sep. si-x. smi. sn. so-d. spi. srr. str. str-i. te. trx. val. vr-a.

CATARACT. acon. aga. alli. amm-ca. amm-cl. anm. arn. art-v. as-o. atp. au. ba-ca. bry. buf. ca-ca. ca-pa. ca-s. can. cap. cch. chd. chi. clv. con. cro. cub. dig. dl-s. dt. euph. euphr. glp. gui. hg. hyo. k-o. kre. ly-b. lyc. mg-ca. mn-ca. n-x. na-ca. na-cl. p. pb. pol. ppv. pul. rs. rut. s. sa-a. sang. sb-t. sep. si-x. smc. smi. sn. so-d. spi. srr. (str). str-i. te. trx. val. vr-a.

Reticulated. k-o. pb.

COLOR, **Black.** anm. atp. ca-ca. can. chi. clv. (con). dig. gui. hg. hyo. n-x. p. pb. pul. rs. rut. s. sb-t. si-x. so-d. spi. (str).

Green. cch. p. pul.

Grey. ba-ca. can. chd. con. euphr. hyo. k-o. mg-ca. n-x. ppv. pul. rut. s.

Red. buf.

White. atp. buf. cub.

SWELLING. cch.

FUNDUS.

atp. p.
COLOR **Green.** p.
Red. atp.

ORBIT.

acon. æth. aga. al-o. alm. alo. amm-cl. anan. anm. aps. arn. art-v. as-o. asc. atp. au. ba-a. ba-ca. bar. ber. bi-na. bry. buf. c-bis. ca-a. ca-ca. ca-o. ca-s. cac. cch. chd. chi. chio. cit-c. cl-hx. con. crn. crot. crt. crt-c. cu. cu-asi. cy-hx. dig. dl-s. dph. elaps. euph-a. f-hx. frm. frm-s. gel. glo. glp. hg. hg-i. hg-s. hll. hur. hyo. i. jan. itu. k-ca. k-i. k-o. kd-o. lau-c. lct. led. li-ca. lo-cœ. ly-b. lyc. men. mg-ca. mg-cl. mg-sa. mgs. mn-ca. morph. morph-a. mrl. msc. myris. n-x. na-ca. na-cl. na-sa. narth. ner. nic. nuph. ol-a. os. ox-x. p. p-x. pæo. par. pau. pb. pet. phy. pol. pru-l. pt. ptv. pul. qu-sa. rho. rs. rut. s. s-x. sb-s. se. sep. si-x. smc. smi. smr. sn. snp-n. so-d. spi. spo. sr-ca. srr. str-i. thu. trg. trn. u-na. val. vr-a. vr-v. vrb. ziz. zn. zng.

BORING. ca-ca. ca-s. cch. ol-a. srr.
BRUISED. crt. cu. pol. rs.
BURSTING. buf. buf-s. gel. morph. morph-a. pb.
COLDNESS. sep.
CONTRACTIVE. spi. vrb.
CRAMPY. aga.
CUTTING. chi. srr.
DRAWING. cch. mn-ca. s. sn. val.
EMPTINESS, **Feeling of.** s. sep.
FALSE SENSATIONS, **Wind.** sep.
GNAWING. hyo.
HEAT. men. nic. s. trn.
HEAVINESS. crot. crt-c. glo. hur. nuph.
ITCHING. buf-s. p.
MOTION IN, **Whirling.** ly-b.

PRESSING. acon. al-o. alo. anm. arn. as-o. atp. au. ba-ca. c-bis. ccs. chd. chi. chio. cit-c. con. crt. cy-hx. dph. frm-s. gel. glp. hll. hur. hyo. k-ca. k-o. lct. led. ly-b. msc. narth. ner. nic. p. p-x. pæo. par. pb. pol. pru-l. qu-sa. rho. rut. s. sb-s. sep. si-x. smc. sn. spi. sr-ca. str-i. trg. val. vr-a.

SHOOTING. acon. æth. au. ca-ca. glo. k-o. lau-c. ly-b. p-x. rho. rs. sb-s. val. ziz.

SMALL **Feeling.** par. trg.
SMARTING. (chd). glo. pt. si-x.
TEARING. acon. al-o. atp. au. bi-na. ca-ca. cl-hx. con. dph. mg-ca. mrl. p. phl. s-x. sep. smc. spi.
TENSIVE. men. pt. spi. thu.
THROBBING. amm-cl. ba-ca. ca-ca. dig. mgs. sn. trn.
TINGLING. ly-b.
UNDEFINED. alo. anan. atp. chd. chi. con. crt-c. gel. hg. i. jan. (ly-b). na-ca. nuph. ox-x. p. pb. pru-l. pul. se. spi. trg.

ORBIT CIRCUMFERENCE.

anm. aps. arn. ca-ca. cch. cl-hx. crn. li-ca. ly-b. mrl. na-cl. na-sa. narth. p. p-x. phl. phy. rho. rs. s. so-d. str-i. val. zng.
BRUISED. rs.
BURSTING. na-sa.
CONTRACTIVE. crn. so-d.
DRAWING. s. val. zng.
HEAVINESS. crn.
ITCHING. p.
PRESSING. anm. arn. mrl. str-i.
SHOOTING. p-x.
TEARING. ca-ca. cch. cl-hx. mrl.
UNDEFINED. anm. aps. (ly-b). p. phy.

ORBIT SUPERIORLY.

acon. al-o. alo. amm-cl. ba-ca. bar. ber. bry. ca-a. ca-ca. ca-o. cac. chd. chi. chio. cis. cu-asi. elaps. frm. glo. hg. hg-i. hg-s. hll. hur. hyo. jcr. k-bicr. k-i. kd-o. li-ca. mg-ca. mg-sa. mrl. msc. myris. na-cl. na-sa. ner. nic. ol-a. os. p-x. par. pet. phl. phy. pt. rs-r. rut. sep. smc. sn. snp-n. str-i. vr-v. zn.
BORING. ca-a. ca-ca. ca-o. myris.
CONTRACTIVE. myris.
CUTTING. hg-s.
FALSE SENSATIONS, **Foreign Body.** mg-sa.
GNAWING. hyo. pt.
NUMBNESS. mrl.
PRESSING. alo. hur. hyo. mg-sa. mrl. myris. ner. par. phy. pt. rut. zn.

Like a Plug. smc.
SHOOTING. acon. alo. ba-ca. ber. ca-a. hur. mrl. nic. ol-a.
SMARTING. hg-s. pt.
SWELLING, **Feeling of.** hg-s.
TEARING. al-o. kd-o. mg-ca. mrl. os. phl.
TENSIVE. mrl. pt.
UNDEFINED. chi. hg. ner. sep. snp-n. zn.

ORBIT INFERIORLY.

aps. art-v. au. euph-a. hg-i. hg-s. k-i. mg-cl. na-sa. p. phy. smi. thu.
BRUISED. mg-cl. smi.
GNAWING. k-i.
PRESSING. art-v.
TEARING. p.

ORBIT EXTERNALLY.

au. f-hx. led. li-ca. narth. pt. ptv. sn.
BRUISED. ptv.
PRESSING. led. narth.

ORBIT INTERNALLY.

cit-c. hg. k-bicr. lch. mn-ca. p-x. sep. si-x. thu.
COLDNESS. p-x.
CRAMPY. mn-ca.
PRESSING. cit-c.
SHOOTING. p-x.
SWELLING. hg.
TEARING. mn-ca.

ORBIT POSTERIORLY.

au. dig. rs. smr.
CRAMPY. au.

PRESSING. au
SHOOTING. dig.
UNDEFINED. rs. smr.

ORBITAL INTEGUMENTS.

acon. æsc. æth. aga. al-o. alli. alo. amb. amm-cl. anm. aps. arn. art-v. as-h. as-o. asc. atp. ba-ca. ber. bi-na. br. bry. buf. c-bis. ca-a. ca-ca. ca-s. can. can-i. cb-a. cb-v. cch. chi. cic, cit-c. cle. clv. cmc. cn-sa. con. cph. cr-o. crd. crn. cro. crt. crt-c. cth. cu. cyc. delph. dig. dl-s. dph. dro. dt. elaps. ery. euphr. evo. f-hx. fe. glo. glp. grp. grt. gui. hæm. hg. hg-bicl. hg-s. hll. hpm. hur. hyo. i. irs. jat. jnp-s. k-bicr. k-ca. k-na. k-o. klm. lac-ac. lac-f. lct. lo-cœ. ly-b. lyc. mg-ca. mgs-ar. mgs-au. mn-ca. morph-a. mrl. mtr. myris. n-x. na-ba. na-ca. na-cl. narth. ner. nic. ol-a. p. p-x. par. pau. pb. ped. phl. phy. pln. pod. pru-l. pt. rn-b. rn-s. rs. rs-r. rut. s. s-x. sa-l. se. sep. si-x. smc. smi. sn. so-d. spi. spi-m. spo. spo-f. sr-ca. str. str-i. thu. trg. trn. trx. vi-t. vr-a. vr-s. vtx. woo. zn. zng.

COLOR **Dark**. acon. aga. anm. art-v. as-h. as-o. ber. bi-na. buf. c-bis. ca-ca. ca-s. cch. chi. clv. cn-sa. cph. crn. cu. cyc. dl-s. dph. dt. ery. fe. grp. hæm. hg. hg-bicl. hg-s. hpm. hur. irs. jat. jnp-s. k-ca. lyc. mrl. mtr. myris. n-x. na-ca. ner. p. p-x. pb. pod. ptv. rs. rs-r. s. sa-l. sep. smc. sn. spi. spo-f. sr-ca. str. str-i. trg. trn. trx. vr-a. vr-s. woo.

Green. (myris). vr-a.

Red. ca-s. ery. hg. na-ba. rs. si-x. sr-ca.

Yellow. crt-c. n-x. spi. str.

CREEPING. as-o. sep.

DRAWING. f-hx.

ERUPTIONS, **Boils**. s.

Pimples. ca-s. dl-s. euphr.

Scabs. grp. hg.

Tubercles. p.

Undefined. as-o. ca-ca. ca-s. con. dl-s. hg. ner. pet. s. si-x. str-i. vtx.

HEAT. as-o. cic. glo. p. rs-v.

HEAVINESS. lac-f.

ITCHING. amb. aps. as-o. ber. can-i. cb-v. con. cr-o. lyc. p. smi. trg.

MOVEMENTS, **Convulsions**. cic. dph. rut.

PRESSING. arn. elaps. lac-f. mg-ca. phl.
SHOOTING. æth. ber. br. spo.
SMARTING. æth. ber. br. cr-o. mgs-au. n-x. ped.
STIFFNESS. klm.
SWELLING. alli. aps. as-o. elaps. fe. hg-s. n-x. p. pul. rhe. rs. rs-v. spi-m. spo.
Œdematous. aps. rs. rs-v.
Red. rs.
TEARING. amb. i. lyc.
TENSIVE. al-o. myris.
UNDEFINED. aps. n-x. p.

ORBITAL INTEGUMENTS SUPERIORLY.

(**Eyebrows**).

acon. æth. aga. al-o. alli. alo. amb. amm-cl. aps. arn. art-v. as-h. as-o. asc. atp. ba-ca. ber. br. bry. ca-a. ca-pa. ca-s. can. cb-a. chi. cic. cit-c. cle. con. cph. crd. cro. crt. crt-c. cth. cu. delph. dig. dl-s. dro. dt. elaps. eryn. euph. evo. f-hx. fe. glo. glp. grp. grt. gui. hg. hll. hur. hydr. hyo. i. jcr. jnp-s. k-ca. k-i. k-na. k-o. lac-ac. lau-c. lch. li-ca. ly-b. mg-ca. mgs-ar. mn-ca. morph-a. mrl. msc. n-x. na-cl. narth. ner. ol-a. p-x. par. pau. pb. pet. phl. phy. pln. ppv. pru-l. pt. rho. rn-b. rn-s. rs. rs-r. rs-v. rut. s. sb-s. sb-t. se. sep. si-x. smc. sn. so-d. spi. spo. sr-ca. str. str-i. thu. trg. trn. trx. vi-t. vr-v. vtx. zn. zng.
BORING. ca-a.
COLOR **Red.** elaps.
CONTRACTIVE. hll. n-x. so-d.
CRAMPY. hll. narth.
CREEPING. rn-b.
CUTTING. crd. dro.
DRAWING. (alo). atp. cic. dro. grt. hll. k-o. mgs-ar. narth. pru-l. rs.
ERUPTIONS, **Boils.** na-cl.
Hard. gui. rn-b.
Hot. sn.
Itching. na-cl. se.
Pimples. gui. hur. rn-s. sn. trx.
  Hot. sn.
  Pressing. sn.
Pressing. se. sn.
Pustules. thu.
Scabs. f-hx. sep.

Tubercles. k-o. sb-s.
Undefined pain. sb-s.
White. sb-s.
Undefined. as-o. ba-ca. cle. dl-s. hll. i. k-na. k-o. na-cl. par. s. se. sep. si-x. thu.
Undefined Pain. sb-s.
Urticaria. f-hx.
Vesicles. se.
White. sb-s.
GNAWING. hyo. vtx.
HAIRS, **Color White**. as-h.
Fall out. aga. hll. k-ca. pb. se.
HEAT : acon. aga. alli. aps. as-o. atp. ber. bry. cit-c. dig. dro. elaps. hg. k-ca. s. sb-t. spi. thu.
HEAVINESS. con.
ITCHING. æth. aga. al-o. alli. aps. ber. chi. k-na. k-o. mgs-ar. na-cl. ol-a. par. s. sb-t. se. si-x. vtx.
MOVEMENTS, **Convulsions.** al-o. art-v. crt-c. glp. grt. hll. ol-a. rut. sep. sr-ca.
Downwards. cb-a.
Feeling of. can. ol-a.
Upwards, drawn. lch.
NUMBNESS. as-h.
PECKING. pet.
PRESSING. aga. amb. arn. br. ca-s. cb-a. chi. crt. cth. evo. fe. hyo. k-o. morph-a. mrl. ner. p-x. par. phy. rn-b. s. str-i. zng.
SHOOTING. aga. alli. aps. as-o. ba-ca. ber. ca-a. cb-a. cic. cph. crt. elaps. f-hx. glp. hll. ly-b. mn-ca. pet. thu. vi-t. zn.
SMARTING. ber. glo. gui. k-o. par. pet. pt. vtx.
SWELLING. aps. k-ca.
Feeling of. par.
TEARING. al-o. amm-cl. arn. atp. mg-ca. mrl. rs. smc.
TENSIVE. con. dro. ly-b. par. pt.
THROBBING. k-ca. k-o. pet. sr-ca. zn.
TINGLING. cro.
UNDEFINED. delph. hydr. ner. pau. spi.
WRINKLED. dt. str.

ORBITAL INTEGUMENTS INFERIORLY.

æsc. aps. as-h. as-o. atp. atrop. bi-na. bry. cmc. crn. cro. cu. dt. f-hx. glo. hg-s. lct. lo-cœ. mn-ca. mtr. myris. n-x. na-cl.

ner. p. pau. pb. pb-a. pln. ptv. pul. rs. rs-r. rut. s-x. sep. si-x. spi. spo. str. teu. trn. vtx.

COLOR **Dark.** as-h. as-o. bi-na. crn. cu. dt. glo. myris. p. rs. rs-v. trn.

Yellow. n-x. spi.

CONTRACTIVE. cro.

HEAT. cro. f-hx. mn-ca.

ITCHING. vtx.

MOVEMENTS, **Convulsions**. sep.

SHOOTING. rs.

SMARTING. vtx.

SWELLING. aps. as-o. bry. cmc. dt. lct. mtr. ner. p. pln. pul. rs-v. str.

Œdematous. lct.

Red. ner. sep.

ORBITAL INTEGUMENTS EXTERNALLY.

f-hx. spi. spo.

SWELLING. spi.

EYELIDS.

ach. acon. æsc. æth. ag. ag-na. aga. al-o. alli. alm. amb. amm-ca. amm-cl. amph. anan. anm. aph. aps. arn. art-v. arum-t. as-o. asr. ast. atp. atrop. au. ba-ca. ba-cl. bap. ber. bi-na. br. bru. bry. buf. bz-x. c-bis. ca-a. ca-ca. ca-o. ca-pa. ca-s. can. can-i. cap. cast. cb-a. cb-v. cch. ccs. chd. chi. chio. chlor. cic. cit-c. cl-hx. cle. clv. cmc. cmf. co. con. cop. cph. cr-o. crn. cro. crot. crt-c. cth. cu. cub. cy-hx. cyc. dig. dl-s. dph. dph-i. dro. dt. elaps. erig. ery. eryn. eupat. euph. euphr. f-hx. fe. fe-mgs. fe-pa. frm. glo. glp. gn-l. grc. grp. grt. gui. gym. hæm. hg. hg-s. hll. hpm. hur. hydr. hyo. i. ind. irs. itu. jat. jnp-s. k-bicr. k-ca. k-cla. k-i. k-na. k-o. klm. kre. krm. lac-ac. lac-c. lac-d. lac-f. lam. lau-c. lct. led. lpd. lpt. ly-b. lyc. men. mg-ca. mg-cl. mgs. mgs-ar. mgs-au. mn-ca. morph-a. mph. mrl. msc. mtr. myris. n-x. na-ba. na-ca. na-cl. na-sa. naj. narth. ner. ni-ca. nic. ol-a. os. ox-x. p. p-x. pæo. par. pb. pet. phl. phy. physo. pim. pln. pnx. pol. ppv. pru-l. pso. ptv. pul. pul-n. qu-sa. rhe. rho. rn-b. rn-s. rs. rs-r. rut. s. s-x. sa-a. sa-l. sang. sb-s. sb-t. se. sep. si-x. smb. smc. smi. smr. sn. so-d. so-o. so-t. spi. spi-m. spo. spo-f. sr-ca. srr. stc. str. str-i.

stry. te. teu. thu. til. trg. trn. trx. tx-b. u-na. urg. urt. val. vi-o. vi-t. vin. vp-r. vr-a. vr-s. vrb. vsp. vtx. woo. ziz. zn. zng.

ADHESION **of.** ach. acon. æth. ag-na. aga. al-o. amm-ca. amm-cl. aps. art-v. arum-t. as-o. atp. au. ba-ca. bry. ca-a. ca-ca. ca-s. cast. cb-a. cb-v. cch. ccs. chd. cic. cl-hx. co. con. cop. cro. dig. dl-s. dro. dt. erig. (eryn). euph. euphr. fe. glp. grc. grp. grt. (gym). hg. (hydr). i. k-bicr. k-ca. (k-na). k-o. kre. led. lpt. ly-b. lyc. mg-ca. mg-cl. mgs-ar. mgs-au. mn-ca. mrl. mtr. myris. n-x. na-ba. na-ca. na-cl. na-sa. ni-ca. ol-a. p. p-x. pb. phy. pol. pru-l. pt. pul. pul-n. rhe. rho. rs. rs-r. rut. s. s-x. sb-s. sep. si-x. smi. sn. spi. spo. str. str-i. thu. trn. trx. (u-na). vr-a. ziz. zn.

BRUISED. as-o. chlor. s.

BURSTING. aps. woo.

COLDNESS. al-o. asr. br. chlor. grp. hur. k-ca. p-x. rs-r.

COLOR **Dark.** as-o. clv. dig. dro. hur. k-ca. n-x. spo-f. tx-b.

Red. acon. ag. alli. (alm). anan. aps. as-o. atp. atrop. au. ba-ca. ba-cl. ber. bi-na. bry. buf. ca-ca. ca-s. can. cb-v. chlor. cl-hx. cmc. cmf. con. cu. dig. dl-s. dt. euph. euphr. fe. gel. grp. hg. hll. hur. hyo. i. irs. k-bicr. k-i. k-o. kre. lau-c. lpd. lyc. mg-cl. mgs. mgs-au. mtr. na-ca. na-cl. ni-ca. p-x. par. pb. pso. pul. rho. rs. rs-r. s. sa-a. sb-s. sep. (si-x). smi. so-t. spi. spo. srr. str. str-i. thu. trg. vin. vr-a. vr-s. woo. zn.

White. acon.

Yellow. acon.

CONTRACTIVE. ber. chi. crot. dl-s. euphr. lpt. ner. pb. physo. rs. sn. str. vi-t.

CRAMPY. crot. vi-o.

CREEPING. art-v. chi. k-bicr. pol.

CUTTING. ca-ca.

DISCHARGE **Hard.** k-o. p-x. (sb-s).

Mucus. acon. æth. ag-na. aga. amm-cl. (aps). ba-ca. bry. ca-a. ca-ca. dro. erig. euph. euphr. fe. grt. hg. hydr. i. k-bicr. (k-ca). k-i. k-o. kre. lct. led. lpt. lyc. mg-ca. mgs-ar. mgs-au. mrl. mtr. n-x. na-ca. (p-x). phy. pol. pul. pul-n. rhe. rs. (sb-s). spi. str. str-i. vr-a. ziz.

Pus. dl-s. dt. rs. rut. str-i. trx.

Yellow. aga. ziz.

DRAWING. ber. cch. grp. mgs-ar. p. p-x. pt. pul. rhe. str.

DRYNESS. acon. al-o. anm. arn. art-v. as-o. asr. ber. bry. cb-v. chi. cph. cyc. dl-s. dph-i. euph. glp. grp. hpm.

k-bicr. mg-cl. mgs. mgs-ar. mgs-au. mn-ca. mrl. mtr. myris. pul. rs. s. smi. srr. str. vr-a.

ERUPTIONS **Dry**. kre.
Encysted Tumors. ca-ca. thu.
Erythema circumscripta. ery.
Granulations. k-bicr.
Herpes. ery. kre. woo.
Dry. kre.
Hot. smi. woo.
Itching. smi.
Pimples. pet. s. smi.
Pustules. ca-ca. con. lyc. pt. rs. s. se.
Feeling of. trn.
Scabs. buf. hg. lyc.
Scales. kre. pul.
Dry. kre.
Shooting. smi.
Smarting. hg-s.
Spongy. (alm).
Styes. amb. aps. au. ca-s. con. cub. dig. dl-s. fe. k-o. lyc. men. mgs-au. pul. rs. sep. si-x. sn. val.
Tubercles. (alm). bry. dl-s. k-i. k-o. rn-s.
Spongy. (alm).
Ulcers. buf. cch. cro. dl-s. k-i. led. lyc. na-cl. p. pul. rs. si-x. spi. str. str-i.
Undefined. ca-s. hg. k-bicr. sep.
Urticaria. chlor. smi.
Hot. smi.
Itching. smi.
Shooting. smi.
Vesicles. mgs-ar. rs. se.

EVERSION. (alm). aps. atp. hg. spi. str-i.

GNAWING. str-i. vtx.

HÆMORRHAGE. arn. atp. (ery.)

HAIRS **Falling out**. al-o. aps. buf. chlor.
Inverted.(al-o). na-ba. rs. spi. zn.
Feeling. (te).
Irregular. chlor. na-ba.

HARDNESS. acon. bry. dl-s. n-x. rn-s. spi. thu.
Feeling of. dl-s. spi.

HEAT. acon. aga. al-o. alli. amb. aph. aps. art-v. as-o. asr. atp. ber. bry. buf. bz-x. ca-ca. ca-pa. cap. cb-v. ccs. chd. chlor. cit-c. cle. con. cro. glo. grp. hg. hydr. itu. k-bicr. k-ca.

k-i. k-o. kre. lau-c. lct. lyc. mgs-au. mrl. n-x. narth.ner. ni-ca. p. p-x. pæo. par. phl. phy. pnx. pol. pru-l. pul. pul-n. rn-s. rs. rs-r. s. sb-t. sep. spi. si-x. smi. sn. so-t. spi. stc. str. thu. trg. vi-o.

HEAVINESS **see** UPPER LIDS.

INVERSION. (alm).

ITCHING. acon. al-o. amb. anm. aps. art-v. as-o. atp. ber. bry. c-bis. ca-a. cb-v. chi. cit-c. cro. crot. (cu). cyc. dl-s. dph. dro. euph. euphr. grt. hg. hg-s. hur. i. k-bicr. k-i. k-o. kre. lau-c. lyc. mgs. mgs-ar. mgs-au. mrl. na-ca. na-cl. narth. ner. ol-a. p. pæo. par. pb. pet. pul. rs. rs-r. s. sb-t. sep. si-x. smr. spi. spo. str. til. trg. trn. tx-b. vin. vr-a. vtx. zn.

LOOSENESS, **Feeling of.** spi.

MOVEMENTS. **Closing.** acon. æth. ag. ag-na. aga. al-o. alm. alo. amm-ca. amm-cl. aps. arn. art-v. arum. as-o. atp. atrop. ba-ca. bap. bru. bry. c-bis. ca-ca. ca-pa. ca-s. can. cb-a. cb-v. chd. chi. chlor. cit-c. cl-hx. cld. cof. (cop). cph. cro. crt. cth. cu. cy-hx. dig. dl-s. dph. dt. elaps. ery. euph. fe. gel. glo. glp. grt. hg. (hg-bicl.) hg-s. hll. hur. hyo. (hyp). ind. jnp-s. k-na. k-o. kre. lac-ac. lac-c. lac-f. lau-c. lch. li-ca. lpd. ly-b. lyc. (mg-cl). mg-sa. mgs-au. mrl. mtr. myris. na-ca. na-cl. (na-sa). narth. ner. ox-x. p-x. pb. phl. physo. pnx. ppv. pru-l. pt. ptv. qu-sa. rs. rs-r. rut. s. s-x. sa-l. sb-t. sep. smb. snp-n. spi. (spo). srr. (stach). str. str-i. thu. trx. tx-b. urg. vi-o. vi-t. vr-a. vr-s. vrb. zn.

Spasmodically. acon. al-o. amb. anm. as-o. atp. br. bry. ca-ca. (ca-i). ca-s. chd. chi. cic. con. cop. cro. (crot). cyc. dl-s. dt. euph. euphr. fe. (grp). hæm. hg. hg-bicl. hyo. (hyp). ind. k-ca. kre. (lyc). mrl. mtr. n-x. na-ba. na-ca. na-cl. nic. p. pb. pru-l. pt. (rho). rs. s. sb-t. sep. si-x. spi. spo. str-i. sym. urg. vi-o. vi-t.

Convulsions. æsc. aga. al-o. amb. anan. anm. art-v. as-o. ast. atp. ber. bry. c-bis. ca-ca. chd. cph. cro. crot. cth. cu. (dt). glp. grt. hg. hll. hyo. i. ind. jat. k-bicr. k-o. kre. lac-f. men. mgs-ar. mtr. na-ca. na-cl. ol-a. pb. pet. pol. ppv. pt. pul. rhe. rho. rs. rut. s. se. sep. si-x. smc. so-d. str. str-i. thu. vi-o. vr-a. vrb. woo.

Opening Wide (**spasmodically**). acon. alm. anm. atp. bru. bry. chi. cit-c. cof. con. cph. (cu). cy-hx. (dl-s). dol. dt. dt-t. eupat-p. f-hx. fe. glp. hll. hyo. lau-c. lch. lyc. mtr. na-cl. narth. p-x. pb. pod. ppv. pru-l. s. sb-s. sb-t. smb. (spo). str-i. urg. vr-a.

Outwards Drawn. cph. cro. mtr. rhe. rut.

Winking. ag-na. aga. amm-ca. anan. ast. atp. buf. ca-ca. ca-s. cb-a. chd. chi. con. cro. (cu). dl-s. dph. euphr. f-hx. glo. k-o. lau-c. mrl. (myris). n-x. p-x. pet. ppv. (pt). sb-s. smc. sn. spi.

NUMBNESS. mrl. pb.

PARALYSIS. acon. ag-na. aga. al-o. amb. amm-ca. anan. anm. art-v. as-o. atp. ba-ca. bar. br. bry. ca-ca. ca-s. cap. cb-a. cb-v. chd. chlor. con. cro. cu. cy-hx. dro. (dt). elaps. eug. euph. fe. gel. grp. hg. hll. hyo. k-ca. k-o. li-ca. lpd. ly-b. lyc. men. mg-ca. mg-cl. mrl. mtr. myris. n-x. na-ba. na-ca. na-cl. nic. p. pæo. pb. pet. physo. pnx. pol. ppv. pul. rs. s. s-x. sa-l. sep. si-x. so-d. spi. srr. str. thu. trg. trn. vi-t. vr-a. zn.

Closing Difficult. acon. cy-hx. eug. myris. na-ba. ppv. (sa-l).

Opening Difficult. acon. ag-na. aga. (al-o). amb. amm-ca. anan. anm. art-v. as-o. atp. ba-ca. bap. br. bry. ca-ca. ca-s. cap. cb-a. cb-v. chd. chlor. con. cro. cu. cy-hx. dro. (dt). elaps. euph. fe. gel. hg. hll. hyo. k-ca. k-o. li-ca. ly-b. lyc. men. mg-ca. mg-cl. mrl. mtr. myris. n-x. na-ba. na-ca. na-cl. nic. p. pæo. pb. ped. pet. physo. pnx. ppv. ptv. pul. rs. s. s-x. sa-l. sep. si-x. so-d. spi. srr. str. thu. trg. trn. vi-t. vr-a. zn.

PRESSING. al-o. amb. amm-ca. aps. art-v. atrop. bry. ca-s. can. cro. cu. cyc. dt. euph. grp. k-ca. lyc. mph. msc. myris. n-x. na-cl. pol. rhe. s. si-x. smi. sn. spi. spo. str. vr-a.

SHOOTING. acon. aps. arn. as-o. ber. cyc. hg. hll. hur. k-bicr. lau-c. mgs-ar. mgs-au. narth. p-x. s. so-t. spi. str-i. trx. tx-b. vr-a. zng.

SMALL. can-i. kre. pb. rho.

Feeling. gui. kre.

SMARTING. acon. æth. aps. atrop. ber. bry. ca-ca. ca-s. cb-v. (chd). cit-c. cle. cmf. co. cr-o. cro. cth. dig. dro. frm. glp. k-ca. k-o. kre. lau-c. led. mgs-au. ol-a. p-x. pet. phy. pln. pnx. pul. pul-n. rs. rs-r. s. si-x. so-t. spi. str. str-i. thu. trn. val. vr-a. vr-v. vtx. ziz. zn.

STIFFNESS. al-o. chlor. klm. men. rs. s. spi. vr-a.

SWEAT. ca-pa.

SWELLING. acon. ag. ag-na. aga. al-o. alli. anan. aps. arn. as. as-o. atp. au. ba-ca. ba-cl. bry. buf. ca-ca. ca-s. cch. chd. chlor. cl-hx. cln. clv. con. cph. crot. cu. cyc. dt. euph. euphr. fe. grp. hg. hg-bicl. hll. hyo. i. k-bicr. k-ca. k-o. kre. lyc. mg-ca. mg-cl. mn-ca. mtr. n-x. na-ca. ni-ca. p.

pb. phy. pol. pso. pul. rho. rs. rs-r. rut. s. sa-a. sb-t. sep. spi-m. spo. srr. str. str-i. thu. til. urt. urt-u. val. vp-r. woo.

Bag-like. k-ca.

Dark. phy.

Hard. acon. thu.

Œdematous. aps. as-o. crot. i. k-bicr. k-i. pb. phy. rs-r. sa-a. urt. urt-u.

Red. acon. phy. thu.

Watery. pul.

Feeling of. acon. ber. (ccs). chd. cro. cyc. gel. hg-s. k-o. men. myris. rs. rs-r. sa-l. thu. val. vr-v.

TEARING. ber. bry. can. cch. i. k-na. mg-ca. pb. smc. str. zn.

TENSIVE. acon. as-o. cth. dl-s. hg-s. lyc. mrl. myris. n-x. s. s-x.

THROBBING. buf. cch. cph. cro. euphr. hur. k-ca. men. mg-ca. mgs-ar. mtr. rhe. rs. rs-r. s. woo.

TINGLING. art-v. pol.

UNDEFINED. as-o. atrop. ca-ca. (ca-s). (cb-a). chi. grp. (hg). (k-bicr). lyc. mgs-ar. mn-ca. p. pb. pnx. rs. s. si-x. spi. (spo-f). str-i. val. zn.

WRINKLED. (chio).

UPPER EYELID.

acon. æth. ag. ag-na. aga. al-o. alli. alo. amb. amm-ca. amm-cl. amph. anan. anm. aps. arn. art-v. arum-t. as-o. asr. atp. au. ba-ca. ba-cl. bap. ber. br. bru. bry. buf. c-bis. ca-ca. ca-o. ca-s. can. can-i. cap. cb-a. cb-v. cch. chd. chi. chio. cic. cit-c. cl-hx. cld. cle. cmf. co. cof. con. cop. cph. crd. crn. cro. crot. crt-c. cth. cu. cy-hx. cyc. dig. dl-s. dph. dph-i. dro. dt. elaps. ery. eug. euph. euphr. f-hx. fe. fe-mgs. frm. gel. glo. glp. gn-l. grp. grt. hæm. hg. hg-s. hll. hur. hyo. ind. jnp-s. k-bicr. k-ca. k-cla. k-i. k-na. k-o. kre. krm. lac-ac. lac-c. lac-d. lac-f. lau-c. lch. li-ca. lpd. lpt. ly-b. lyc. men. mg-ca. mg-cl. mgs-ar. mgs-au. mn-ca. morph-a. mrl. msc. mtr. myris. n-x. na-ba. na-ca. na-cl. na-sa. naj. narth. ner. nic. ol-m. os. ox-x. p. p-x. pæo. par. pb. pet. phl. physo. pim. pnx. pol. ppv. pru-l. pt. ptv. pul. qu-sa. rhe. rho. rs. rs-r. rut. s. sang. sb-s. sb-t. sep. si-x. smb. smc. smi. sn. so-d. so-o. so-t. spi. spo. srr. str. str-i. stry. te. teu. thu. trg. trn. trx. tx-b. urg. vi-o. vi-t. vr-a. vr-s. vr-v. vrb. vsp. vtx. ziz. zn.

COLDNESS. grp.

COLOR, **Dark**. str-i.
Red. acon. ca-s. hg. k-bicr. k-o. s. teu. zn.
CONTRACTIVE. bry. dl-s. euphr.
CREEPING. asr. par.
CUTTING. thu.
DRYNESS. acon. arn. cb-v. glp. n-x. str-i. vr-a.
ERUPTIONS, **Hard**. dl-s.
Herpes. bry. rs. sep.
Hot. c-bis.
Itching. c-bis.
Pimples. ca-s. cth. lyc. msc. n-x. s.
Pustules. c-bis. ca-s. chd.
Hot. c-bis.
Itching. c-bis.
Rhagades. anan.
Scabs. co.
Styes. al-o. fe. hg. k-o. p-x. pul. s. trg. ziz.
Tubercles. dl-s. k-i. k-o. n-x.
EVERSION. anan. atp. str-i.
HARDNESS. acon.
HEAT. alli. bry. ca-ca. can-i. co. k-bicr. lyc. p. p-x. trg.
HEAVINESS. acon. al-o. anan. aps. arum-t. as-o. atp. ba-ca. ber. br. c-bis. ca-ca. ca-o. ca-s. can. chd. cit-c. cl-hx. cph. cr-o. crn. cro. crot. crt-c. dig. dl-s. dph. dph-i. ery. euph. euphr. fe. frm. gel. glo. grp. grt. hg. hg-s. hll. hur. ind. jnp-s. k-bicr. k-na. k-o. lac-c. lac-d. lac-f. lpd. ly-b. lyc. mrl. mtr. na-ca. na-sa. narth. ner. ol-m. ox-x. p-x. phl. physo. pnx. ppv. pru-l. pt. ptv. pul-n. qu-sa. rs. rs-r. s. sep. si-x. spi. spo. str. str-i. thu. trn. trx. tx-b. vi-o. vi-t. vr-a. vr-s. vr-v. zn.
ITCHING. alli. art-v. ba-ca. bry. cb-a. dl-s. f-hx. glp. k-bicr. lyc. n-x. na-ba. si-x. vtx.
MOVEMENTS, **Convulsions.** aga. al-o. amph. arum-t. as-o. asr. atp. bry. ca-ca. cb-a. cl-hx. con. crd. cro. cy-hx. jnp-s. lau-c. lch. mg-cl. mn-ca. mrl. par. rho. s. so-t. vr-a.
Feeling of. lch.
Upward drawn. acon. lch.
NUMBNESS. narth.
PRESSING. ca-s. can. cb-a. cb-v. chd. dl-s. fe-mgs. k-o. lac-f. lyc. msc. mtr. na-ba. narth. p. rhe. s. si-x. sn. spi. str. trx. vr-a.
SHOOTING. ba-ca. br. ca-o. ca-s. cb-a. cyc. glp. mgs-ar. mn-ca. sang. si-x. spi. trg. vr-a.

SMALL. na-ba.
SMARTING. ca-s. co. crn. gn-l. k-o. pim. trg. vtx.
STIFFNESS. hg-s. krm. rs. spi. vr-a.
SWELLING. acon. al-o. aps. (as-o). bry. ca-s. cyc. hg. hg-bicl. k-bicr. k-ca. k-o. mg-cl. morph-a. msc. myris. n-x. na-ca. s. sep. si-x. str-i. teu. thu. zn.
Feeling of. al-o. can-i. k-o. vi-o.
TEARING. al-o. can. k-ca. k-o.
TENSIVE. acon. amm-ca. cth.
THROBBING. ba-ca. br. cl-hx. lau-c. mn-ca.
UNDEFINED. as-o. ca-o. cmf. cth. k-cla. lpt. pnx. spi.

LOWER EYELID.

ag. aga. al-o. alm. amm-cl. aps. arn. as-o. asc. asr. atp. au. bry. c-bis. ca-ca. ca-s. cb-v. cch. chd. chi. cic. cit-c. clv. cro. cth. dig. dph. dro. euph. euphr. fe. fe-mgs. fe-pa. glo. grp. hur. i. ind. jnp-s. k-bicr. k-i. k-o. lam. lau-c. led. lyc. mg-ca. mgs. mgs-au. mn-ca. mtr. myris. na-ca. na-cl. ner. ol-a. p. p-x. pet. phy. pol. ppv. pru-l. pul. rn-b. rph. rs. rut. s. s-x. sep. si-x. sn. spi. spo. trg. zn.
COLOR, **Dark.** glo.
Red. as-o. atp. bry. dig. glo. grp. k-i. lau-c. mg-ca. na-cl. p-x. s. sep. si-x. trg.
CUTTING. spi.
DRAWING. grp. rut.
DRYNESS. pet.
ERUPTIONS, **Pimples.** al-o.
Pustules. na-cl. pol.
Styes. grp. p. pol. rs.
Tubercles. au. bry. ca-ca. thu.
Undefined pain. bry.
Ulcers. cch. na-cl.
Undefined pain. bry.
HEAT. chd. ind. k-bicr. k-o. ner.
HEAVINESS. k-o.
ITCHING. k-o. lam. ner. ol-a. pet. rut. s-x.
MOVEMENTS, **Convulsions.** amm-cl. cic. cth. grp. hg. i. ind. k-i. lyc. mg-ca. mgs. p-x. pol. rut. s. sep.
Downwards drawn. phy.
PRESSING. bry. cit-c. cro. sep.
SHOOTING. al-o. aps. cro. cth. dph. jnp-s. s-x.
SMARTING. al-o. asc. ca-ca. led. rs. s-x.

SWELLING. as-o. atp. au. bry. ca-ca. dig. euphr. fe-mgs. glo. mg-ca. mgs-au. p-x. ppv. rs. sep. trg. u-na.
Œdematous. bry. hur. rph. u-na.
Feeling of. cit-c.
TEARING. mg-cl.
TENSIVE. myris.
THROBBING. atp. mg-ca. pol.

TARSAL EDGES.

acon. æth. ag. ag-na. alm. amm-ca. anan. aps. arn. art-v. arum-t. as-o. ast. atp. ba-ca. ber. bry. c-bis. ca-ca. ca-s. can-i. cb-v. cch. ccs. chd. chlor. cle. cln. cmc. con. cth. dig. dl-s. dph. dt. eupat. euphr. grp. grt. hg. hg-bicl. hg-s. hur. ind. jat. jnc. k-bicr. k-na. k-o. kre. krm. lac-d. lau-c. lch. li-ca. lo-cœ. lyc. mgs-ar. mgs-au. mph. mrl. mtr. myris. na-ba. na-cl. narth. ni-ca. ox-x. p. p-x. pd. pnx. pol. pru. pru-l. ptv. pul. rhe. rn-s. rs. rs-r. s. sb-t. se. sep. si-x. smc. spi. spo-f. srr. str. str-i. trn. val. vr-s. woo. zn.
COLDNESS. p-x.
COLOR, **Dark**. spo-f.
Red. acon. æth. ag. as-o. ast. atp. c-bis. ca-ca. cb-v. cch. chd. cle. cmc. dig. dl-s. dt. eupat. euphr. grp. hur. k-bicr. mgs-au. mrl. na-ba. pul. spi. val. vr-s. woo.
DISCHARGE, **Foam**. ber.
Hard. ag-na. ca-ca. dl-s. grp. k-na. ox-x. pol. s.
Mucus. æth. aps. hg. pol. str-i.
Pus. as-o. euphr. mrl. pul.
White. ber.
DRYNESS. arn. as-o. cln. mtr. pd. rs.
ERUPTIONS, **Granulations**. aps.
Feeling of. k-bicr.
Itching. ca-ca. se.
Moist. ca-ca.
Pimples. na-cl.
Scabs. con. hg. sb-t. srr. woo.
Tubercles. hg-s. srr.
Ulcers. anan. cle. con. euphr. hg. mrl. na-ba. s. spi. woo.
Undefined. ca-ca.
Vesicles. se.
GNAWING. str-i.
HARDNESS. na-ba. rs. spi. spo-f.

HEAT. aps. art-v. as-o. bry. c-bis. cch. ccs. dph. hg. hg-bicl. k-bicr. k-o. lau-c. mph. ni-ca. pol. ptv. pul. rn-s. rs-r. **str.**

ITCHING. acon. amm-ca. art-v. bry. ca-ca. can-i. cb-v. chd. chlor. con. dl-s. grt. hg. hur. jat. jnc. k-bicr. kre. mgs-ar. narth. pnx. pru. rs-r. se. str. trn.

PRESSING. se. smc.

SHOOTING. dph. hur. narth. ni-ca.

SMALL. woo.

Feeling. lac-d.

SMARTING. acon. aps. arn. bry. ccs. cle. cln. cth. dig. hur. jat. kre. lau-c. li-ca. na-ba. pnx. rs-r. s. spi. str. str-i. **val.**

SWELLING. ag. arum-t. con. kre. lch. na-cl. ni-ca. pul. s.

Feeling of. ccs. val.

TEARING. bry. cle.

UNDEFINED. as-o. p.

UPPER TARSAL EDGE.

art-v. ba-ca. dl-s. hg-s. krm. lo-cœ. mgs-ar. myris. pol. pru-l. rhe. (spi).

COLOR **Red.** myris.

DRAWING. pru-l.

ERUPTIONS, **Vesicles.** mgs-ar.

FALSE SENSATIONS, **Sand.** (spi).

HEAT. art-v. pol. rhe.

ITCHING. art-v. ba-ca. dl-s.

PRESSING. rhe.

SHOOTING. hg-s.

SMARTING. krm.

LOWER TARSAL EDGE.

alm. ber. chd. dph. hur. ind. jnp-s. mtr. na-cl. pul. rut. sep. thu.

COLOR **Red.** chd. ind. mtr. pul.

CREEPING. ber.

DRAWING. ber.

ERUPTIONS, **Pimples.** na-cl. thu.

HEAT. dph. sep.

ITCHING. dph. rut.
SHOOTING. dph. jnp-s.
SMARTING. ber.
SWELLING. chd. mtr. pul.
THROBBING. ber.

EYELIDS, INNER SURFACE.

æth. ag-na. arn. as-o. atp. ba-ca. ber. ca-o. chd. chlor. cit-c. co. con. dig. eupat. glp. hg-bicl. hur. hydr. ind. k-bicr. k-o. lo-i. mrl. mtr. n-x. na-ba. (na-sa). ol-a. p-x. pol. ppv. pul. pul-n. rhe. rs. rs-r. s. smr. so-t. spo-f. str-i. thu. vr-a. zn. zng.

APPEARANCE **Velvety**. con.
COLDNESS. p-x.
COLOR, **Red**. ag-na. as-o. atp. ba-ca. ber. ca-o. chlor. con. cph. dig. glp. hg-bicl. hydr. k-bicr. mrl. na-ba. ol-a. ppv. pul. rs. rs-r. s. smr. so-t.
Yellow. dig.
CREEPING. chi.
DISCHARGE, **Mucus**. æth. pol. str-i.
Tenacious. eupat.
DRYNESS. arn. mtr. n-x. ol-a. s.
ERUPTIONS, **Blisters**. (na-sa). thu.
Granulations. k-bicr.
Pimples. hur.
Ulcers. na-ba.
HARDNESS. spo-f.
HEAT. ber. con. pul-n. rhe. s.
ITCHING. k-o. vr-a.
PRESSING. n-x. rhe.
SHOOTING. zng.
SMARTING. arn. lo-i. s. vr-a.
SOFTNESS. rs. thu.
SWELLING. æth. con. rs.
Red. rs.
TENSIVE. s.
WRINKLED. ag-na. zn.

UPPER EYELIDS, INNER SURFACE.

co.
SMARTING. co.

LOWER EYELIDS, INNER SURFACE.

chd. ind. rs.
COLOR, **Red**. chd. ind.
SMARTING. rs.

PUNCTA LACHRYMALIA.

acon. aps. as-o. atp. grp. hg-s. hur. na-cl.
ITCHING. hur.
OCCLUSION. acon. as-o. atp. grp. na-cl.
SMARTING. hur.

PUNCTA LACHRYMALIA.—UPPER EYELID.

hg-s.
SHOOTING. hg-s.

CANTHI.

acon. æsc. æth. ag. ag-na. aga. al-o. amm-ca. amm-cl. anan. aps. arn. art-v. arum-t. as-o. as-ters. asr. atp. au. ba-a. ba-ca. ber. bi-na. bru. bry. buf. bz-x. ca-a. ca-ca. ca-s. cast. cb-a. cb-v. cch. chd. chi. cic. cit-c. cl-hx. cle. cof. con. cop. cot. cph. cr-o. crd. crot. crt. crt-c. dig. dl-s. dph. elaps. ery. eug. euph. euphr. f-hx. fe-mgs. frm. glo. glp. grc. grp. grt. gui. hæm. hg. hg-a. hg-s. hll. hyo. i. ind. irs. k-bicr. k-ca. k-cla. k-i. k-na. k-o. kre. lac-d. lam. lau-c. lch. led. lo-cœ. ly-b. lyc. men. mg-ca. mg-cl. mgs. mgs-ar. mgs-au. mrl. msc. mtr. n-x. na-ba. na-ca. na-cl. ner. ni-ca. ol-a. p. p-x. par. pb. pb-a. pet. phl. phy. pnc. pol. ppv. pru. pru-l. pt. pul. rho. rn-b. rn-s. rs. rs-r. rut. s. s-x. sa-l. sang. sb-s. sb-t. sep. si-x. smc. smi. sn. so-o. spi. spo. sr-ca. str. str-i. teu. thu. til. trg. trn. trx. urg. val. vi-t. vr-a. vr-s. zn.
BORING. thu.
COLOR, **Dark.** pb.
Red. acon. ag-na. aga. al-o. as-o. [bi-na. bru. crt. euphr. grc. hg-a. hg-s. ly-b. mg-ca. mtr. na-cl. p. pul. s. str. str-i.
CRAMPY. msc.
CREEPING. cop. pt.

DISCHARGE, **Hard**. aga. bi-na. ca-ca. cof. cph. dig. dl-s. euph. grp. gui. k-o. pol. sb-s. str. thu.

Mucus. as-ters. bi-na. ca-a. cof. dig. dl-s. euphr. grp. hll. k-bicr. k-i. k-o. kre. lch. lyc. mtr. n-x. na-ca. par. pol. sb-s. vi-t.

Pus. art-v. buf. dl-s. grp. grt. mtr. pul. str.

Thin. pet.

White. lch.

Yellow. k-bicr. str.

DRYNESS. euph.

ERUPTIONS, **Ulcers.** buf. euph. hg. k-ca. na-cl. p. s. sb-s.

HEAT. aga. al-o. amm-cl. asr. au. ba-ca. buf. ca-ca. cb-v. cle. dl-s. hg-a. hll. k-na. mg-ca. mrl. na-ca. na-cl. ol-a. p. p-x. par. pnc. pul. s. sep. si-x. sn. sr-ca. str. thu.

ITCHING. æth. ag. ag-na. aga. al-o. aps. arn. art-v. ber. bru. bry. bz-x. ca-a. ca-ca. cb-v. cl-hx. cle. con. crt. crt-c. euph. f-hx. hg-a. hll. hyo. i. k-bicr. k-ca. k-o. lam. lyc. mg-ca. mgs. na-ba. na-cl. pb-a. pnc. pru. pt. pul. s. vr-a.

LACHRYMATION. pet. thu.

MOVEMENTS, **Closing Spasmodically**. crot.

Convulsions. crt. hyo.

PRESSING. aga. ca-a. cb-v. cch. dl-s. grt. hll. mg-cl. msc.

SCRAPING. pru-l.

SHOOTING. aga. al-o. ber. ca-a. ca-ca. con. crot. dl-s. mgs-ar. na-cl. p-x. pet. sb-t. sn. vr-a.

SMARTING. al-o. aps. asr. ber. cast. cb-v. cch. cl-hx. dl-s. dph. fe-mgs. hg. hll. hyo. k-ca. mgs-ar. pb. pnc. rn-b. rn-s. s. sb-s. sep. si-x. str. thu.

SWELLING. aga. ca-a. si-x.

Feeling of. rs.

TEARING. cast. hyo. men.

TENSIVE. ner.

THROBBING. ca-ca. k-cla.

UNDEFINED. aga. si-x.

EXTERNAL CANTHUS.

acon. æth. aga. alo. amm-cl. anan. art-v. arum-t. as-o. asr. ba-ca. ber. bry. ca-a. ca-ca. ca-s. cb-a. cb-v. cch. chd. chi. cl-hx. co. con. cot. cph. crt-c. dig. dl-s. euph. euphr. fe-mgs. frm. glo. grc. grp. hg. hg-s. hyo. k-bicr. k-ca. k-na.

lau-c. lch. lct. lo-cœ. lyc. mgs. mgs-ar. mn-ca. msc. mtr. n-x. na-ba. na-ca. na-cl. ni-ca. p. p-x. pnc. pol. pru-l. pul. rn-b. rn-s. rs. rs-v. rut. s. s-x. sa-l. sb-s. sep. si-x. smc. smi. sn. spi. spo. sr-ca. stach. str. str-i. thu. til. trn. trx. urg. vr-s.

COLDNESS. asr. ni-ca.

COLOR, **Red**. ber. ca-ca. grp. hg. k-bicr. rn-b. s. str.

CONTRACTIVE. euph.

CUTTING. ca-s.

DISCHARGE, **Hard**. chi. cph. dl-s. vr-s.

Mucus. al-o. as-o. ba-ca. ca-s. cch. chi. cph. dl-s. lyc. mgs-ar. na-cl. pul. rut. sep. str-i. vr-s.

ERUPTIONS, **Rhagades**. grp.

Ulcers. anan. ca-a. ca-ca. lyc. sb-s. zn.

FALSE SENSATIONS, **Sand**. aga. al-o. ba-ca. con. crt-c. n-x. str-i.

Water. ni-ca.

HÆMORRHAGE. grp.

HEAT. art-v. cb-a. dig. dl-s. k-bicr. k-ca. k-na. pnc. s. sep. spi. sr-ca. urg.

ITCHING. æth. art-v. bry. euph. hg-s. hyo. lo-cœ. mgs. na-ba. pnc. pul. s. sb-s. sep. til. trn. urg.

LACHYMATION. arum-t.

MOVEMENTS, **Closing**. grp. stach.

Convulsions. ba-ca. lau-c. na-cl.

NUMBNESS. acon.

PRESSING. ba-ca. ca-ca. chi. con. dl-s. lch. n-x. p-x. pul. s-x. str-i.

SHOOTING. ba-ca. ca-a. dl-s. hg-s. k-ca. s. str-i.

SMARTING. ag-na. ca-ca. ca-s. cb-a. cb-v. cch. co. dig. grc. grp. k-bicr. k-ca. k-na. lau-c. lct. lyc. mgs-ar. mn-ca. mtr. rn-b. rs. sep. str. str-i. zn.

SWELLING. anan. grp. rn-b.

TEARING. amm-cl. dl-s. str-i.

TENSIVE. dl-s. grt.

THROBBING. ba-ca. lau-c.

UNDEFINED. (fe-mgs). rs-r.

INTERNAL CANTHUS.

æsc. æth. ag-na. aga. al-o. anan. arn. art-v. as-o. asr. atp. au. ba-a. ba-ca. ber. br. bru. bry. buf. ca-a. ca-ca. ca-s. cb-a. cb-v. chd. cic. cit-c. cl-hx. cle. cof. con. cr-o. crd. dig. dl-s. dph. elaps. ery. eug. euphr. glo. glp. grc. grp. grt.

hæm. hg. hg-cy. hg-s. hll. hyo. ind. irs. k-bicr. k-cla. k-i. k-na. k-o. lac-ac. lac-d. lct. led. lo-cœ. lyc. men. mg-ca. mg-cl. mgs. mgs-ar. mgs-au. msc. mtr. n-x. na-ba. na-ca. na-cl. ner. ni-ca. nic. ol-a. p. p-x. par. pb. pet. phl. phy. ppv. pru-l. pul. rho. rs. rs-r. rut. s. s-x. sa-l. sang. sb-s. sb-t. sep. si-x. smc. smi. sn. so-o. spi. spo. sr-ca. str. str-i. teu. thu. trg. trx. val. vr-a. zn.

COLOR, **Dark**. au. pb. smi.

Red. ag-na. aga. au. ber. cle. eug. glo. grp. grt. hæm. hg. mg-ca. na-ca. rs. str. teu. val.

CONTRACTIVE. anan. eug.

CRAMPY. eug.

DISCHARGE, **Hard**. dl-s. euphr. hll. par. rs.

Mucus. aga. al-o. art-v. cof. con. dl-s. euphr. hyo. lyc. mg-ca. ni-ca. p. pul. rho. rs. rut. sb-s. si-x. thu. zn.

Pus. buf. ca-ca. grp. na-cl. p.

Tenacious. lac-ac.

Thin. k-i.

DRYNESS. al-o. asr. ber. mtr. na-cl. rs. str.

ERUPTIONS, **Blisters**. k-bicr.

Boils. bry.

Pustules. bry.

Soft. bry.

Rhagades. zn.

Soft. bry.

Styes. na-cl. s. sn.

Ulcers. buf.

FALSE SENSATIONS, **Pellicle**. k-o.

Sand. al-o. dig. (spi.) trx.

HEAT. æsc. aga. art-v. asr. au. ba-ca. ber. buf. ca-ca. dig. glo. glp. grp. hll. irs. k-bicr. k-o. mg-ca. na-cl. nic. p. p-x. par. pet. phl. pru-l. rho. sb-t.

ITCHING. æth. art-v. atp. br. bru. ca-a. con. cr-o. dl-s. dph. glo. grc. grt. ind. k-o. led. lyc. mg-ca. mgs. mgs-ar. n-x. na-ba. na-cl. ol-a. p-x. pb. phl. phy. pul. rs-r. rut. sep. sn. spi. sr-ca. str. str-i. zn.

MOVEMENTS, **Closing Spasmodically**. eug.

Convulsions. k-cla.

PRESSING. ber. cb-a. lyc. na-cl. p-x. pet. pul. rho. rs-r. trg. zn.

SCRAPING. pru-l.

SHOOTING. aga. anan. arn. atp. ca-a. ca-ca, cle. con. crd. dl-s. elaps. eug. grp. grt. ind. men. na-ca. p-x. phl. pru-l. pul. sb-t. sn. vr-a.

SMARTING. al-o. atp. bry. cl-hx. con. cr-o. dig. dl-s. dph. grp. grt. hg-s. hll. ind. k-ca. k-o. lct. mg-ca. mgs-au. ni-ca. ol-a. p. phy. pul. rut. s. sb-t. sep. spi. str. teu. zn.
SWELLING. ag-na. aga. ca-ca. hg. k-i. na-cl. pet. ppv.
TEARING. atp. k-na. men.
TENSIVE. ba-a. grt. hg-cy. ner.
THROBBING. ca-ca.
UNDEFINED. al-o. atp. dig. k-i. na-cl. so-o. trg.

CARUNCULA LACHRYMALIS.

ag-na. aga. (alm). bry. ca-ca. dl-s. hæm. hur. k-bicr. ppv. pul. str. zn.
COLOR, **Red**. ag-na. hæm. hur.
ERUPTIONS, **Spongy**. (alm).
Tubercles. (alm).
Spongy. (alm).
SWELLING. ag-na. aga. ppv.

LACHRYMAL GLAND.

aga. anan. arn. br. (cu). dl-s. grp.
ERUPTIONS, **Ulcers.** anan.
PRESSING. arn. dl-s.
SWELLING. aga. grp.
TEARING. dl-s.
UNDEFINED. (fe-mgs).

LACHRYMAL BONES.

hg. k-bicr. lch. si-x.
SWELLING. hg.

LACHRYMAL SAC.

(alm). ca-ca. chd. dl-s. f-hx. grp. na-ca. na-cl. pet. pul. rut. s. si-x. sn. trg.
ERUPTIONS, **Abscess**. na-ca. pul.
Fistula. (alm). ca-ca. chd. dl-s. f-hx. grp. pet. pul. rut. s. si-x. sn. trg.
SWELLING. na-cl. pet.
UNDEFINED. na-cl.

I. C. GENERAL CHARACTER, SEQUENCE, and DIRECTION.

PERIODICAL.

acon. amb. amm-ca. aph. arn. as-o. atp. ba-ca. ber. c-bis. ca-ca. ca-s. cac. chd. chi. clv. con. cro. dig. dl-s. dt. euphr. fe-mgs. grp. hg. hyo. k-bicr. k-na. k-o. lyc. n-x. na-ca. na-cl. na-sa. narth. ni-ca. p. pæo. pb. pet. phl. physo. pnx. pul. rho. rn-s. rs. rut. s. sb-s. sb-t. sep. si-x. smb. smc. smi. spi. spo-f. srr. str. thr. vr-a. vr-s. woo.

OBJECTS IMAGINARY. **Vibrations.** thr.

Visions Terrible. smb.

PHOTOPHOBIA. as-o. na-cl. si-x.

SIGHT IMPAIRED. acon. amm-ca. atp. ba-ca. ca-ca. cac. chd. chi. clv. con. cro. dig. dl-s. dt. euphr. fe-mgs. grp. hg. hyo. k-na. k-o. lyc. na-ca. na-cl. p. pb. pet. physo. pul. rs. rut. s. sb-s. sb-t. sep. si-x. smc. spi. srr. vr-a. woo.

EYEBALL. **Color, Red.** as-o. k-o. na-cl.

Discharge. s.

Dryness. rho.

Heat. amb. amm-ca. as-o. narth. rho. spi. vr-s.

Lachrymation. as-o. na-cl.

Pressing. arn. ca-s. s. si-x.

Small. sep.

Tearing. as-o. ber. ca-ca.

Tensive. spi.

Throbbing. ca-ca. p.

IRIS. **Pupils Contracted.** na-cl.

ORBIT CIRCUMFERENCE. **Pressing.** arn.

ORBIT SUPERIORLY. **Shooting.** ber.

ORBITAL INTEGUMENTS. **Pressing.** phl.

EYELIDS. **Adhesion of.** s.

Heat. aph.

Movements, Closing Spasmodically. na-cl.

UPPER EYELIDS. **Itching.** pæo.

EYELIDS, INNER SURFACE. **Color, Red.** as-o.

Pressing. n-x.

CANTHI. **Smarting.** rn-s.

PERIODICAL—ALTERNATE DAYS.

amb. as-o. smi.
EYEBALL. **Heat.** amb.
Lachrymation. smi.

PERIODICAL—EVERY DAY.

as-o. fe-mgs. spi.
OBJECTS IMAGINARY. **Blue.** fe-mgs.
Bright. fe-mgs.
Circles. fc-mgs.
  Blue. fe-mgs.
  Bright. fe-mgs.
  Zigzags. fe-mgs.
Zigzags. fe-mgs.
SIGHT IMPAIRED. fe-mgs.

PERIODICAL—FROM 4 A.M. TO 3 P.M.

spi.

PERIODICAL.—FROM 10 A.M. TO 3 P.M.

as-o.

PERIODICAL—EVERY NIGHT.

(dt).

PERIODICAL.—EVERY FORENOON.

dt. na-cl. p. s.
OBJECTS IMAGINARY. **Veil.** dt.
SIGHT IMPAIRED. dt.
EYEBALL. **Color Red.** na-cl.
Lachrymation. na-cl.
Throbbing. p.
EYELIDS. **Adhesion of.** s.
Movements, Closing Spasmodically. na-cl.

PERIODICAL—AT 7 A.M.

na-cl.
PHOTOPHOBIA. na-cl.
IRIS. **Pupils Contracted.** na-cl.

PERIODICAL—EVERY NOON.

vr-a.

PERIODICAL—EVERY AFTERNOON.

as-o. asr. ca-ca. (dt). rho. s. si-x.
EYEBALL. **Pressing**. s. si-x.
EYELIDS. **Heat**. aph.

PERIODICAL—FROM 3 TO 4 P.M., TO 9 TO 10 P.M.

ca-ca.
EYEBALL. **Tearing**. ca-ca.

PERIODICAL—AT 4 P.M.

as-o.
PHOTOPHOBIA. as-o.
EYEBALL. **Color, Red.** as-o.
Heat. as-o.
Lachrymation. as-o.
EYELIDS, INNER SURFACE. **Color Red.** as-o.

PERIODICAL—AT 5 P.M.

asr.
EYEBALL. **Color, Red**. asr.
Lachrymation. asr.
CANTHI. **Heat**. asr.

PERIODICAL—AT 6 P.M.

rho.
EYEBALL. **Heat**. rho.

PERIODICAL—EVERY HALF-HOUR.

hg.
SIGHT IMPAIRED. hg.

PERIODICAL—SYNCHRONOUS **with** PULSE.

pnx. si-x.
OBJECTS **Appear Moving Up and Down.** si-x.
Vibrating. pnx.

GRADUALLY INCREASE **and** DECREASE.

as-o. dig. k-bicr. lyc. myris. na-cl. ner.
OBJECTS IMAGINARY. **Vibrations Bright**. dig.
PHOTOPHOBIA. na-cl.
SIGHT IMPAIRED. lyc.
EYEBALL. **Color, Red.** na-cl.
Lachrymation. na-cl.
IRIS. **Pupil Contracted.** na-cl.
ORBIT SUPERIORLY. **Contractive**. myris.
Pressing. ner.
EYELIDS. **Movements, Closing Spasmodically.**—na-cl.

GRADUALLY COME, SUDDENLY GO.

pul.

SUDDENLY COME, GRADUALLY GO.

hg-s.

SUDDENLY COME **and** GO.

dig. hg-s. na-ba.
EYEBALL. **Cutting**. na-ba.

CHANGING CHARACTER **or** PLACE **in** EYES.

aga. amb. atp. ba-ca. ber. bru. ca-a. ca-ca. ca-s. can. cb-a. ccs. chd. chio. cic. cl-hx. con. cot. cro. crot. cu. cy-hx. dl-s. dt. (ery). eryn. f-hx. gn-l. grp. jnp-s. k-bicr. k-ca. k-o. kre. lam. lau-c. men. mg-ca. mgs. mgs-ar. msc. n-x. na-ba. na-cl. na-sa. ner. p. p-x. pb. pnx. pol. pru-l. pul. qu-sa. s. sb-t. sep. si-x. smb. smc. smi. sn. spi. spo. sr-ca. str-i. thu. trg. trn. trx. u-na.
OBJECTS APPEAR **Blue then Grey**. atp.
Blue then White. atp.
Bright then Red. atp.
Red then Blue. atp.
OBJECTS IMAGINARY. **Plain White to which Spots Bright descend, then Plain Bright to which Spots White descend**. p-x.
Vibrations Bright Red, then Flames Red. f-hx.

SIGHT IMPAIRED. **Presbyopia then Myopia.** dt.

EYEBALL. **Coldness then False Sensations, Sand.** f-hx.

then Shooting. mgs-ar.

Color Red then Lachrymation. grp.

Drawing then Lachrymation. grp.

Eruptions, Blisters then Granulations. sb-t.

False Sensations, Wind (cold) **then Sand.** f-hx.

Heat then Coldness. chd.

then Color Red. sr-ca.

then Shooting. sr-ca.

Itching then Color Red. kre.

then False Sensations, Sand. kre.

then Heat. cb-a. k-bicr. kre.

then Lachrymation. cb-a. k-o.

then Pressing. ca-ca. cb-a. kre. trg.

then Smarting. kre.

then Undefined. k-bicr.

Lachrymation then Dryness. s.

Movements Convulsions then Itching. na-cl.

Pressing then Color Red. kre.

then Lachrymation. ca-s. grp. kre.

Hot. grp. kre.

then Shooting. k-ca.

Shooting then Color Red. n-x.

then Pressing. spo.

Smarting then Lachrymation. s.

Tearing then Lachrymation. mg-ca.

Undefined then Color Red. crot.

IRIS. **Pupils Contracted then Dilated.** aga-p. atp. can. cic. cl-hx. cu. dl-s. jnp-s. k-o. lam. lau-c. men. pb. pnx. pol. pul. smb. smc. sn. trx.

Dilated then Contracted. aga. atp. ca-a. cy-hx. ner. p-x. qu-sa.

ORBIT. **Shooting then Pressing.** ba-ca.

TARSAL EDGES. **Sensitive then Drawing.** ber.

then Throbbing. ber.

Tingling then Drawing. ber.

then Throbbing. ber.

EYELIDS, INNER SURFACE. **Smarting then Dryness.** s.

CANTHI. **Color Red then Itching.** bru.

OBJECTS IMAGINARY, **then** SIGHT IMPAIRED. p.

Mist Red then EYEBALL **Lachrymation.** (ery).

Flames Red then EYEBALL **Lachrymation.** spi.
,, **then** IRIS **Pupils Dilated.** spi.
SIGHT IMPAIRED **then** SIGHT DAZZLED. na-cl.
then EYEBALL **Appearance Dim.** dt.
then ,, **Color Red.** kre.
then ,, **Lachrymation.** ca-ca. dt. kre. p-x. spi.
then ,, ,, **Hot.** kre.
then ,, **Pressing.** dt.
then ,, **Smarting.** dt.
then IRIS **Pupils Dilated.** spi.
EYEBALL **Heat then** OBJECTS IMAGINARY, **Flames Red.** spi.
Shooting then ,, **Mist.** k-ca.
Appears Staring, then SIGHT IMPAIRED. cic. msc.
Heat then. ,, spi.
Lachrymation then ,, cro.
Pressing then ,, ,, cro. (sep).
Shooting then ,, ,, k-ca.
Undefined then ,, ,, con. cro.
Color Red then LENS **Cataract.** atp. n-x.
Appearance Staring then IRIS **Pupils Contracted.** msc.
Itching, then EYELIDS **Adhesion of.** k-bicr.
Sensitive, then UPPER EYELIDS **Shooting.** gn-l.
Undefined then ,, ,, gn-l
Gnawing, then CANTHI **Discharge.** kre.
Heat then ,, ,, kre.
Itching then ,, ,, kre.
ORBIT **Shooting, then** EYEBALL **Lachrymation, Feeling of.** ba-ca.
Pressing, then ORBIT SUPERIORLY **Pressing Down.** chio.
EYELIDS **Movements Closing, then** OBJECTS IMAGINARY, **Flames Red.** spi.
then SIGHT IMPAIRED. spi.
Adhesion then EYEBALL **Lachrymation.** smi. str-i.
Movements Closing then ,, **Appearance Staring.** lau-c.
,, **then** ,, **Upward-looking.** lau-c.
Opening Spasmodically then ,, **False Sensations, Sand.** f-hx.

EXTERNAL CANTHUS **Pressing then** EYELIDS **Adhesion**. pul.
INTERNAL CANTHUS **Heat then** LOWER EYE-LID **Heat**. k-bicr.

ALTERNATING **in** CHARACTER **or** PLACE **in** EYES.

ba-a. ba-ca. buf. c-bis. ca-ca. can. chi. cic. cl-hx. clf. crb-x. cro. lyc. physo. pnx. si-x. smi. so-n. str-i. thu.
OBJECTS APPEAR **Near and Distant**. cic.
PHOTOPHOBIA **with** EYEBALL **Color Red**. si-x.
,, **with** ,, **Lachrymation**. si-x.
SIGHT IMPAIRED. **Myopia with Presbyopia**. lyc.
,, ,, **with** EYEBALL **Pressing**. cro.
EYEBALL **Color Red with** PHOTOPHOBIA. si-x.
Lachrymation with ,, si-x.
Pressing with SIGHT IMPAIRED. cro.
IRIS. **Pupils Contracted and Dilated**. ba-a. ba-ca. buf. can. chi. cic. cl-hx. clf. crb-x. physo. pnx. so-n. str-i.
EYELIDS. **Heat with Pressing**. smi.

ALTERNATELY **in** EITHER EYE.

acon. amb. atp. chio. cu. glp. lyc. na-sa. rn-b.
EYEBALL. **Dryness**. atp.
Heat. acon. atp. cu.
Pressing. na-sa. rn-b.
Shooting. lyc.
Smarting. cu.
Tearing. amb.
Tensive. glp.
ORBIT SUPERIORLY. **Undefined**. chio.

RIGHT **then** LEFT.

aga. alm. *as-o. ber. chd. *chi. chio. cot. cph. cro. cund. fe-mgs. hg-bini. hg-s. *k-ca. lac-ac. lch. menth. mg-cl. n-x. *na-cl. *s. sep. str-i.
OBJECTS IMAGINARY. **Blue**. fe-mgs.
Bright. fe-mgs.
Circles. fe-mgs.
Blue. fe-mgs.
Bright. fe-mgs.
Red. fe-mgs.
Zigzags. fe-mgs.

Red. fe-.mgs
Zigzags. fe-mgs.
SIGHT IMPAIRED. *chi.
EYEBALL. **Boring**. ber.
Color Red. *as-o. cph. hg-bini. n-x.
False Sensations, Sand. lch.
Movements, Convulsions. aga. lac-ac.
Pressing. *as-o. chd. menth.
Shooting. ber. chd.
Smarting. cot.
Tearing. chd.
Undefined. str-i.
LENS. **Cataract**. *p.
ORBIT SUPERIORLY. **Drawing**. chio.
Smarting. hg-s.
Swelling, Feeling of. hg-s.
ORBITAL INTEGUMENTS. **Swelling**. *k-ca.
EYELIDS. **Movements, Convulsions**. cro.
LOWER EYELIDS. **Itching**. alm.
EYELIDS, INNER SURFACE. **Color Red**. cph.
INTERNAL CANTHUS. **Itching**. mg-cl.
FORWARDS. **Orbit Superiorly Pressing**. na-cl.
DOWNWARDS. **Orbit Superiorly Pressing**. chio.
TO HEAD—ANTERIORLY. **Eyeball Boring**. ber.
Shooting. ber.
RIGHT OBJECTS IMAGINARY, **Pyriform body**, **then** LEFT OBJECTS APPEAR **Confused**. cund.
then LEFT OBJECTS IMAGINARY, **Mist**. cund.
RIGHT EYEBALL **Shooting then** LEFT EYEBALL **Color Red**. n-x.

LEFT then RIGHT.

aga. ba-ca. *cph. *cro. *crot. dig. f-hx. glo. *li-ca. *mg-ca. na-cl. *na-cl. na-sa. rs. *rs. smi. *spi. thu. *zn.
OBJECTS, FALSE APPEARANCE of. **Part Visible**. *li-ca.
OBJECTS IMAGINARY. **Vibrations Bright**. dig.
SIGHT IMPAIRED. *li-ca.
EYEBALL **Color Red**. *spi.
Eruptions, Pterygium. *zn.
Heat. na-cl.
Itching. na-sa.

Lachrymation. aga. ba-ca. *spi.
Appearance of. *cro.
Feeling of. ba-ca. *cro.
Pressing. ba-ca. smi. *spi.
Shooting. *cph. *spi. thu.
LENS. **Cataract.** *mg-ca.
ORBIT. **Pressing.** thu.
Tensive. thu.
EYELIDS. **Movements Closing.** ba-ca.
Swelling. *rs.
UPPER EYELIDS. **Swelling.** *crot. rs.
Œdematous. *crot. rs.
Red. *crot. rs.
TARSAL EDGES. **Discharge Pus.** *crot. rs.
White. *crot. rs.
Yellow. *crot. rs.
FORWARDS. **Eyeball Pressing.** *spi.
Shooting. *spi.
EYEBALL to JAW. **Undefined.** f-hx.
LEFT SIGHT DAZZLED **then** RIGHT OBJECTS IMAGINARY, **Veil Crooked.** *na-cl.
LEFT INTERNAL CANTHUS **Bruised, then** LEFT ORBIT SUPERIORLY **Bruised.** glo.

ANTERO—POSTERIORLY—FORWARDS. (**Within—Outwards**).

acon. al-o. alli. alo. anan. asr. ast. atp. au. ber. br. bry. ca-ca. ca-o. ca-s. can. can-i. cb-v. cl-hx. cmc. con. crd. (cro). crt-c. cth. dl-s. dro. (dt). gel. glo. glp. gui. gym. hll. k-i. k-na. k-o. lau-c. lch. led. ly-b. lyc. mg-ca. mg-cl. mg-sa. mgs-ar. mrl. mtr. n-x. na-ba. na-ca. na-cl. narth. p. p-x. pan. par. pol. ppv. pru-l. pso. ptv. pul. rho. rn-b. rs. s. sang. scu. sep. si-x. snc. spi. str. str-i. thu. trg. val. vi-t. zng.

EYEBALL. **Pressing.** (**as if eyes would come out, &c.**) acon. al-o. alo. anm. asr. atp. au. ber. bry. ca-ca. ca-o. ca-s. can. can-i. cb-v. cmc. con. crd. crt-c. cth. dl-s. glo. gui. gym. hll. k-i. k-na. k-o. lau-c. lch. led. lyc. mg-ca. mg-cl. mg-sa. mgs-ar. mrl. mtr. na-cl. narth. p. p-x. par. pol. pru-l. pso. ptv. pul. rn-b. rs. sang. scu. sep. si-x. spi. str. str-i. thu. trg. val. zn.

Shooting. anm. au. ca-ca. cl-hx. dro. gel. na-ca. s. sep. si-x. val. vi-t.

Tearing. alli. anm. atp. ca-ca. p-x. si-x

Tensive. glp.
Undefined. ast.
EYEBALL SUPERIORLY. **Pressing**. au.
EYEBALL INTERNALLY. **Pressing**. au.
ORBIT. **Tearing**. atp.

ANTERO—POSTERIORLY—BACKWARDS.

(Without—Inwards.)

acon. aga. amb. aps. arn. ast. atp. au. bap. bi-na. bry. ca-ca. ca-s. can. chd. chi. chio. cit-c. (con). cor. dph. dt. grp. hæm. hg-s. hyp. k-ca. k-o. kre. lac-f. ly-b. mn-ca. na-ba. na-sa. p. p-x. pb. pet. pnx. s. sa-l. si-x. smc. spi. teu. zn.

EYEBALL. **Drawing**. ast. ca-s. ly-b. pb. s. si-x.
Pressing. acon. aga. amb. ast. atp. au. bap. bi-na. bry. ca-ca. can. chd. cit-c. cor. hæm. hg-s. k-ca. k-o. kre. na-ba. p-x. pnx. smc. spi. teu. zn.
Like a Plug. chi.
Shooting. aps. arn. atp. p. pet.
ORBIT. **Pressing**. atp. chd.
UPPER EYELIDS. **Pressing**. acon.

VERTICALLY—DOWNWARDS.

ath. atp. au. bap. bry. cb-a. cb-v. chd. chi. chio. cit-c. gel. hll. k-o. lac-f. ner. par. rn-b. s. smc. snp-n. spi. trg. zn. zng.

EYEBALL. **Pressing**. ath. bap. cb-v. chd. chio. rn-b. s. smc. snp-n.
Scraping. pul.
Shooting. cb-a.
EYEBALL INTERIORLY. **Pressing**. chio.
ORBITAL INTEGUMENTS. **Pressing**. lac-f.
EYELIDS. **Swelling**. as-o.
TARSAL EDGES. **Cutting**. zng.
ORBITAL INTEGUMENTS SUPERIORLY **to** TARSAL EDGES. **Cutting**. trg.

VERTICALLY.—UPWARDS.

acon. amm-cl. arn. atp. bi-na. chio. cmc. euph-a. krm. nic. vr-s.
EYEBALL. **Boring**. ber.
False Sensations, Sand. amm-cl.
Pressing. arn. bi-na. chio.
Shooting. ber.
Undefined. acon.
EYEBALL INTERIORLY. **Pressing**. chio.
EYEBALL **to** ORBITAL INTEGUMENTS SUPERIORLY. **Undefined.** acon.
EYEBALL **to** EYELIDS. **Drawing**. chd.
UPPER TARSAL EDGE **to** ORBIT. **Shooting**. nic.

LATERALLY—LENGTHWAYS.

cr-o. dro. gel. na-ba. p-x.
EYEBALL. **Shooting**. gel.
EYELIDS. **Shooting**. p-x.

LATERALLY—OUTWARDS (**To External Canthi**).

alo. arn. bap. (con). euph-a. hg-s. i. lch. na-ca. p-x. rs.
EYEBALL. **Drawing**. arn.
Pressing. bap. p-x.
ORBIT SUPERIORLY. **Cutting**. hg-s.
ORBITAL INTEGUMENTS SUPERIORLY. **Drawing**. alo.

LATERALLY—INWARDS (**To Internal Canthi**).

cub. nic. pet. rho. s-x. spo.
EYEBALL. **Shooting**. cub.

OBLIQUELY.

dro.

ALTERNATING **with** HEAD.

atp. dt. phl. trg.
OBJECTS IMAGINARY. **Vibrations.** trg.
Zigzags. trg.
SIGHT IMPAIRED. phl.

EYEBALL. **Appearance Wild.** dt.
ORBIT. **Pressing—Backwards.** atp.
Tearing—Forwards. atp.

ALTERNATING **with** EARS.

atp. cic.
OBJECTS FALSE APPEARANCE **of. Black.** cic.
Multiplied. cic.
ORBIT. **Pressing—Backwards.** atp.
Tearing—Forwards. atp.

ALTERNATING **with** FACE.

kre.

ALTERNATING **with** ABDOMEN.

cic. euphr. hg-bini. kre.
EYEBALL. **Color Red.** hg-bini.
Heat. hg-bini.
Movements, Convulsions. cic.
Undefined. euphr.

ALTERNATING **with** URINARY ORGANS.

kre.

ALTERNATING **with** GENITAL ORGANS.

kre.

ALTERNATING **with** CHEST.

kre. rn-b.
EYEBALL. **Pressing.** rn-b.

ALTERNATING **with** BACK.

hg-bini.
EYEBALL. **Color Red.** hg-bini.
Heat. hg-bini.

ALTERNATING **with** ARMS.

atp. hg-bini.
SIGHT IMPAIRED. atp.
EYEBALL. **Color Red.** hg-bini.
Heat. hg-bini.

ALTERNATING **with** LEGS.

atp.
SIGHT IMPAIRED. atp.

To HEAD.

acon. aga. anan. as-o. atp. ba-ca. ber. br. buf. ca-o. cb-v. cch. ccs. cic. cit-c. cmc. cmf. crt-c. cth. euph-a. glo. grp. hg-s. hur. k-o. kre. lac-ac. lac-f. lch. li-ca. ly-b. lyc. nic. par. pau. phy. s. sang. spi. spo-f. thu. trg. trn. u-na. vr-v. woo.
EYEBALL. **Boring.** ber.
Cutting. cit-c.
Drawing. aga. crt-c. grp.
Heaviness. glo.
Pressing. aga. cit-c. kre. nic.
Shooting. ber. ca-o. s. spi. thu. trg.
Tensive, like a thread. par.
Throbbing. br. ccs.
Undefined. acon. ccs. spo-f. woo.
ORBIT, CIRCUMFERENCE. **Shooting.** k-o.
ORBIT, SUPERIORLY. **Shooting.** pau.
Throbbing. buf.
EYELIDS. **Swelling.** as-o.
INTERNAL CANTHUS. **Contractive.** anan.
Shooting. anan.

To HEAD—ANTERIORLY.

acon. aga. atp. ber. br. ca-o. ccs. cit-c. cth. hur. lac-ac. lac-f. ly-b. lyc. sang. spo-f. trg. vr-v.
EYEBALL. **Boring.** ber.
Drawing. aga.
Pressing. aga. cit-c.
Shooting. ber. ca-o.
Throbbing. br.
Undefined. ccs. spo-f.
ORBIT. **Undefined.** hur.
ORBIT SUPERIORLY. **Shooting.** acon. cth.

To HEAD—SUPERIORLY.

cmf. kre. phy. trg.
EYEBALL. **Pressing.** kre.
Shooting. trg.
Undefined. cmf.

To HEAD—TEMPLES.

acon. ba-ca. br. ccs. crt-c. glo. hg-s. lac-f. lch. li-ca. spo-f.
EYEBALL. **Drawing.** crt-c.
Heaviness. glo.
Throbbing. ccs.
Undefined. spo-f.
ORBIT SUPERIORLY. **Shooting.** acon.

To HEAD—LATERALLY.

cit-c. trn.
EYEBALL. **Pressing.** cit-c.

To HEAD—POSTERIORLY.

cch. ccs. cic. cmc. cmf. lch. nic. spi. thu. u-na.
EYEBALL. **Pressing.** nic.
Shooting. spi. thu.

To EARS.

ba-ca. dl-s. elaps. hg-s. li-ca.

To NOSE.

alli. ba-ca. ca-o. chd. cit-c. k-o. ni-ca. sa-l.
EYEBALL. **Drawing.** chd.
ORBIT SUPERIORLY. **Tearing.** ca-o.

To NOSE—ROOT.

chd.
EYEBALL. **Drawing.** chd.

To NOSE—POINT.

sa-l.

To FACE.

acon. aga. ca-o. cl-hx. cor. f-hx. jcr. k-bicr. lyc. i. mgs. spi.
ORBIT. **Shooting.** acon.
UPPER EYELIDS. **Drawing.** cl-hx.
Shooting. cl-hx.
INTERNAL CANTHUS. **Tearing.** ca-o.

To FACE—JAWS.

mgs.

To FACE—UPPER JAW.

aga. f-hx. k-bicr.

To FACE—LOWER JAW.

jcr.

To FACE—UPPER LIP.

ca-o.

To TEETH.

acon. hg-bicl. lac-ac. lyc.
ORBIT. **Shooting**. acon.

To TEETH—UPPER.

hg-bicl.

To ABDOMEN.

mgs.

To CHEST.

mgs.

To BACK.

as-o. mgs. rs. trg.

To BACK—NECK.

trg.
EYEBALL. **Tensive like a Thread.** trg.

To LEGS.

mgs.

To LEGS—HIPS.

mgs.

To WHOLE BODY.

acon. cit-c.
EYEBALL. **Undefined.** cit-c.
EXTERNAL CANTHUS. **Numbness.** acon.

I D. RIGHT SIDE, (**Right Eye**).

acon. æsc. aga. al-o. alli. alm. alo. amb. amm-ca. amm-cl. amph. anan. aps. arn. arum-t. asc. asr. ast. atp. atrop. au. bap. bar. ber. br. bry. buf. c-bis. ca-a. ca-ca. ca-pa. cac. cb-a. cb-v. cch. ccs. chd. chio. cic. cis. cit-c. cl-hx. cld. cle. cmc. cmf. cof. con. cop. cot. cph. cr-o. crb-x. cro. crt. cth. cu. cund. cyc. delph. dig. dl-s. dro. dt. elaps. ele. erig. ery. eug. f-hx. fe-mgs. fe-pa. frm. gel. glo. glp. grp. gui. gym. hg. hg-bini. hg-i. hg-s. hur. hyp. i. irs-f. jcr. k-bicr. k-ca. k-i. k-na. k-o. klm. kre. krm. lac-ac. lac-f. lau-c. lch. li-ca. lo-cœ. lo-i. lpd. ly-b. lyc. mg-ca. mg-cl. mg-sa. mgs. mll. mn-ca. mrl. mtr. myris. n-x. na-ba. na-ca. na-cl. na-sa. naj. narth. ner. ni-ca. nic. ol-a. p. p-x. pæo. par. pau. pb. pet. phl. phy. pim. pnc. pnx. pol. ppv. pru-l. pso. pt. ptv. pul. qu-sa. rho. rn-b. rs. rs-r. rs-v. rut. s. s-x. sa-l. sang. sb-s. sb-t. sep. si-x. smc. smi. sn. so-o. so-t. spi. spi-m. spo. spo-f. sr-ca. str. str-i. te. teu. thr. thu. trg. trn. trx. tx-b. u-na. urg. urt. val. vi-t. vr-a. vr-s. vsp. xan. ziz. zn. zng.

OBJECTS, FALSE APPEARANCE **of. Blue.** ni-ca.
Confused. eug. rs-r.
Multiplied. (mtr).
Small. thu.

OBJECTS IMAGINARY. **Black.** cund. p. (qu-sa). (si-x).
Blue. cund. elaps.
Bright. ca-ca. cit-c. na-sa. ol-a.
Circles. cit-c.
Crystals with Black tips. cund.
Curls. cund.
Feathers. al-o.
Figures. myris.
  At side of Visual Ray. myris.
Green. na-sa.
Halo. cmc.
  Red. cmc.
Horns Black. cund.
Leaf White. na-sa.

Low down. cit-c.
Mist. au. cit-c. cund. mg-ca. na-sa. ol-a.
Moving. cund.
Moving with Eye. ca-ca. (qu-sa).
Near Eye. na-sa.
Pyriform body. cund.
  Blue. cund.
  Red. cund.
Red. cmc. cund.
Serpentine bodies. cund.
  Black. cund.
  Moving. cund.
Moving. cund.
Side of Visual Ray at. cit-c. myris.
Spots, Black. (qu-sa). (si-x).
      Moving with Eye. (qu-sa).
  Bright. cit-c. ol-a.
    Low down. cit-c.
    Moving with Eye. ca-ca.
    Side of Visual Ray, at. cit-c.
  Low down. cit-c.
  Moving with Eye. ca-ca.
  Side of Visual Ray, at. cit-c.
Star Bright. ca-ca. na-sa.
    Moving with Eye. ca-ca.
    Near Eye. na-sa.
   Green. na-sa.
    Near Eye. na-sa.
   Moving with Eye. ca-ca.
   Near Eye. na-sa.
    Yellow. na-sa.
    Near Eye. na-sa.
Threads. con. cund. pol.
Veil Black. p.
  Blue. elaps.
  Crooked. na-cl.
  White. elaps.
Vibrations. chd. dig. trg.
  White. elaps. na-sa.
  Yellow. na-sa.

SIGHT IMPAIRED. aps. (atp). cit-c. con. cph. cro. cund. elaps. eug. k-o. krm. mg-ca. n-x. na-ca. na-sa. ol-a. p. qu-sa. rut. str-i. trn.

EYEBALL. **Boring**. ber. cof.
Bruised. ly-b. ptv. smi.
Bursting. lau-c.
Coldness. asr. cro. dt. li-ca. par. pt. s.
Color Dark. k-bicr.
Red. al-o. aps. atp. ca-ca. cb-a. ccs. con. cot. cph. dt. eug. hg-bini. hg-s. hur. lac-f. lau-c. n-x. p. sep. vr-a. zn.
Contractive. krm. n-x. spi. urg.
Like a Cord. amph.
Cutting. (atp). cl-hx. s. vi-t. zn.
Discharge Hard. sb-s.
Mucus. al-o. aps. euph. k-na. p.
Undefined. s.
Drawing. arn. ccs. crt. cth. hg-s. vr-s.
Dryness. atp. cr-o. ppv. sa-l.
Eruptions, Styes. ca-ca. cth. na-cl.
False Sensations, Hair. nic.
Mucus. euph.
Pellicle. k-o.
Sand. amph. dt. lo-cœ. lyc. pt. rs. sep. sr-ca. teu. zn.
Water. dt.
Wind. asr. cro.
Gnawing. kre.
Hard. cit-c.
Heat. alo. amb. aps. cu. dig. dro. k-bicr. lo-cœ. ly-b. na-sa. pb. rs-v. sang. sep. spi. te. teu.
Heaviness. aps. lpd. trn.
Itching. aga. asc. chd. dt. f-hx. lch. ly-b. na-sa. spi. zn.
Lachrymation. aps. atp. br. cb-v. con. crb-x. dt. ery. hg-bini. hg-s. k-o. lac-f. lo-cœ. na-sa. (s). sa-l. sang. sep. so-t. te. teu. (trg).
Hot. atp. k-na. na-sa. spi.
Motion in, Jumping, like something. dt.
Passing round, like something. rs.
Undulation. pt.
Movements, Convulsions .æsc. krm. lac-ac. sa-l. thu. trg. zn.
Squinting. (alm). dt. hyo. pb. spi-m.
Inwards. (alm). hyo. pb.
Paralysis. k-o.
Pressing. aga. alo. arum-t. au. bry. cch. ccs. chd. cit-c. cmf. con. crt. f-hx. glo. glp. k-o. klm. myris. na-sa. pul. rho. rn-b. rs. smi. spi. spo. thu. trg. val. zn.

Projecting. arn.
Feeling. cmc.
Shooting. acon. aga. as-o. atp. ber. c-bis. ca-a. ca-ca. chd. cic. cld. cyc. grp. gym. hur. k-ca. k-o. lac-f. li-ca. lpd. mg-cl. mn-ca. n-x. na-cl. pso. rho. s. spi. spo. str-i. trg. trn. trx. vi-t. zn.
Hot. rho.
Smarting. al-o. anan. aps. cmc. cot. cu. gym. k-i. kre. krm. lo-cœ. lo-i. lyc. na-ca. p. pb. pim. pt. rho. rn-b. rs. sep. (trg). urt.
Swelling. anan. ele. k-ca. p.
Chemosis. vsp.
Œdematous. chio.
Veins of. mg-ca.
Feeling of. cmc.
Tearing. aga. amb. as-o. ca-a. cch. cro. hyp. k-ca. lyc. mg-cl. mrl. pnc. thu. val.
Tensive. au. glp. k-o. zn.
Throbbing. atp. bry. c-bis. pet. thr. thu. trg.
Undefined. anan. bap. erig. f-hx. gel. (hg-bini). mll. na-sa. sa-l. sang. str-i. trn. urt. vsp. vr-v. zn.
EYEBALL SUPERIORLY. **False Sensations, Sand.** lo-cœ. spi.
Pressing. ast. dl-s.
Shooting. cot.
Swelling. br. si-x.
Undefined. alli.
EYEBALL INFERIORLY. **Crampy.** aga.
Pressing. sep.
EYEBALL EXTERNALLY. **Bruised.** vr-a.
Color Dark. k-bicr.
False Sensations, Sand. dt.
Heat. p-x. sn.
Shooting. p-x.
Smarting. sn.
EYEBALL INTERNALLY. **Color Red.** ca-ca. ery. mtr.
Heat. trx.
Swelling. ca-ca.
Undefined. li-ca.
EYEBALL POSTERIORLY. **Pressing.** glo. sep.
Undefined. spo-f.
EYEBALL INTERIORLY. **Drawing.** vr-s.
Pressing. glo.
Shooting. as-o. lac-f.

Smarting. rn-b.
Undefined. as-o. li-ca.
EYEBALL CIRCUMFERENCE. **Undefined**. gel.
EYEBALL CENTRE. **Shooting**. lac-f.
CORNEA. **Eruptions Pustule**. dig.
With Red Areola. dig.
Ulcers. aps.
Opacity. (rs).
IRIS. **Color Discolored**. atp. (rs).
Green. (rs).
Pupil Contracted. atp. nic.
Dilated. atp. mn-ca. p-x. pru-l. rho.
Insensible. (rs).
Irregular. (rs).
LENS. **Cataract**. amm-ca. con.* (rs). s.
ORBIT. **Boring**. frm. lo-cœ.
Drawing. atp. li-ca. sn.
Heaviness. hur.
Pressing. acon. atp. f-hx. glo. glp. ppv. sn. thu.
Shooting. f-hx. glo. nic.
Smarting. hg-i.
Tearing. k-ca. zn.
Tensive. thu.
Throbbing. hur. li-ca. trg.
Undefined. hg-i. hur. ziz.
ORBIT CIRCUMFERENCE. **Drawing**. li-ca.
Tearing. cl-hx.
Throbbing. li-ca.
ORBIT SUPERIORLY. **Boring**. elaps. ol-a.
Bruised. glo.
Bursting. dl-s. na-cl.
Contractive. acon.
Drawing. chio. k-i. li-ca.
Heaviness. cac.
Motion in, Undulation. pt.
Pressing. amm-cl. bry. vr-v.
Shooting. bry. cis.
Smarting. hg-s.
Swelling, Feeling of. hg-s.
Tearing. acon. amm-cl. bar. k-i. phl.
Throbbing. amm-cl. li-ca. na-cl. sn.
Undefined. chio. dl-s. jcr. (na-cl). pet. rs-r.
ORBIT INFERIORLY. **Pressing**. na-sa. phy. thu.
Shooting. na-sa.

Softness, Feeling of. na-sa.
Undefined. (au). hg-i. (thu).
ORBIT EXTERNALLY. **Crampy.** pt.
Drawing. li-ca.
Tearing. au.
Throbbing. li-ca.
ORBIT INTERNALLY. **Boring.** thu.
Swelling. k-bicr. si-x.
Throbbing. k-bicr.
ORBITAL INTEGUMENTS. **Color Red.** dt.
Heat. k-bicr.
Swelling. dt.
Tearing. cch.
Tensive. myris.
ORBITAL INTEGUMENTS SUPERIORLY. **Bruised.** pt.
Contractive. bry. rho.
Crampy. aga.
Creeping. phl. rn-b.
Drawing. k-i.
Eruptions, Boils. ca-pa. i.
Hard. gui.
Pimples. asc. gui.
Hard. gui.
Smarting. asc.
Undefined pain. gui.
Smarting. asc.
Undefined pain. gui.
Heat. f-hx. hg.
Itching. aps. f-hx. rho. spi.
Movements, Convulsions. k-ca.
Numbness. ppv.
Pressing. dig. grp. k-ca. lau-c. ol-a. thu. zn.
Shooting. mn-ca. nic. ol-a. thu. trn.
Smarting. aps.
Swelling, Feeling of. aps.
Tearing. bar. k-ca. phl.
Tensive. i.
Undefined. chd. delph. jcr. li-ca. str.
ORBITAL INTEGUMENTS INFERIORLY. **Color Dark.** s-x.
Contractive. si-x.
Cutting. atrop.
Drawing. lo-cœ.
Movements, Convulsions. n-x.

Shooting. pau.
Swelling. myris.
Tearing. teu.
EYELIDS. **Adhesion of**. ca-ca. euph. k-na. na-ba. na-ca. p. s.
Color Red. k-ca. k-o. p. pol. s. vsp.
Discharge Mucus. sb-s.
Pus. s.
Drawing. cb-v.
Heat. hg. k-na. narth. ner. s. sn.
Itching. aps. asc. cro. k-na. na-ca. p.
Movements, Closing. (chi). dig. (grp). k-o. mg-cl. (pb). pnx. (vr-a). zn.
Spasmodically. hyp. lyc.
Convulsions. s. trg.
Open wide. buf. dl-s. na-cl.
Winking. pt.
Paralysis, Opening difficult. myris.
Shooting. aps. s. sn.
Smarting. k-na. s.
Swelling. k-o. lyc. p. pol. (sep). vsp.
Red. vsp.
Feeling of. trx.
Tensive. myris. ner.
UPPER EYELID. **Boring**. ptv.
Color Red. acon. crot. na-ca. rs. sep.
Drawing. cb-v.
Eruptions. **Boils**. ca-pa.
Herpes. trn.
Pimples. trn.
Pustules. cth. lyc.
Vesicles. br.
Hardness. acon. rs.
Heat. alli. cit-c. cle. cmf. ner. p-x. rs. s. sn. spi.
Heaviness. p-x. pnx.
Itching. al-o. aps. p. pæo. pru-l. rs. rs-r. vsp. zn.
Movements, Convulsions. al-o. aps. atp. ba-ca. bar. ca-ca. cch. chd. chi. cit-c. cop. frm. krm. lac-ac. n-x. na-cl. par. pb. pnc. pol. rho. smi. thu. trn.
Feeling of. dt.
Numbness. naj.
Paralysis. al-o. pnx. rs.
Pressing. chd. hyo. lyc. na-ca. na-cl. p. p-x. pol. rs. thu. trg. trx.

Shooting. bar. chd. cyc. irs-f. pæo. rs. sn. spi.
Hot. os.
Smarting. bar. rs. zn.
Swelling. acon. cmf. crot. k-ca. k-o. na-ca. p. rs. sep. vsp.
Air-like. p.
Hard. acon.
Œdematous. atp. crot. rs.
Red. acon.
Feeling of. rs.
Tearing. al-o. ba-ca. zn.
Tensive. acon.
Throbbing. cth. mn-ca. p. s.
Undefined. xan.
LOWER EYELID, **Contractive.** rs.
Cutting. cit-c.
Eruptions Pustules. chio.
Styes. fe-pa. pol. so-o.
Ulcers. na-cl.
Heat. alm. cit-c. pru-l. rn-b. si-x. sn.
Itching. alm. hg-s. hur. krm.
Movements, Convulsions. aga. ars. cth. krm. narth.
Pressing. hg-s. p-x.
Scraping. si-x.
Shooting. ·cth. hg-s. sn. zn.
Smarting. aps. c-bis. dro. na-cl. rn-b. si-x.
Swelling. chio.
Œdematous. chio.
Throbbing. asr. pol. pru-l. rho. rs.
TARSAL EDGES. **Discharge.** crot. rs.
Pus. crot. rs.
White. crot. rs.
Yellow. crot. rs.
Heat. narth.
Itching. k-ca.
Scraping. p.
UPPER TARSAL EDGE. **Discharge.** s
Hard. s.
Dryness. li-ca.
Eruptions, Tubercles. thu.
Vesicles. pol.
Warts. sb-t.
Itching. spi.
Shooting. spi.
Smarting. li-ca. lo-cœ.

Swelling. s.
Tingling. par.
LOWER TARSAL EDGE. **Eruptions, Pimples**. au.
 Smooth. au.
 Tubercles. au.
  Smooth. au.
Heat. alm.
Itching. alm.
Smarting. hur.
EYELIDS, INNER SURFACE. **Color Red**. cph.
Shooting. cit-c.
CANTHI. **Discharge, Mucus**. gui.
Itching. asc.
Movements, Convulsions. lch.
Scraping. pru-l.
Undefined. sa-l.
EXTERNAL CANTHUS. **Bruised**. vr-a.
Coldness. asr.
Color Red. na-ba.
Cutting. k-i.
Discharge, Mucus. euph. na-ba. sb-s.
Dryness. thu.
Eruptions, Pustules. alo.
False Sensations, Sand. s-x. (spi).. thu.
Heat. dl-s. glo. na-ca. ol-a. sn. spi.
Itching. al-o. bry. ca-ca. euph. frm. na-cl. tx-b. urg.
Movements, Convulsions. pol. ppv.
Pressing. cb-v.
Shooting. cl-hx. dl-s. k-ca. rn-s. sn.
Smarting. ag-na. cb-v. cch. cot. frm. p. rn-b. rn-s. rs.
Swelling. br.
Tearing. au.
Undefined. sa-l.
INTERNAL CANTHUS. **Boring**. thu.
Coldness. li-ca.
Color Red. amm-ca. ery. mg-ca. pet. pt. sb-t. zn.
Creeping. pt.
Discharge, Mucus. na-ca. zn.
 Pus. zn.
Dryness. al-o.
Eruptions, Styes. na-cl.
False Sensations, Sand. bar. rho. s-x. thu. trx.
Hæmorrhage. mtr.

Heat. au. cit-c. cle. f-hx. gel. hg-s. hur. mg-ca. narth. pru-l. sb-t. trx.

Itching. al-o. au. ca-ca. cl-hx. f-hx. hg-s. k-o. lpd. mg-cl. nic. p.

Movements, Convulsions. krm. s-x. sn.

Pressing. amph. cb-v. chd. cic. dl-s. hg-s. hll. ppv. rho. smc. sn. trx. zn.

Shooting. chd. cit-c. f-hx. hg-s. mg-cl. pru-l. spi. thu.

Smarting. cb-v. cl-hx. k-bicr. mg-ca. mg-sa. s. sb-t. sep. sn.

Swelling. pet. si-x. smi.

Tearing atp. krm. lyc.

Throbbing. chd. rs-r. s-x.

Undefined. k-o. sa-l. sang.

CARUNCULA. **Smarting**. bry.dl-s. k-bicr. pul. str. zn.

Swelling. ca-ca.

LACHRYMAL GLAND. **Swelling**. br. si-x.

LACHRYMAL BONE. **Swelling**. k-bicr. si-x.

Throbbing. k-bicr.

LACHRYMAL SAC. **Swelling**. si-x.

PERIODICAL. **Eyeball Shooting**. c-bis.

Smarting. rho.

Throbbing. c-bis.

Eyeball Externally. **Bruised**. vr-a.

Eyeball Posteriorly. **Undefined.** spo-f.

External Canthus. **Heat.** dl-s.

SUDDENLY COME **and** GO. **Eyeball Pressing.** dig.

ALTERNATING **in** EYE. **Eyeball Shooting with Throbbing**. c-bis.

Throbbing with Sensitiveness. thu.

CHANGING CHARACTER **or** PLACE. **Objects Imaginary, Mist, then Star Bright Green Yellow Near Eye.** na-sa.

Eyeball Contractive, then Lachrymation. aga.

then Smarting. aga.

False Sensations, Pellicle, then Shooting. k-o.

Shooting, then Heat. p-x.

Tensive, then Shooting. k-o.

Throbbing then Sensitive. thu.

Orbit Inferiorly, Sensitive then Pressing. na-sa.

Shooting-Backwards then „ na-sa.

Softness, Feeling of then „ na-sa.

Lower Eyelid. Swelling, then Eruptions, Pustules. chio.

Objects Imaginary, Star Bright Green Yellow Near Eye, then Eyeball Pressing. na-sa.

Sight Impaired, then Objects Imaginary, Star Bright Green Yellow Near Eye. na-sa.

Eyeball Pressing, then Sight Impaired. sep.

Moving Body in, then Orbit Superiorly Sensitive. cb-a.

Smarting, then External Canthus Smarting. cot.

Eyelids, Movements, Winking, then Orbit Superiorly Sensitive. cb-a.

Pressing-Forward, then Orbit Circumference, Pressing. na-ba.

Upper Eyelid, Movements, Drawn-Down, then Orbit Superiorly Sensitive. cb-a.

Eyeball to Jaw Shooting, then Eyeball to Abdomen, Chest, Neck, Legs, Drawing. mgs.

FORWARDS. **Eyeball, Pressing.** cmc. pul. str-i. zng.

Shooting. rho.

Tearing. ly-b.

Orbit, Pressing. ppv.

Orbit Superiorly, Pressing. dl-s.

Lower Eyelid, Tearing. na-ca.

BACKWARDS. **Eyeball, Pressing.** cit-c.

Shooting. atp. grp. hyp. lac-f.

Undefined. sa-l.

Orbit Inferiorly, Shooting. na-sa.

Orbital Integuments Superiorly, Shooting. mn-ca.

DOWNWARDS. **Eyeball, Pressing.** au. bry. cit-c.

Shooting. gel.

Orbit, Drawing. atp.

Orbit Superiorly, Pressing. chio.

Eyelids, Swelling. vsp.

UPWARDS. **Eyeball, Boring.** ber.

Drawing. vr-s.

Shooting. ber.

Upper Eyelid, Pressing. krm.

INWARDS. **Eyeball, False Sensations, Sand.** s-x.

Shooting. rho.

Orbital Integuments Superiorly, Shooting. nic.

ALTERNATING **with** HEAD. **Orbit, Pressing.** atp.
To HEAD. **Eyeball, Drawing.** trg.
Shooting. s. trg.
Orbital Integuments Superiorly, Drawing. cb-v.
To FOREHEAD. **Eyeball, Shooting.** lac-f. trg.
Tearing. lac-f.
Throbbing. ly-b.
Orbit Superiorly, Undefined. vr-v.
To VERTEX, **Eyeball, Shooting.** trg.
To TEMPLE. **Eyeball, Shooting.** lac-f.
Throbbing. lac-f.
Orbital Integuments Superiorly, Undefined. li-ca.
Punctum Lachrymale, Undefined. hg-s.
To OCCIPUT. **Eyeball, Pressing.** nic.
Shooting. cic. spi.
Throbbing. ccs.
Undefined. cmc. cmf.
Orbit, Shooting. u-na.
To EAR. **Orbital Integuments Superiorly, Undefined.** li-ca.
Eyelids, Boring. elaps.
External Canthus, Heat. dl-s.
Internal Canthus, Drawing. hg-s.
To NOSE. **Eyeball, Undefined.** alli.
External Canthus, Drawing. k-o.
To TIP **of** NOSE. **Internal Canthus, Undefined.** sa-l.
To FACE. **Internal Canthus, Tearing.** i.
To UPPER JAW. **Eyeball, Undefined.** f-hx.
To LOWER JAW. **Eyeball, Drawing.** jcr.
To ABDOMEN. **Eyeball, Drawing.** mgs.
To CHEST. **Eyeball, Drawing.** mgs.
To NECK. **Eyeball, Drawing.** mgs.
To HIP. **Eyeball, Drawing.** mgs.
DIAGONALS **with** OTHER ORGANS. cld. cro. dro. frm. li-ca. n-x. na-sa. thu. trg. trn.
With LEFT HEAD. **Eyeball, Shooting.** trn.
With LEFT EAR. **Eyeball, Dryness.** thu.
Heat. dro.
Itching. na-sa.
Shooting. n-x.
Lower Tarsal Edge, Heat. thu.

With LEFT TEETH. **Eyeball, Tearing.** cro.
With LEFT GENITALS. **Eyeball, Dryness.** thu.
Lower Tarsal Edge, Heat. thu.
With LEFT ARM. **Eyelids, Movements, Convulsions.** trg.
With LEFT LEG. **Eyeball, Shooting.** cld.
Eyelids, Movements, Convulsions. trg.
Before LEFT HEAD. **Eyeball, Pressing.** trg.
Before LEFT EAR. **Orbit, Boring.** frm.
Before LEFT LEG. **Eyeball, Pressing.** trg.
After LEFT HEAD **Orbital Integuments Superiorly, Undefined.** li-ca.

I. E. LEFT SIDE (**Left Eye**).

ach. æsc. ag. ag-na. aga. al-o. alli. alm. amm-cl. amph. aps. arn. art-v. as-o. asc. asr. ast. atp. au. ba-a. ba-ca. ba-cl. bar. blt. br. bry. c-bis. ca-a. ca-ca. cb-a. cb-v. cch. ccs. chd. chi. chio. cis. cit-c. cl-hx. cle. cnv-d. con. cop. cor. cot. cph. cr-o. crb-x. cro. crt. crt-c. cth. cu. cu-asi. cund. cyc. dl-s. dph. dro. dt. ecb. elaps. ele. eryn. (eupat). euph. euph-a. euphr. f-hx. frm. frm-s. glo. glp. grc. gym. hg. hg-bini. hg-bicl. hg-s. hll. hur. hydr. i. itu. jat. jnp-s. k-bicr. k-ca. k-cla. k-na. k-o. klm. krm. lac-cg. lac-d. lac-f. lau-c. lch. lct. led. li-ca. lo-cœ. lo-i. lpd. lyc. men. mg-ca. mg-sa. mgs. mgs-au. mim. msc. myris. n-x. na-ba. na-cl. na-sa. narth. ner. ni-ca. nic. ol-a. ox-x. p. p-x. pan. pau. pb. pb-a. pd. ped. pet. phl. phy. plb. pln. pod. pol. pru-l. pt. ptv. pul. rhe. rho. rmx. rn-b. rs. rs-r. rut. s. s-x. sa-l. sa-mgs. sang. sb-s. se. (sep). si-x. smc. smi. sn. snc. snp. snp-n. so-o. so-t. spi. spo. sr-ca. str. str-i. stry. te. teu. thu. trg. trn. trx. tx-b. u-na. urg. urt. vi-t. vr-a. vr-s. vr-v. zn. zng.

OBJECTS FALSE. APPEARANCE **of. Black.** na-cl.
Confused. cund.
Multiplied. atp. (mtr).
Small. pet.
White. cop. rn-b.
OBJECTS IMAGINARY. **Black.** aga. atp. ca-ca. k-o s. zn.
Blue. dt.
Bright. cph. dig. dt. str. vr-a.
Brown. aga.

Circles Black. s.
Bright. cph.
Variegated. cph.
Far off. dt.
Green. zn.
Grey. lch.
Halo Green. zn.
Variegated. atp.
Mist. ag-na. cund. ly-b. pt. s.
Moving. k-o. lch.
Moving with Eye. s.
Rays. atp.
Side of Visual Ray at. dt. str.
Spots Black. aga. atp. ca-ca. k-o. s.
Moving. k-o.
Moving with Eye. s.
Blue. dt.
Bright. dt. vr-a.
Far off. dt.
Side of Visual Ray at. dt.
Brown. aga.
Far off. dt.
Grey. lch.
Moving. lch.
Moving. k-o. lch.
Moving with Eye. s.
Side of Visual Ray, at. dt.
Stripe Black. zn.
Variegated. atp. cph.
Veil. smi.
Vibrations Bright. dig. dt. str.
Side of Visual Ray at. str.
SIGHT DAZZLED. na-cl.
SIGHT IMPAIRED. ag-na. amm-cl. as-o. atp. ca-ca. cb-a. hg. ly-b. na-ba. na-cl. narth. pt. rmx. rn-b. si-x. smi.
EYEBALL. **Appearance Dim.** as-o. chd. s.
Boring. ber. euph-a. s.
Bruised. s. str.
Bursting. mg-ca.
Coldness. æsc. nic. trn.
Color Red. al-o. alli. as-o. atp. cnv-d. cop. eryn. glo. hg-bini. hur. led. mim. pau. pb. phy. plb. pod. rn-b. rs. str. str-i. te. teu. thu. trg.

Contractive. ag. amph. jnp-s. lch. lpd. n-x. ppv.
Vertically. lch.
Crampy. chd. cit-c. k-cla.
Creeping. na-sa.
Cutting. cr-o. cund. i. s.
Discharge Corrosive. u-na.
Mucus. cb-a. cb-v. eryn.
Pus. eryn. na-sa. pb. (spi). u-na.
Drawing. alli. alo. f-hx. nic. pt. s.
Dryness. sa-mgs.
Eruptions, Granulations. eryn.
Pterygium. ca-ca.
Pustules. k-bicr.
Styes. dl-s. lyc. pul.
False Sensations, Hairs. k-na. trn.
Mucus. aps.
Pellicle. s.
Sand. al-o. as-o. cb-a. dl-s. dt. f-hx. hur. k-bicr. mg-sa. na-sa. ox-x. p-x. rhe. rs. sa-mgs. smi. zng.
Water, Cold. trn.
Gnawing. s.
Heat. æsc. al-o. bry. c-bis. chd. cit-c. crb-x. cu. dro. glo. gym. k-ca. klm. led. myris. na-ba. s. spo. trx. vr-s.
Heaviness. acon. pd. trn.
Itching. ag-na. aps. ca-ca. chd. elaps. f-hx. hg-bicl. hur. na-sa. sn. spi. sr-ca.
Lachrymation. alli. amph. chd. dt. euph. hg-s. k-ca. lac-f. lpd. (ly-b). pau. phy. plb. pul. rs-r. rut. s. s-x. (sep). si-x. snp. stry. thu. trg. u-na.
Cold. trg.
Hot. al-o. ca-ca. spi.
Feeling of. hg-s.
Movements, Convulsions. aga. al-o. aps. as-o. lac-cg. **se**. trg. zn.
Squinting. art-v. ca-ca. cyc.
Inwards. art-v. ca-ca. cyc.
As if Turned Round. chi.
Numbness. s.
Pressing. acon. al-o. as-o. asr. c-bis. cb-v. ccs. chd. chio. cit-c. cle. eryn. hg-bini. hydr. lch. na-sa. ner. pan. pol. rn-b. s. smi. sn. spi. str-i. teu. urt. vr-v. zng.
Shooting. æsc. al-o. alli. atp. ber. br. chd. chi. cis. dro. dt. elaps. frm-s. glo. hg-bini. hur. i. k-bicr. lac-f. mgs

myris. pau. phy. pul. s. sb-s. si-x. sn. snc. snp. snp-n. spi. spo. trn. vr-v. zn.

Smarting. ag-na. al-o. cb-v. cot. cu. (eupat). lac-f. mg-ca. n-x. ner. p. pod. rn-b. s. si-x. snp-n. u-na. vi-t. zn.

Stiffness. ca-ca.

Swelling. cb-v. ele. eryn.

Chemosis. atp.

Veins of. atp. pru-l.

Feeling of. aga. chd. cit-c. rs. rs-r.

Tearing. au-cl. cb-v. cch. chd. dro. k-ca. ni-ca. ol-a. pb. s. smc. spo.

Tensive. dro. glp. lyc. nic. sn. spi.

Laterally like a Thread. s.

Throbbing. as-o. ca-ca. cl-hx. hur. lau-c. na-cl. pb.

Undefined. alli. au. br. cb-v. (eupat). gym. hg-bini. lac-cg. lyc. pd. ppv. s. sa-l. sang. snp-n. str-i.

EYEBALL SUPERIORLY. **False Sensations, Sand.** dl-s. hg. phy.

Heat. thu.

Pressing. as-o. chd. sr-ca. thu.

Shooting. as-o. i. snc.

EYEBALL INFERIORLY. **False Sensations, Sand.** men.

Pressing. aps.

Shooting. zn.

Smarting. zn.

EYEBALL EXTERNALLY. **Boring.** i.

False Sensations, Sand. rs.

Heat. spi.

Pressing. i. spo.

EYEBALL INTERNALLY. **Color Red.** k-bicr

Eruptions, Pustule. k-bicr.

White with Red Areola. k-bicr

Heat. thu.

Pressing. rut.

EYEBALL POSTERIORLY. **Crampy.** au.

Pressing. au.

Undefined. asc. pd.

EYEBALL INTERIORLY. **Drawing.** alli.

Pressing. cis. chd. pol.

Smarting. lac-f.

Swelling, Feeling of. chd.

Undefined. lac-cg.

EYEBALL CIRCUMFERENCE. **Heat.** æsc. spo.
Shooting. æsc.
EYEBALL ROUND CORNEA. **Color Red.** thu.
EYEBALL CENTRE. **False Sensations, Sand.** rs.
Shooting. k-bicr. lac-f.
CORNEA. **Color Dark.** k-bicr.
White. k-bicr.
Eruptions, Pustules. k-bicr. p.
With Red Areola. k-bicr.
Opacity. atp. k-bicr.
Shooting. k-bicr.
CHAMBERS **of** EYE. **Discharge, Pus.** atp.
IRIS. **Pupil Contracted.** ag-na. as-o. rho.
Dilated. cb-a. dt. nic. rho.
Insensible. ag-na.
Irregular. nic. s.
LENS. **Cataract.** mg-ca.
ORBIT. **Contractive.** spi.
Gnawing. s.
Heat. cit-c.
Heaviness. hur.
Pressing. aga. aps. bry. cit-c. spi. thu.
Shooting. ba-ca. itu.
Smarting. cu-asi.
Tearing. aga.
Tensive. thu.
Throbbing. as-o. ba-a. bry. glo. hur. sn.
Undefined. asc. li-ca. s.
ORBIT CIRCUMFERENCE. **Bruised.** na-cl.
Pressing. na-cl. narth. rho.
Shooting. aps. rho.
Tearing. phl.
Undefined. narth. os.
ORBIT SUPERIORLY. **Boring.** cu-asi.
Crampy. p-x.
Drawing. al-o. chio. sn.
Pressing. msc. myris. p-x. sn. str-i.
Like a Plug, &c. hll. na-sa.
Shooting. hur. k-bicr.
Smarting. cu-asi.
Tearing. chd.
Throbbing. myris.
Undefined. chio. frm. hg-i. k-bicr. msc.

ORBIT INFERIORLY. **Boring.** euph-a.
Bruised. alm.
Pressing. aps.
Smarting. hg-s.
Swelling, Feeling of. hg-s.
Tearing. na-sa.
Throbbing. na-sa.
ORBIT EXTERNALLY. **Heat.** f-hx.
Throbbing. sn.
ORBIT INTERNALLY. **Broken, as if.** lch.
Bruised. lch.
Creeping. sep.
ORBITAL INTEGUMENTS. **Drawing.** pt. spo.
Heat. aps. dl-s.
Itching. aps.
Pressing. dl-s. dph.
Shooting. spo.
Swelling, Feeling of. aps.
ORBITAL INTEGUMENTS SUPERIORLY. **Boring.** (ca-a).
Bruised. pln.
Contractive. p-x.
Crampy. arn.
Creeping. cro.
Drawing. ca-a. n-x. rho.
Eruptions, Granulations. eryn.
  Hard. rn-s.
  Pimples. k-ca. rho. rn-s.
    Hard. rn-s.
  Scabs. spo.
      Undefined Pain. spo.
      Yellow. spo.
  Tubercles. thu.
  Undefined Pain. spo. thu.
  Yellow. spo.
Heat. aga. alli. aps. men. narth. str.
Itching. br. pru-l. vi-t. vr-v.
Movements, Convulsions. k-o. zn.
  Downwards—Drawn. elaps.
    Feeling of. ol-a.
Pressing. acon. ca-a. jnp-s. msc. sb-s. thu. trx.
Shooting. aps. (ca-a). ol-a. rs-r. sb-s. thu. vi-t. zn.
Smarting. aps. dro. k-ca. ner.

Tearing. jnp-s. thu. trg. zn.
Tensive. hll.
Throbbing. aga.
Undefined. amm-cl. chd. crt-c. elaps. lac-cg. msc. rs-v. (thu).

ORBITAL INTEGUMENTS INFERIORLY. **Drawing**. atp.
Heat. hg-s. pb-a. rut.
Itching. na-cl. spo.
Movements, Convulsions. æsc.
Shooting. pb. ptv. spo.
Smarting. na-cl. ptv.

ORBITAL INTEGUMENTS EXTERNALLY. **Itching**. f-hx.
Movements, Convulsions. f-hx.
Tensive. spo.

EYELIDS. **Adhesion of**. cb-a. cb-v. chd. eryn. gym. k-ca. na-ba. na-sa. pb. rs. (spi). u-na.
Bruised. s.
Color, Red. atp. s. u-na.
Cutting. s.
Discharge, Mucus. k-ca.
Dryness. zn.
Eruptions, Styes. elaps. s.
Smarting. s.
Smarting. s.
Heat. al-o. asr. dro. rs-r. trx. zn.
Itching. aps. chi. hur. na-ca. ped.
Movements, Closing. atp. buf. chd. (chi). euph. grp. na-sa. (pb). sep. thu. tx-b. urg. (vr-a).
Spasmodically. rho. spo.
Convulsions. cb-v. k-o. lyc. mg-ca. p. phl. s. sb-s. trg.
Paralysis. ag-na. al-o. ba-cl. pb.
Opening Difficult. al-o.
Shooting. tx-b.
Smarting. aps. k-o.
Swelling. aga. arn. atp. cb-v. p. s..
Tensive. dro. ner.
Throbbing. cro.

UPPER EYELID. **Color, Red**. arn. atp. chio. crot. crt. lch. rs. so-o.
Contractive. so-t.

Cutting. dl-s. hg.
Dryness. crt. zn.
Eruptions, Blisters. arn.
Pimples. hg. trg.
Pustules. chd.
Scabs. te.
Styes. u-na.
Tubercles. lch.
Undefined Pain. hg-s.
Vesicles. arn. lch.
Hairs feel Inverted. te.
Heat. bar. bry. ca-a. chd. crt. hg-bicl. k-o. lau-c. men. phl. zn.
Heaviness. cit-c. k-o.
Itching. alli. bry. chd. chi. chio. lch. mg-cl. ner. pb. te.
Movements, Convulsions. ach. cb-v. cl-hx. dph. jat. lac-f. mg-ca. narth. ni-ca. nic. ol-a. rho. rs. sr-ca.
Pressing. as-o. (chd). jnp-s. narth. te. zn.
Shooting. ag. aga. au. ba-ca. bar. chd. cro. krm. ner. spi. zn.
Smarting. au. c-bis. dro. k-o. phl. te.
Swelling. asr. chio. cit-c. crot. p. rs. te. trg. urg.
Œdematous. as-o. chio. crot. rs. te.
Red. te.
Tearing. ba-ca. hg-bicl.
Tensive. ach. men.
Throbbing. asr. rs. so-t. stry.
Undefined. (atp).
Wrinkled. chio.
LOWER EYELID. **Color, Dark.** arn.
Red. ca-ca.
Contractive. cro.
Creeping. aga.
Drawing. bar. cch.
Eruptions, Pimples. bry.
Pustules. al-o.
Styes. cch. p. rs.
Heat. cro. hg. k-o. phl. sep. sn. spo.
Itching. aga. al-o. alm. euph. grc. hur. phl. trg.
Movements, Convulsions. amm-cl. ccs. chi. hg. hur. lyc. mg-ca. sep. thu. zn.
Downwards-Hanging. grp.

Pressing. mgs-au. p-x. rs. zn.
Shooting. ca-ca. cro. hg-s. k-i. p. rs-r.
Smarting. hur. phl.
Swelling. ca-ca. cch. hg.
  Œdematous. arn.
  Feeling of. rs-r.
Tearing. ba-ca. na-ca. phl.
Tensive. bar. phl.
Throbbing. ca-ca. chi. cth.
Undefined. cro.
TARSAL EDGES. **Color Red.** atp. hur.
Discharge Pus. atp. crot. rs.
  White. crot. rs.
  Yellow. crot. rs.
Heat. atp. chd.
Itching. bry. hur.
Pressing. atp.
Swelling. atp.
Undefined. aps.
UPPER TARSAL EDGE. **Heat.** cit-c.
  Itching. zn.
  Pressing. pol.
  Shooting. cit-c.
LOWER TARSAL EDGE. **Cutting.** spi.
  Eruptions, Ulcers. cch.
  Pressing. zn.
EYELIDS, INNER SURFACE. **Color Red.** cit-c.
  Eruptions, Ulcers. cit-c.
  Shooting. cit-c.
LOWER EYELIDS, INNER SURFACE. **Shooting.** chd.
PUNCTUM LACHRYMALE. **Color Red.** atp. hur.
Discharge, Pus. atp.
Heat. atp.
Itching. hur.
Pressing. atp.
Smarting. hur.
Swelling. atp.
Undefined. aps.
CANTHI. **False Sensations, Sand.** aga.
Itching. chd. lo-i.
Pressing. si-x.
Shooting. ag. blt.

Smarting. hll. lct.
Swelling. aga.
EXTERNAL CANTHUS. **Color Red**. rn-b. str.
Contractive. euph.
Discharge, Hard. rs.
Mucus. rs. str.
Drawing. spo.
Dryness. thu.
Eruptions, Dry. tx-b.
Herpetic. tx-b.
Red Areola with. tx-b.
Ulcers. k-ca.
False Sensations, Sand. aps. rs. str-i.
Heat. aga. chd. pru-l. thu. trx.
Itching. ca-a. ca-ca. cb-v. cl-hx. rs.
Movements, Convulsions. na-cl. ni-ca. p.
Pressing. aga. smc. thu.
Shooting. amph. chd. elaps. n-x. ni-ca. ol-a. pru-l. spo trx. urg.
Smarting. bry. cl-hx. k-ca. rn-b. sep.
Swelling. rn-b.
Tearing. chi.
Tensive. spo.
Throbbing. na-cl.
Undefined. sa-l.
INTERNAL CANTHUS. **Bruised**. glo.
Bursting. au.
Color Red. atp. ca-ca. chd. hg-s. na-ba. pru-l. rs. sep.
Contractive. aga.
Creeping. ach.
Discharge, Mucus. na-ba. rs.
Drawing. spo.
False Sensations, Sand. aga. chd.
Heat. asr. chd. cle. con. rs-r. sep. sn.
Itching. aps. bar. cb-v. chd. f-hx. k-o. lch. lo-cœ. na-cl. os. pru-l. sep. spi.
Movements, Closing. aga.
Convulsions. lac-d.
Pressing. aga. euphr. si-x. sn.
Scraping. pb.
Shooting. aga. al-o. au. blt. ca-ca. cb-a. chd. cle. ecb. hg-s. n-x. na-ca. pru-l. rs-r. sn. spo. thu.
Smarting. aps. cb-a. cb-v. dl-s. lo-cœ. ox-x. rs-r. sa-l.

Swelling. aga. hg-s. sep. sn.
Feeling of. rs.
Tearing. ni-ca.
Undefined. atp. hg-s. hur. lac-d. sa-l.
CARUNCULA. **Swelling**. aga.
LACHRYMAL BONE. **Broken as if**. lch.
Bruised. lch.
PERIODICAL. **Objects Imaginary, Mist**. s.
Eyeball, Creeping. na-sa.
Shooting. spi.
Tearing. ni-ca.
Orbit Superiorly, Undefined. k-bicr.
ALTERNATE DAYS. **Sight Impaired**. as-o.
Eyeball, Appearance Dim. as-o.
Color Red. as-o.
Pressing. as-o.
Throbbing. as-o.
FROM 4 A.M. TO 3 P.M. **Eyeball, Color Red**. spi.
Lachrymation Hot. spi.
Undefined. spi.
FROM 10 A.M. TO 3 P.M. **Orbit Superiorly, Throbbing**. as-o.
EVERY NIGHT. **Eyeball, Pressing-Forward**. (dt).
EVERY NOON. **Objects Imaginary, Spots Bright**. vr-a.
EVERY AFTERNOON. **Eyeball, Pressing-Forward**. (dt).
GRADUALLY INCREASE and DECREASE. **Sight Impaired**. as-o.
Eyeball, Appearance Dim. as-o.
Color Red. as-o.
Pressing. as-o.
Throbbing. as-o.
Orbit Superiorly, Shooting. k-bicr.
Throbbing. as-o.
Undefined. k-bicr.
SUDDENLY COME and GO. **Orbit Inferiorly, Smarting**. hg-s.
Swelling, Feeling of. hg-s.
SUDDENLY COME, GRADUALLY GO. **Orbit Inferiorly Smarting**. hg-s.
Swelling, Feeling of. hg-s.

CHANGING CHARACTER or PLACE. **Eyeball, Color Red, then Discharge Pus.** eryn.

Drawing then Pressing. rho.

False Sensations, Hair, then Pressing. ccs.

Pressing, then Discharge Pus. eryn.

Shooting, then Lachrymation. snp.

then Numbness. s.

Swelling, then Discharge Pus. eryn.

Tearing then Shooting. thu.

Eyeball Superiorly, Throbbing, then Pressing. amb.

Tingling, then ,, amb.

Orbit, Shooting, then Pressing. ba-ca.

Upper Eyelids, Swelling, then Color Red. chio.

then Itching. chio.

then Wrinkled. chio.

Punctum Lachrymale, Heat then Pressing. atp.

Internal Canthus, Itching then Pressing. pru-l.

Eyeball, Color Red, then Eyelids, Adhesion of. eryn.

Lachrymation, then ,, u-na.

Pressing, then ,, eryn.

Swelling, then ,, eryn.

Orbit, Shooting, then Eyeball, Lachrymation, Feeling of. ba-ca.

then Eyelids, Movements, Closing. ba-ca.

FORWARDS. **Eyeball, Drawing.** alo.

Pressing. al-o. (dt). gym. lau-c.

Shooting. pan. sep. snc.

Tearing. chd.

Orbit Superiorly, Drawing. alo.

BACKWARDS. **Eyeball, Shooting.** chio. dt.

DOWNWARDS. **Eyeball, Pressing.** bry. chd. ner. spi.

Orbit Superiorly, Pressing. chio.

UPWARDS. **Eyeball, Boring.** ber.

Shooting. ber. br.

Throbbing. br.

Orbit Inferiorly, Boring. euph-a.

Orbital Integuments Inferiorly, Drawing. atp.

External Canthus, Shooting. cmc.

LENGTHWAYS. **Eyeball, Cutting**. cr-o. na-ba.
Heat. dro. na-ba.
Tearing. dro.
Tensive. dro. na-ba.
Eyelids, Heat. dro.
Tensive. dro.
OUTWARDS. **Eyeball, Cutting**. i.
False Sensations, Sand. rs.
Shooting. i.
Orbit Superiorly, Shooting. k-bicr.
Orbit Inferiorly, Boring. euph-a.
Orbit Internally to Eyeball, Bruised. lch.
INWARDS. **Orbital Integuments, Drawing**. spo.
Shooting. spo.
OBLIQUELY. **Orbit Superiorly, Cutting**. dro.
To HEAD. **Eyeball, Shooting**. atp.
Orbit, Boring. euph-a.
To FOREHEAD. **Eyeball, Tearing**. ccs.
Undefined. lac-cg.
Orbit Superiorly, Shooting. ber.
Tearing. ber.
Upper Eyelid, Shooting. br.
Throbbing. br.
To VERTEX. **Eyeball, Shooting**. phy.
To TEMPLE. **Eyeball, Undefined**. ba-ca.
Orbit Internally, Bruised. lch.
Upper Eyelid, Shooting. br.
Throbbing. br.
To SIDE **of** HEAD. **Eyeball, Shooting**. trn.
To OCCIPUT. **Eyeball, Tearing**. cch.
Orbit Internally, Bruised. lch.
To EAR. **Eyeball, Undefined**. ba-ca.
To NOSE. **Internal Canthus, Tearing**. ni-ca.
To FACE. **Eyeball, Shooting**. mgs.
Undefined. f-hx.
Orbit, Drawing. cor.
Pressing. spi.
Orbit Superiorly, Undefined. k-bicr.
To JAWS. **Eyeball, Shooting**. mgs.
To UPPER JAW. **Eyeball, Shooting**. aga.
Orbit Superiorly, Undefined. k-bicr.
To TEETH. **Eyeball, Undefined**. lac-cg.

To NECK. **Orbit, Undefined.** rs.
DIAGONALS **with** OTHER ORGANS. ber. f-hx. pet. trg.
With RIGHT FACE. **Eyeball, Drawing.** f-hx.
With RIGHT ARM. **Eyeball, Undefined.** trg.
Before RIGHT EAR. **Eyeball, Undefined.** pet.
To RIGHT HEAD. **Orbit Superiorly, Shooting.** ber.

SECTION II. CONDITIONS.

A. AGGRAVATIONS.

DAY. (**Sunrise to Sunset**).

ag-na. al-o. amb. amm-ca. as-o. au. c-bis. cop. cro. dt. ery. euphr. grc. hur. k-bicr. lct. led. ly-b. lyc. na-cl. na-sa. p. p-x. pul. sb-t. sep. smi. sn. so-d. str-i. vr-s. zn.

OBJECTS, FALSE APPEARANCE **of**. amm-ca. ly-b.
Black. amm-ca.
Inverted. ly-b.
Moving. amm-ca.
OBJECTS IMAGINARY. ag-na. sb-t.
Bright. sb-t.
Figures. ag-na.
Flashes, Bright. sb-t.
PHOTOPHOBIA. grc. na-cl. (p-x). sep.
SIGHT IMPAIRED. amm-ca. as-o. lct. sn. so-d.
EYEBALL. al-o. as-o. au. c-bis. dt. ery. euphr. k-bicr. lyc. p. pul. smi. str-i. zn.
Appearance, Dim. (as-o).
Color, Dark. (c-bis).
Red. (as-o). (dt). na-cl.
Discharge. ery. p. (vr-s).
Mucus. ery. p. (vrs).
False Sensations. (al-o). (dt). k-bicr.
Sand. (al-o). (dt). k-bicr.
Heat. k-bicr. (lct).
Itching. (euphr).
Lachrymation. al-o. (dt). lyc. na-cl. smi. (str-i). zn.
Hot. str-i.
Movements. (cop). (na-cl).
Convulsions. (cop).
Pressing. (as-o). k-bicr. (na-sa). (pul).
Shooting. (hur).
Sunken. c-bis.
Tearing. amb.
Throbbing. (as-o). (cro). p.
Undefined. (au).

EYEBALL EXTERNALLY. dt.
IRIS. lct. na-cl.
Pupils Contracted. na-cl.
Dilated, lct.
ORBIT. na-sa. pul.
ORBIT SUPERIORLY. na-sa.
ORBITAL INTEGUMENTS. amb. c-bis.
Color, Dark. c-bis.
Tearing. amb.
EYELIDS. cro. hur. lct. na-cl. vr-s.
Adhesion of. vr-s.
Heat. lct.
Movements, Closing. na-cl.
Spasmodically. na-cl.
Throbbing. cro.
TARSAL EDGES. hur.
Shooting. hur.
CANTHI. vr-s.
EXTERNAL CANTHUS. vr-s.
Discharge, Mucus. vr-s.
RIGHT. cop. dt. pul.
Eyeball, Color Red. dt.
Lachrymation. dt.
Pressing. pul.
Eyeball Externally, False Sensations, Sand. dt.
Orbit, Pressing. pul.
Upper Eyelid, Movements, Convulsions. cop.
LEFT. al-o. as-o. au. na-sa.
Sight Impaired. as-o.
Eyeball, Appears Dim. as-o.
Color Red. as-o.
False Sensations, Sand. al-o.
Pressing. as-o.
Throbbing. as-o.
Undefined. au.
Orbit Superiorly, Pressing. na-sa.

FORENOON. (**Morning, Sunrise to Noon**).

ach. acon. ag-na. aga. al-o. alli. alm. amb. amm-ca. amm-cl. aps. art-v. arum-t. as-o. atp. ba-ca. ber. bry. ca-a. ca-pa. ca-s. cap. cb-a. cb-v. ccs. chd. chi. cit-c. cl-hx. cmf. cof. con. cop. cr-o. cro. cth. dig. dl-s. drm. dro. dt. elaps.

erig. ery. eug. euph. fe-mgs. frm. frm-s. gel. glo. glp. grc. grp. gua. gym. hg. hg-i. hll. hydr. k-bicr. k-ca. k-na. k-o. kre. krm. lch. lct. led. li-ca. lpd. ly-b. lyc. mg-ca. mg-cl. mg-sa. mgs. mgs-ar. mgs-au. mn-ca. mph. mrl. mtr. myris. n-x. na-ba. na-ca. na-cl. na-sa. ni-ca. ol-a. ox-x. p. p-x. par. pb. pet. phl. phy. pnx. pod. pol. pru-l. pt. pul. pul-n. rhe. rho. rn-b. rs. rs-r. rut. s. s-x. sb-s. sb-t. se. sep. si-x. smc. smi. spi. spo. sr-ca. str. str-i. te. thu. trg. trn. trx. urg. val. vr-a. vr-s. ziz. zn.

OBJECTS, FALSE APPEARANCE **of**. dig. ery. gel. gua. lpd. ly-b. lyc. mg-ca. mtr. p.

Inverted. gua.

Moving. ery. gua. lpd. ly-b. lyc. mg-ca. p.

Circularly. ery. lpd. ly-b. lyc. mg-ca.

From Below Upwards. gua.

Downwards. lpd.

Vibrating. p.

Multiplied. gel.

White. dig.

OBJECTS IMAGINARY. ag-na. amm-cl. ba-ca. ca-ca. ca-s. cb-v. cit-c. dt. ery. fe-mgs. frm-s. hg. k-o. lch. lct. ly-b. na-ba. ni-ca. pul. trg. zn.

Blue. dt. fe-mgs.

Bright. ag-na. ca-ca. ca-s. cb-v. cit-c. dt. ery. fe-mgs. na-ba. pul. trg.

Circles. cit-c. fe-mgs. pul.

Blue. fe-mgs.

Bright. cit-c. fe-mgs. pul.

Red. fe-mgs.

Zigzags. fe-mgs.

Flames. ag-na. ca-s. ery.

Flashes, Bright. ag-na. ery.

Halo. trg.

Mist. amm-cl. ba-ca. (cit-c). frm-s. k-o. lct. ly-b. ni-ca. trg. zn.

Red. fe-mgs.

Spirits. ca-s.

Spots. ca-ca. dt. ery. lch.

Blue. dt.

Bright. ca-ca. dt. ery.

Yellow. lch.

Threads. (ery).

Veil. dt.

Vibrations, ca-ca. cb-v. cit-c. (dt). na-ba.
Bright. ca-ca. cb-v. cit-c. (dt). na-ba.
Water. hg.
Yellow. lch.
Zigzags. fe-mgs.

PHOTOPHOBIA. (dt). k-na. na-sa. phy. pnx. sb-s. si-x. str. str-i.

SIGHT DAZZLED. s.

SIGHT IMPAIRED. amm-cl. ba-ca. bry. cap. cb-v. chd. cit-c. drm. dt. ery. glp. k-o. lct. ly-b. lyc. mtr. na-ba. na-cl. na-sa. ni-ca. p. pet. pul. s. s-x. sep. str. trg. trn. val. zn.

EYEBALL. ach. ag-na. aga. al-o. alli. amb. amm-ca. amm-cl. aps. art-v. as-o. atp. ba-ca. ber. bry. ca-a. ca-ca. cap. cb-a. cb-v. chd. cl-hx. cmf. con. cr-o. cro. dig. dl-s. ery. eug. euph. frm. frm-s. glp. grc. grp. gym. hg. hll. k-bicr. k-ca. k-na. k-o. kre. krm. lch. led. li-ca. ly-b. lyc. mg-ca. mg-cl. mn-ca. mph. mrl. mtr. myris. na-ca. na-cl. na-sa. ni-ca. ox-x. p. p-x. par. pb. phl. pod. pol. pru-l. pt. pul. rs. s. s-x. sb-s. sb-t. se. sep. si-x. smc. smi. spi. str. str-i. te. thu. trg. trn. trx. val. zn.

Appearance Dim. mtr.
Boring. aps.
Bruised. (smi).
Bursting. (na-sa).
Color Red. (acon). atp. bry. (ery). eug. (hg). rs. sep. (str).
Discharge. ach. ag-na. aga. al-o. amm-cl. art-v. as-o. atp. ba-ca. ber. bry. ca-a. (cb-a). cb-v. chd. cl-hx. (cof). dig. dl-s. (euph). glp. grp. hg. (hll). k-bicr. k-ca. k-na. k-o. kre. krm. led. ly-b. lyc. mg-ca. mg-cl. mn-ca. mrl. na-ca. na-cl. ni-ca. ox-x. p. (p-x). par. pb. pol. pru-l. pul. rs. s. s-x. sb-s. sep. si-x. str. str-i. trx. zn.
Hard. atp. (hll). p-x. (sb-s).
Pus. atp.
Drawing. myris. pol.
Dryness. ag-na. ber. dl-s. (grp). lch. (li-ca). lyc. mg-ca. (mg-cl). (mgs). (mgs-ar). p. si-x.
False Sensations. k-na. na-cl. pul. (s-x). si-x.
Sand. k-na. na-cl. pul. (s-x). si-x.
Gnawing. (str-i).
Hardness. (acon).
Heat. ag-na. al-o. (alm). amm-cl. cap. cl-hx. frm-s. (glp). grc. grp. (hg). (k-bicr). k-na. krm. lch. mg-ca. mph.

(n-x). na-sa. (ol-a). (phl). (pol). pul. s. sep. (**si-x**). (smi). (sr-ca). val.

Heaviness. (glo). k-bicr. (sep).

Itching. (alm). amm-ca. (dl-s). frm-s. grp. (hg). (k-o). (na-cl). (sep). (te).

Lachrymation. al-o. amm-cl. ca-ca. cap. cb-v. (con). cr-o. (dig). (dl-s). (ery). hg. k-bicr. k-na. k-o. (kre). krm. lch. mg-ca. (na-cl). na-sa. ni-ca. p. phl. pru-l. s. sep. te. zn.

Hot. con. dig. dl-s. kre. na-cl.

Appearance of. ca-ca.

Movements. (ca-pa). cit-c. (cop). (li-ca). mgs-au. (na-cl). (pod). (s). (sep). (spo).

Convulsions. mgs-au. (s).

Squinting, Feeling of. pod.

Paralysis. (ag-na). (amb). art-v. (ba-ca). (ca-s). (con). (k-ca). (mg-ca). (n-x). (na-ba). (ni-ca). (pet). s-x. (si-x).

Pressing. ach. ag-na. aga. amb. atp. bry. ca-ca. cmf. dl-s. (glp). grp. (k-ca). k-na. k-o. (lct). lyc. mph. (na-ba). pt. sb-t. (spi). (str).

Scraping. (si-x).

Shooting. (alli). aps. (bry). (cb-a). (con). cro. hll. na-sa. (p). sb-s. se. (sep). smc. (str-i). thu. (trn).

Smarting. al-o. amm-ca. (cb-a). gym. (hll). k-bicr. (k-o). (krm). li-ca. rs. (si-x). str. (str-i). (te). val.

Stiffness. ca-ca.

Swelling. (acon). ba-ca. (ca-ca). chd. (elaps). k-bicr. (k-ca). mtr. (phy). (rs-r). (s). sep. (te).

Dark. (phy).

Hard. (acon).

Œdematous. (te).

Red. (acon). (te).

Feeling of. cmf. (k-o). mg-ca. ni-ca. (val).

Tearing. lyc. mg-ca. (na-sa). (pb). smc. (str-i).

Tensive. (acon). (s-x).

Throbbing. (na-sa). pb.

Undefined. (alli). (chi). cmf. ery. frm. (hg-i). (k-bicr). na-ca. p-x. s. (sep). smi. (trg). zn.

EYEBALL SUPERIORLY. cmf.

Undefined. cmf.

EYEBALL INTERNALLY. ery.

EYEBALL ANTERIORLY. sb-s.

Shooting. sb-s.

EYEBALL INTERIORLY. cmf.

Undefined. cmf.

IRIS. pnx. pul. val.
Pupil Contracted. pnx.
Dilated. pul. val.
ORBIT. bry. chi. hg-i. k-bicr. k-ca. lct. na-sa. smi.
Pressing. k-ca. lct.
ORBIT CIRCUMFERENCE. na-sa.
Bursting. na-sa.
ORBIT SUPERIORLY. bry. chi. hg-i. k-bicr.
Undefined. chi.
ORBIT INFERIORILY. na-sa. smi.
Bruised. na-sa.
ORBITAL INTEGUMENTS. elaps. na-cl.
Swelling. elaps.
ORBITAL INTEGUMENTS SUPERIORLY. na-cl.
Itching. na-cl.

EYELIDS. ach. acon. ag-na. aga. alm. amb. aps. art-v. as-o. atp. ba-ca. ca-ca. ca-pa. ca-s. ccs. chd. cit-c. con. cop. dig. dl-s. erig. glo. grp. hg. hg-s. hydr. k-bicr. k-ca. k-o. kre. led. li-ca. mg-ca. mg-cl. mgs. mgs-ar. mn-ca. mtr. n-x. na-ba. na-cl. na-sa. ni-ca. p. p-x. pb. pet. phl. phy. pol. pul. pul-n. rs. rs-r. s. s-x. sb-s. sep. si-x. smi. spo. str. str-i. te. thu. trn. val. ziz. zn.

Adhesion. ach. aga. as-o. atp. ca-ca. ccs. chd. cop. dig. dl-s. erig. grp. hydr. k-bicr. k-ca. k-o. kre. led. mg-ca. mn-ca. mtr. na-sa. ni-ca. p. phy. pul. pul-n. rs. (s). (sb-s). si-x. smi. str. str-i. thu. trn. ziz. zn.

Discharge. k-bicr. mg-ca. si-x.
Hard. p-x.
Dryness. grp. mg-cl. mgs. mgs-ar.
Heat. grp. k-bicr. n-x. phl. smi.
Movements, Closing. ca-pa. (cop). li-ca. (na-cl). (s). sep. (spo).
Spasmodically. cop. na-cl. s. sep. (spo).
Paralysis. ag-na. amb. art-v. ba-ca. ca-s. con. k-na. mg-ca. n-x. na-ba. ni-ca. pet. s-x. si-x.
Swelling. ba-ca. chd. k-ca. s.
Feeling of. k-o.
Tearing. pb.
Tensive. s-x.
Undefined. sep.

UPPER EYELIDS. acon. ag-na. amb. art-v. ba-ca. ca-s. cit-c. con. glo. k-ca. k-na. mg-ca. n-x. na-ba. ni-ca. pet. s-x. sep. si-x. str. te.

Color Red. acon.
Heaviness. glo. sep.

Pressing. str.
Swelling. acon.
Tensive. acon.
LOWER EYELID. alm. aps. ca-ca. rs-r. si-x.
Itching. alm.
Swelling. ca-ca. rs-r.
TARSAL EDGES. alm. hg. hg-s. li-ca. pol. str. str-i. val.
Color Red. hg.
Gnawing. str-i.
Heat. hg-s. pol.
Itching. hg.
Smarting. str. str-i. val.
Swelling, Feeling of. val.
UPPER TARSAL EDGE. pol.
Heat. pol.
LOWER TARSAL EDGE. alm.
CANTHI. aga. as-o. cb-a. cof. con. dl-s. ery. hll. k-bicr. k-o. lyc. ni-ca. ol-a. p. pul. s. s-x. sb-s. sep. si-x. sr-ca. str. str-i. zn.
Smarting. si-x.
EXTERNAL CANTHUS. as-o. ol-a. pul. s-x. sb-s. sr-ca. str. str-i.
Discharge. as-o. pul. str. str-i.
Heat. sr-ca.
Shooting. str-i.
Tearing. str-i.
INTERNAL CANTHUS. aga. cb-a. cof. con. dl-s. ery. hll. k-bicr. k-o. lyc. ni-ca. p. pul. sb-s. sep. str. zn.
Discharge. aga. cof. dl-s. lyc. ni-ca. p. pul. sb-s. zn.
  Hard. hll.
Dryness, str.
Heat. k-bicr.
Itching. dl-s. sep.
RIGHT **then** LEFT. alm.
Lower Eyelid, Itching. alm.
TO FACE. k-bicr.
RIGHT. acon. alli. alm. aps. bry. cit-c. ery. eug. euph. glp. hg-i. k-o. krm. li-ca. na-ba. na-sa. ol-a. s. s-x. sb-s. sep. si-x. spi. trn.
Sight Impaired. chd. cit-c.
Eyeball, Color Red. eug.
  Discharge. euph. sb-s.
    Hard. sb-s.

Heat. na-sa.
Itching. k-o.
Lachrymation. ery. na-sa.
Pressing. glp. na-ba. spi.
Shooting. alli. trn.
Smarting. krm.
Undefined. alli.
Eyeball Internally, Color Red. ery.
Orbit Superiorly, Pressing. bry.
Shooting. bry.
Undefined. hg-i.
Eyelids, Adhesion of. s. sb-s.
Discharge, Hard. sb-s.
Movements, Convulsions. s.
Upper Eyelid, Color Red. acon. sep.
Movements, Convulsions. cit-c.
Swelling. acon. sep.
Hard. acon.
Red. acon.
Tensive. acon.
Lower Eyelid, Heat. si-x.
Scraping. si-x.
Smarting. aps.
Upper Tarsal Edge, Dryness. li-ca.
Smarting. li-ca.
Lower Tarsal Edge, Heat. alm.
Itching. alm.
External Canthus, Discharge. sb-s.
False Sensations, Sand. s-x.
Heat. ol-a.
Internal Canthus, Color Red. ery.
Itching. k-o.
Smarting. k-o.

LEFT. alm. cb-a. dt. hll. k-bicr. na-sa. pb. phy. rs. sep. spo. str. te. trg.

Objects Imaginary, Blue. dt.
Bright. dt.
Spots, Blue. dt.
Bright. dt.
Vibrations Bright. dt.
Eyeball, Discharge. cb-a.
Tearing. pb.

Throbbing. pb.
Undefined. trg.
Orbit Superiorly, Undefined. k-bicr.
Orbit Inferiorly, Tearing. na-sa.
Throbbing. na-sa.
Eyelids, Adhesion of. rs.
Movements, Closing. sep.
Spasmodically. spo.
Swelling. phy.
Dark. phy.
Upper Eyelid, Itching. te.
Smarting. te.
Swelling. te.
Œdematous. te.
Red. te.
Lower Eyelid, Itching. alm.
Canthi, Smarting. hll.
Internal Canthus, Color Red. str.
Heat. sep.
Shooting. cb-a.
Smarting. cb-a.
Swelling. sep.
To Face. Orbit, Undefined. k-bicr.

AFTERNOON. (**Evening, Noon to Sunset**).

ach. ag. aga. al-o. alli. alm. alo. amm-ca. amm-cl. amph. aph. aps. art-v. arum-t. asr. (atp). bar. ber. bry. ca-ca. ca-s. can-i. cb-a. cb-v. ccs. chd. chi. cit-c. cl-hx. cmc. cmf. co. con. cop. cor. cph. cr-o. cro. crt. cth. cu. cub. dig. dl-s. dph. dro. dt. ery. eug. euph. euphr. f-hx. fe. frm. frm-s. gel. glo. glp. grc. grp. hg. hg-bini. hg-s. hur. i. ind. k-bicr. k-ca. k-cla. k-i. k-na. k-o. klm. krm. lch. led. ly-b. lyc. mg-ca. mg-cl. mgs. mgs-ar. mgs-au. mn-ca. mph. mrl. myris. n-x. na-ba. na-ca. na-cl. na-sa. narth. ner. ni-ca. nic. ol-a. os. ox-x. p. p-x. pb. pd. pet. pol. pru-l. pt. ptv. pul. pul-n. rhe. rho. rmx. rn-b. rs. rs-r. rut. s. sang. sb-t. scr-m. se. sep. si-x. smc. smi. so-t. spi. spo. spo-f. srr. str. str-i. te. thu. til. trg. trm. trn. trx. u-na. val. vi-t. vr-a. vtx. woo. zn. zng.

OBJECTS, FALSE APPEARANCE **of**. al-o. amm-ca. cb-v. dt. hg. lyc. rs-r. sep.

Confused. dt.
Moving. al-o. amm-ca. hg. lyc. sep.
  Circularly. al-o. amm-ca. sep.
  Vibrating. hg. lyc.
Small. cb-v.
Strange. rs-r.
OBJECTS IMAGINARY. al-o. art-v. ber. can-i. con. cro. dt. ery. eug. f-hx. fe. grp. krm. lch. mn-ca. na-sa. nic. ol-a. p. p-x. sb-t. scr-m. smi. til. trn. val.
Black, ery.
Bright. dt. ery. eug. f-hx. mn-ca. ol-a. sb-t. til. trn. val.
Circles. f-hx. mn-ca.
  Bright. mn-ca.
Cyphers. p-x.
Far off. (dt).
Figures. can-i.
Flames. ery. eug.
Flashes, Bright. ery. f-hx.
Leaf. (na-sa).
  White. (na-sa).
Light. val.
Mist. ol-a. p.
Semicircle. dt.
  Bright. dt.
Spots. dt. ery. krm. ol-a. sb-t.
  Black. ery.
  Bright. dt. ery. ol-a. sb-t.
    Far off. (dt).
  Far off. (dt).
  White. krm.
Stars. trn.
Stripes. dt.
  Bright. dt.
    Vertical. dt.
  Vertical. dt.
Variegated. ery.
Veil. al-o. art-v. ber. cro. fe. lch. nic. ol-a. p. scr-m. (smi).
Vertical. dt.
Vibrations. f-hx. til.
  Bright. f-hx. til.
White. krm. (na-sa).

Zigzags. con. grp.

PHOTOPHOBIA. (atp). ca-s. cb-a. hg. k-bicr. p. p-x. trg. zng.

SIGHT DAZZLED. hg.

SIGHT IMPAIRED. al-o. alm. art-v. ber. cb-a. cro. dph. dt. fe. frm. k-bicr. lch. (na-ba). na-ca. narth. ni-ca. nic. ol-a. (os). p. pul. sang. scr-m. sep. (smi). str-i. thu. trg. trn. woo. zn.

Presbyopia. dt.

Sensation as if Axis of Vision was Moved Backwards and Forwards. os.

EYEBALL. ach. aga. al-o. alli. alo. amm-ca. amm-cl. aps. art-v. arum-t. asr. (atp). bar. bry. ca-ca. ca-s. cb-a. cb-v. ccs. chd. chi. cit-c. cl-hx. cmc. cmf. con. cor. cph. cro. crt. cu. cub. dig. dl-s. dph. (dt). ery. eug. euph. f-hx. fe. frm-s. gel. glo. grc. grp. hg. hg-bini. hg-i. hg-s. i. k-bicr. k-ca. k-cla. k-i. k-o. klm. krm. lch. led. lyc. mg-cl. mn-ca. mph. mrl. myris. na-ba. na-ca. na-cl. na-sa. ni-ca. nic. ol-a. ox-x. p-x. pb. pd. pet. pol. pru-l. pt. ptv. pul. rho. rmx. rn-b. rs. s. sang. sb-t. se. sep. so-t. spi. spo. srr. str-i. te. thu. trg. trn. val. vtx. woo. zn. zng.

Boring. pul.

Bruised. lyc. s.

Bursting. pol.

Coldness. hg-s. lyc. s.

Color, Red. al-o. asr. (atp). chi. cor. cph. dig. (euph). hg-bini. k-cla. lyc. rs. s. (thu). woo. zn.

Contractive. aga. krm. rs. woo.

Creeping. (chi). (cop).

Cutting. ca-ca. hg. (k-i). pul. (s).

Discharge. (aga). ca-s. euph. grc. k-i. (lch). mg-cl. na-ca. (p). pb. (rs). sep.

White. lch.

Drawing. (crt). klm.

Dryness. al-o. (art-v). bar. ca-ca. cit-c. cro. dl-s. (grp). lyc. mn-ca. na-cl. na-sa. ni-ca. pd. pru-l. (pul). (rs). spi. (str-i). trg.

False Sensations. art-v. (bry). ca-ca. ccs. (chd). chi. cor. fe. gel. k-bicr. ni-ca. (nic). (ox-x). sang. (te).

Hairs. sang. (te).

Sand. art-v. (bry). ca-ca. ccs. (chd). chi. cor. fe. gel. k-bicr. ni-ca. (nic). (ox-x). (sang).

Smoke. sang.

Heat. aga. al-o. (alli). amm-ca. amm-cl. (aph). (art-v).

asr. bar. ber. bry. ca-ca. cl-hx. dl-s. eug. (f-hx). (glp). (grp). hg-bini. hg-s. k-bicr. k-i. k-o. krm. led. (mg-ca). mg-cl. mn-ca. mph. na-ba. na-cl. na-sa. ni-ca. nic. ol-a. p-x. pol. pru-l. pul. (pul-n). rho. rs. rut. (s). sb-t. (sep). spi. thu. (trx). vtx. zn.

Heaviness. (cr-o). (s).

Itching. (alli). (bar). ca-ca. (cr-o). cu. (f-hx). fe. grc. grp. (hur). (ind). k-bicr. (mg-ca). (ol-a). (p). pd. pru-l. (pul). rn-b. (rs-r). s. (si-x). srr. (str). (te). (trm).

Lachrymation. alli. asr. (atp). chi. cub. eug. hg. (lyc). (na-sa). ni-ca. (p). (pul). rs. s. sep. so-t. str-i. trg. zn.

Hot. (na-sa). pul.

Appearance of. trg.

Feeling of. myris.

Movements. (al-o). (cro). (dig). (glo). (myris). (na-ca). (na-cl). (s). (smc).

Convulsions. (cro). na-cl). (s).

Drawn-Down Feeling. (ol-a).

Paralysis. cro. i. lyc.

Pressing. (al-o). (alo). (art-v). bry. ca-ca. cb-v. (cit-c). cmc. cmf. con. cor. crt. dl-s. (dt). ery. (f-hx). (glo). (glp). grp. hg-s. klm. led. lyc. mph. (n-x). na-ba. (na-cl). ni-ca. pet. pol. ptv. rn-b. (rs). s. si-x. spo. (str-i). (te). val. zn.

Shooting. ach. (acon). (ag). aps. (bar). (cld). (f-hx). (frm-s). (krm). (lau-c). lyc. (ol-a). p. pru-l. pul. (s). se. spo. thu. (trn). (u-na). zng.

Cold. s.

Smarting. (acon). al-o. cl-hx. cmc. (cr-o). (cro). (dig). dl-s. gel. hg-s. (hur). (k-ca). lyc. (ol-a). (p). p-x. (pul). (rn-b). s. (str). zn.

Swelling. woo.

Feeling of. arum-t. (hg-s). myris.

Tearing. ca-ca. (k-ca). (krm). na-ba. p.

Tensive. (ner).

Throbbing. (na-cl).

Undefined. (ccs). chi. (cmf). dig. dph. (k-cla). lyc. mrl. (pd). pt. rmx. (trn).

EYEBALL INFERIORLY. glp.

Heat. glp.

EYEBALL EXTERNALLY. rn-b.

Pressing. rn-b.

EYEBALL INTERIORLY. al-o.

Smarting. al-o.

CORNEA. thu.

Color Red. thu.
IRIS. thu.
Pupil Dilated. thu.
ORBIT. cit-c. con. glp. hg-s. lau-c. u-na.
Pressing. cit-c. con.
Shooting. lau-c.
ORBIT INFERIORLY. hg-s.
ORBITAL INTEGUMENTS. alli. cr-o. hg-s. k-ca. ol-a. rn-b. s.
Itching. cr-o.
ORBITAL INTEGUMENTS SUPERIORLY. alli. k-ca. ol-a. rn-b. s.
Itching. alli.
Pressing. rn-b.
ORBITAL INTEGUMENTS INFERIORLY. hg-s.
EYELIDS. acon. ag. aga. al-o. alli. aph. art-v. arum-t. (atp). bar. chi. cmf. cr-o. cro. dig. euph. glo. glp. grp. hur. k-cla. k-i. krm. myris. n-x. na-ca. na-cl. ol-a. p. p-x. pul. pul-n. rs. s. smc. str-i. te. thu. trx.
Adhesion of. aga. euph. rs.
Color Red. euph.
Discharge. euph.
Dryness. art-v. glp. rs.
False Sensations, Hair. (te).
Heat. aph. art-v. grp. k-i. p-x. pul. thu.
Itching. p. pul.
Movements, Closing. (al-o). dig. glo. (na-ca).
Spasmodically. al-o. na-ca.
Convulsions. cro. na-cl. s.
Winking. cro. (myris). smc.
Paralysis. cro.
Pressing. art-v. n-x. s.
Shooting. acon. thu.
Smarting. acon. cr-o. cro. pul.
Swelling, Feeling of. myris.
UPPER EYELIDS. ag. al-o. alli. bar. cmf. cr-o. cro. dig. glo. k-cla. krm. na-ca. rs. s. smc. str-i. te.
Dryness. str-i.
Heat. alli.
Heaviness. cr-o. s.
Itching. alli.
Undefined. cmf. k-cla.
LOWER EYELID. arum-t. dig. ol-a.

Itching. ol-a.
Smarting. dig.
Swelling, Feeling of. arum-t.
TARSAL EDGES. (atp). hur. thu.
Color, Red. (atp).
Heat. thu.
Itching. thu.
Shooting. thu.
Smarting. hur.
EYELIDS, INNER SURFACE. chi. pul-n.
Creeping. chi.
Heat. pul-n.
CANTHI. ag. aga. art-v. asr. bar. cl-hx. cop. f-hx. glp. ind. k-i. krm. lyc. mg-ca. na-cl. ner. ol-a. p. pul. rn-b. rs. rs-r. s. str. thu. trm.
Creeping. cop.
Discharge. k-i.
Heat. asr. mg-ca. p-x.
Itching. mg-ca.
EXTERNAL CANTHUS. cl-hx. k-i. lyc. na-cl. pul. rn-b. s.
Heat. s.
Itching. pul.
Shooting. s.
Smarting. lyc.
INTERNAL CANTHUS. aga. art-v. bar. f-hx. glp. ind. krm. na-cl. ner. ol-a. p-x. pru-l. rs. rs-r. str. thu. trm.
Discharge. aga. rs.
Dryness. na-cl.
Heat. art-v. f-hx. glp. p-x. thu.
Itching. ind. ol-a. pru-l. rs-r. str.
Pressing. na-cl.
Smarting. ol-a. str.
Tensive. ner.
CHANGING CHARACTER **or** PLACE. spo.
Eyeball, Shooting then Pressing. spo.
FORWARDS. (dt). pol. str-i. val.
Eyeball, Pressing. pol. str-i. val.
BACKWARDS. cit-c. hg-s.
Eyeball, Pressing. hg-s.
DOWNWARDS. cit-c.
To HEAD. ccs. u-na.
To FOREHEAD. ccs.

Eyeball, Undefined. ccs.
To OCCIPUT. u-na.
RIGHT. al-o. alo. bar. cit-c. cld. crt. f-hx. glo. glp. k-i. krm. lyc. na-sa. nic. ol-a. p. pul. rn-b. rs. sep. si-x. str-i. trn. trn. u-na. zn.
Objects Imaginary. na-sa.
Leaf White. na-sa.
White. na-sa.
Sight Impaired. pul. trn.
Eyeball Discharge. p.
Drawing. crt.
Dryness. pul.
False Sensations, Sand. nic.
Heat. na-sa. ol-a. sep.
Itching. si-x.
Lachrymation. lyc. s.
Hot. na-sa.
Pressing. al-o. alo. cit-c. crt. f-hx. glo.
Shooting. cld.
Smarting. p. zn.
Undefined. trn.
Orbit, Pressing. glp.
Upper Eyelid, Shooting. bar.
Undefined. rs.
External Canthus, Cutting. k-i.
Smarting. rn-b.
Internal Canthus, Heat. pru-l.
Itching. f-hx. trm.
Shooting. f-hx. pru-l.
Tearing. krm.
Forwards. Eyeball, Pressing. str-i.
Backwards. Eyeball, Pressing. cit-c.
Downwards. Eyeball, Pressing. cit-c.
To Occiput. Orbit, Shooting. u-na.
LEFT. aga. al-o. bar. ca-ca. chd. cl-hx. dt. frm-s. hg-s. k-ca. krm. na-ba. na-cl. ol-a. ox-x. pd. rs. s. smi. te. trn. trx. zn.
Objects Imaginary. Bright. dt.
Far off. dt.
Spot Bright. dt.
Far off. dt.
Veil. smi.
Sight Impaired. na-ba. smi.

Eyeball, Cutting. s.
False Sensations, Hairs. te.
Sand. chd. ox-x.
Itching. ca-ca. ol-a.
Movements, Convulsions. al-o.
Pressing. rs. zn.
Shooting. frm-s. ol-a. trn.
Tearing. k-ca.
Undefined. pd.
Orbit Inferiorly, Smarting. hg-s.
Swelling, Feeling of. hg-s.
Orbital Integuments Superiorly, Movements, Drawn-Down Feeling. ol-a.
Smarting. k-ca.
Orbital Integuments Inferiorly, Heat. hg-s.
Eyelids, Heat. trx.
Upper Eyelid, Itching. te.
Pressing. te.
Shooting. ag. krm.
Canthi, Shooting. ag.
External Canthus, Smarting. cl-hx.
Throbbing. na-cl.
Internal Canthus, Itching. bar.
Forwards. Eyeball, Pressing. (dt).

NIGHT. (**Sunset to Sunrise**).

acon. æth. ag. ag-na. al-o. (alm). amm-ca. amm-cl. anm. aps. art-v. as-o. atp. au. ba-ca. ca-ca. ca-s. cast. cb-v. ccs. cd-sa. chd. (cic). cmf. cn-sa. co. cr-o. cro. crt-c. dl-s. dt. ery. eug. euph. euphr. f-hx. fe. fe-mgs. gel. glo. glp. grc. hg. hyo. k-bicr. k-ca. k-o. kre. krm. led. lpd. lyc. mg-cl. mll. mrl. mtr. myris. n-x. na-ca. na-cl. ol-a. p. pb. phy. pol. pul. rho. rn-s. rs. rs-r. rut. s. sb-t. sep. si-x. sn. spo. srr. str. str-i. trn. vr-a. zn.

OBJECTS, FALSE APPEARANCE **of.** amm-ca. dl-s. myris.
Closer Together. myris.
Far, too. myris.
Moving. amm-ca. dl-s.
Circularly. amm-ca. dl-s.
Oblique. myris.

OBJECTS IMAGINARY. acon. amm-ca. dl-s. dt. fe-mgs. na-cl. p. s. spo.
Blue. dt.

Bright. amm-ca. dl-s. (dt). fe-mgs. na-ca. spo.
Circles. fe-mgs.
Blue. fe-mgs.
Bright. fe-mgs.
Red. fe-mgs.
Zigzags. fe-mgs.
Cyphers. s.
Flames. spo.
Flashes, Bright. dt. na-ca.
Green. dt.
Low Down. dt.
Moving. dt.
Moving with Eye. dt.
Red. fe-mgs.
Spots. amm-ca. dt.
Blue. dt.
Bright. amm-ca. dt.
Green. dt.
Low Down. dt
Moving. dt.
Low Down. dt.
Moving. dt.
Stripes. dl-s. dt. na-ca.
Blue. dt.
Moving with Eye. dt.
Vertical. dt.
Bright. dl-s. dt. na-ca.
Vertical. dl-s.
Green. dt.
Moving with Eye. dt.
Vertical. dt.
Moving with Eye. dt.
Vertical. dl-s. dt.
Vertical. dl-s. dt.
Visions. acon. p.
Zigzags. fe-mgs.
PHOTOPHOBIA. gel.
SIGHT IMPAIRED. mll.
EYEBALL. acon. ag-na. al-o. amm-cl. anm. aps. as-o. atp. ca-ca. ca-s. cast. cb-v. ccs. chd. cmf. cn-sa. co. cph. cr-o. dl-s. dt. ery. eug. euph. euphr. fe. gel. glo. glp. grc. hg. k-bicr. kre. krm. led. lyc. mg-cl. ol-a. pb. phy. pul. rho. rn-s. rs. rs-r. s. sep. si-x. sn. srr. str-i. trn. zn.

Appearance Dim. ca-s.
Bruised. anm.
Color Red. ag-na. eug.
Cutting. (cr-o).
Discharge. al-o. aps. (ba-ca). ca-s. cast. cb-v. chd. (cic). cn-sa. (cro). dl-s. (dt). euph. euphr. fe. glp. grc. hg. krm. led. lyc. mg-cl. (n-x). ol-a. phy. (pol). pul. rho. rs. rs-r. (s). sep. si-x. sn. (spo). str-i.
Pus. rho.
Dryness. lyc. s.
Eruptions. (sb-t).
Scabs. (sb-t).
False Sensation. ca-ca. (dt). k-bicr.
Sand. ca-ca. (dt). k-bicr.
Heat. al-o. amm-cl. kre. rs. trn. zn.
Heaviness. (crt-c). (trn).
Itching. (dt). k-bicr. srr. zn.
Lachrymation. amm-cl. (aps). eug. gel. (k-na). rn-s. (s). zn.
Hot. zn.
Movements. acon. (al-o). (aps). (ca-s). (cro). (na-cl).
Convulsions. acon. (al-o). (aps). (cro).
Feeling of. (dt).
Paralysis. (anm). (cb-v). (cro). (lpd). (mrl). (sep).
Pressing. anm. ca-ca. co. (dt). ery. glo. kre. rs.
Shooting. (ag). as-o. (atp). (k-o). (s). (trn).
Smarting. gel. (k-ca). (s). (si-x).
Swelling. pb.
Tearing. (ccs). (k-ca).
Throbbing. as-o.
Undefined. (cmf). co. pb. zn.
EYEBALL, ROUND CORNEA. thu.
Color Red. thu.
IRIS. (alm). pb.
Pupils, Dilated. (alm). pb.
ORBIT. crt-c. k-ca. k-o. zn.
Shooting. k-o.
ORBIT SUPERIORLY. zn.
Undefined. zn.
ORBITAL INTEGUMENTS SUPERIORLY. trn.
EYELIDS. æth. al-o. anm. aps. au. ba-ca. ca-s. cb-v. chd. cro. dl-s. dt. euph. euphr. k-ca. led. lpd. lyc. mg-cl. mrl. na-cl. phy. pul. rs. s. sb-t. sep. si-x. sn. spo. str-i.
Adhesion of. æth. al-o. aps. au. ba-ca. cb-v. chd. cro.

dl-s. dt. euph. euphr. led. lyc. mg-cl. phy. pol. rs. sep. si-x. sn. spo. str-i.

Movements, Closing. (ca-s). (na-cl).

Spasmodically. ca-s. na-cl.

Paralysis. anm. cb-v. cro. lpd. mrl. sep.

Opening Difficult. anm. cb-v. cro. mrl. sep.

Smarting. k-ca. si-x.

UPPER EYELID. al-o. cro. dt.

Movements, Convulsions. al-o. cro.

TARSAL EDGES. dl-s. sb-t.

Discharge. dl-s.

Eruptions, Scabs. sb-t.

EYELIDS, INNER SURFACE. s.

Dryness. s.

Smarting. s.

CANTHI. ag. lyc. pol.

Discharge. lyc. pol.

FORWARDS. (dt).

BACKWARDS. atp.

LENGTHWAYS. cr-o.

To HEAD. ccs. cmf. trn.

To FOREHEAD. ccs.

To SIDE OF HEAD. trn.

To OCCIPUT. cmf.

RIGHT. aps. atp. crt-c. dt. eug. k-ca. n-x. s. trn.

Eyeball, Color Red. eug.

Discharge. aps. n-x. s.

False Sensations, Sand. dt.

Heaviness. trn.

Itching. dt.

Lachrymation. aps.

Undefined. f-hx.

Orbit, Heaviness. crt-c.

Tearing. k-ca.

Orbital Integuments Superiorly, Shooting. trn.

Upper Eyelid, Movements, Convulsions, Feeling of. dt.

Backwards. Eyeball, Shooting. atp.

To Occiput. Eyeball, Undefined. cmf.

LEFT. ag. aps. as-o. cr-o. dt s. trn.

Objects Imaginary, Blue. dt.
Bright. dt.
Spots Blue. dt.
Bright. dt.
Eyeball, Cutting. cr-o.
Lacrymation. s.
Movements, Convulsions. aps.
Pressing. (dt).
Shooting. s. trn.
Canthi, Shooting. ag.
Forwards. Eyeball, Pressing. (dt).
Lengthways. Eyeball, Cutting. cr-o.
To Forehead. Eyeball, Tearing. ccs.
To Side of Head. Eyeball, Shooting. trn.

BEFORE MIDNIGHT. (**Sunset to Midnight**).

al-o. atp. dt. ery. f-hx. frm. k-ca. na-sa. os. os-x. rut. s. sep. smi.

OBJECTS, FALSE APPEARANCE **of.** os-x. smi.
Confused. os-x.
Large, too. os-x.
Red. smi.

OBJECTS IMAGINARY. al-o. dt. ery. k-ca. na-sa. os. rut. s. sep.
Black. dt.
Blue. dt.
Bright. dt. ery. k-ca. (na-sa).
Flashes, Bright. ery.
Green. dt. na-sa. rut.
Halo. al-o. os. rut. s.
Green. rut.
Red. s.
Variegated. os.
Mist. (na-sa). sep.
Moving with Eye. dt.
Near Eye. (na-sa).
Rays. k-ca.
Red. s.
Spots. dt.
Black. dt.
Moving with Eye. dt.

Blue. dt.
Bright. dt.
Moving with Eye. dt.
Stars. (na-sa).
Bright. (na-sa).
Near Eye. (na-sa).
Green. (na-sa).
Near Eye. (na-sa).
Near Eye. (na-sa).
Yellow. (na-sa).
Near Eye. (na-sa).
Stripes. dt.
Blue. dt.
Vertical. dt.
Green. dt.
Vertical. dt.
Vertical. dt.
Variegated. os.
Vertical. dt.
Vibrations. (dt).
Bright. (dt).
PHOTOPHOBIA. dt.
SIGHT IMPAIRED. (na-sa). sep.
EYEBALL. atp. f-hx. na-sa. smi.
Heaviness. (na-sa).
Pressing. na-sa. smi.
Sensitive. (na-sa).
Shooting. (na-sa).
Smarting. atp.
Softness, Feeling of. (na-sa).
Undefined. (f-hx). (frm).
ORBIT. frm. na-sa.
ORBIT SUPERIORLY. frm.
ORBIT INFERIORLY. na-sa.
EYELIDS. na-sa.
UPPER EYELID. na-sa.
Heaviness. na-sa.
BACKWARDS. na-sa.
CHANGING CHARACTER **or** PLACE. na-sa.
Objects Imaginary, Mist, then Star Bright Green Yellow Near Eye. na-sa.
OBJECTS IMAGINARY **then** EYEBALL. na-sa.
SIGHT IMPAIRED **then** OBJECTS IMAGINARY. na-sa.

RIGHT. na-sa.
Objects Imaginary, Bright. na-sa.
Green. na-sa.
Mist. na-sa.
Near Eye. na-sa.
Star. na-sa.
Bright. na-sa.
Near Eye. na-sa.
Green. na-sa.
Near Eye. na-sa.
Near Eye. na-sa.
Yellow. na-sa.
Near Eye. na-sa.
Yellow. na-sa.
Sight Impaired. na-sa.
Eyeball, Pressing. na-sa.
Undefined. na-sa.
Orbit Inferiorly, Pressing. na-sa.
Sensitive. na-sa.
Shooting. na-sa.
Softness, Feeling of. na-sa.
Backwards. Orbit Inferiorly, Shooting. na-sa.
Changing. Objects Imaginary, Mist, then Star Bright Green Yellow Near Eye. na-sa.
Objects Imaginary then Eyeball, Star Bright Green Yellow Near Eye, then Pressing. na-sa.
Sight Impaired then Objects Imaginary, [Star Bright Green Yellow Near Eye. na-sa.
LEFT. dt. frm.
Objects Imaginary, Blue. dt.
Bright. dt.
Spot Blue. dt.
Bright. dt.
Vibrations, Bright. dt.
Orbit Superiorly, Undefined. frm.

AFTER MIDNIGHT. (**Midnight to Sunrise.**)

cph. dt. frm.
OBJECTS IMAGINARY, dt.
Bright. (dt).
Spots. (dt).
Bright. (dt).

EYEBALL. cph.
Undefined. cph. (frm).
ORBIT. frm.
ORBIT SUPERIORLY. frm.
LEFT. dt.
Objects Imaginary, Bright. dt.
Spot Bright. dt.
Orbit Superiorly, Undefined. frm.

In BED.

amb. ca-ca. ca-s. cr-o. dig. dl-s. dt. (ery). hg. hur. k-ca. mg-ca. mgs-ar. mgs-au. na-ca. rn-b. si-x. spo. str.
OBJECTS, FALSE APPEARANCE **of.** dl-s.
Moving. dl-s.
Circularly. dl-s.
OBJECTS IMAGINARY. ca-s. dt. (ery).
Blue. dt.
Bright. ca-s. dt.
Green. dt.
Flames. ca-s.
Moving with Eye. dt.
Spirits. ca-s.
Spots. dt.
Blue. dt.
Bright. dt.
Stripes. dt.
Blue. dt.
Moving with Eye. dt.
Vertical. dt.
Green. dt.
Moving with Eye. dt.
Vertical. dt.
Moving with Eye. dt.
Vertical. dt.
Threads. (ery).
Vertical. dt.
EYEBALL. ca-ca. cr-o. hg.
Cutting. (cr-o). hg.
Itching. (ca-ca). (hur).
Lachrymation. cr-o.
Movements. (dt). (spo).
Convulsions, Feeling of. dt.

Smarting. (hur).
EYELIDS. dt. hur. spo.
Movements, Closing. (spo).
Spasmodically. (spo).
UPPER EYELID. dt.
PUNCTA LACHRYMALIA. hur.
Itching. hur.
Smarting. hur.
LENGTHWAYS. cr-o.
RIGHT. dt.
Upper Eyelid, Movements, Convulsions, Feeling of. dt.
LEFT. ca-ca. cr-o. dt. spo.
Objects Imaginary, Blue. dt.
Bright. dt.
Spots Blue. dt.
Bright. dt.
Eyeball, Cutting. cr-o.
Itching. ca-ca.
Eyelids, Movements, Closing Spasmodically. spo.
Lengthways. Eyeball, Cutting. cr-o.

COLD.

al-o. amm-cl. anth. ca-ca. cl-hx. cle. co. dig. elaps. hg-s. k-ca. k-i. k-na. men. ni-ca. p-x. pul. rs. sb-t. sep. so-d. zn.
PHOTOPHOBIA. k-na.
SIGHT IMPAIRED. k-na.
EYEBALL. amm-cl. anth. cl-hx. cle. co. elaps. hg-s. k-na. men. ni-ca. sb-t. sep. zn.
Color Red. ni-ca. sb-t. sep. zn.
False Sensations. sb-t.
Sand. sb-t.
Heat. amm-cl. cl-hx. k-na. (rs). zn.
Itching. (rs).
Lachrymation. anth. co. dig. k-na.
Movements. (so-d).
Convulsions. (so-d).
Shooting. (rs).
Smarting. zn.
Undefined. cle. co. elaps. hg-s. (men).

EYELIDS. rs. so-d.
Movements, Convulsions. so-d.
UPPER EYELID. rs.
RIGHT. rs.
Upper Eyelid, Heat. rs.
Itching. rs.
Shooting. rs.
LEFT. men.
Eyeball, Undefined. men.

HEAT.

ag-na. alli. bry. cmc. (dt). glo. hg. hg-s. na-sa. pul. rn-b. s. se.
PHOTOPHOBIA. s.
SIGHT IMPAIRED. pul.
EYEBALL. ag-na. alli. bry. cmc. (dt). glo. hg. hg-s. na-sa. s. se.
Appearance Glassy. glo.
Staring. glo.
Cutting. hg. (hg-s).
Heat. na-sa.
Itching. (alli).
Lacrymation. alli. cmc.
Pressing. (dt). (hg-s).
Shooting. s. se.
Smarting. (hg-s).
Swelling, Feeling of. (hg-s).
Undefined. ag-na. bry. cmc.
IRIS. glo.
Pupils Contracted. glo.
ORBIT. hg-s.
ORBIT SUPERIORLY. hg-s.
Cutting. hg-s.
ORBIT INFERIORLY. hg-s.
EYELIDS. alli.
UPPER EYELID. alli.
BACKWARDS. hg-s.
Eyeball, Pressing. hg-s.
FORWARDS. (dt).
OUTWARDS. hg-s.
Orbit Superiorly, Cutting. hg-s
LEFT. alli. (dt). hg-s.

Orbit Inferiorly, Smarting. hg-s.
Swelling, Feeling of. hg-s.
Upper Eyelid, Itching. alli.
Forwards. Eyeball, Pressing. (dt).

OPEN AIR.

acon. æth. aga. al-o. alli. amm-ca. amm-cl. anan. as-o. asr. atp. bry. bz-x. ca-ca. ca-o. cb-v. cch. chd. cl-hx. cle. cmc. co. cof. con. cth. cub. dig. dl-s. dt. ery. euphr. glo. grp. hg. hg-s. hll. k-bicr. k-ca. k-i. k-o. klm. lau-c. led. lpd. lyc. men. mgs-au. mll. mrl. n-x. na-cl. na-sa. ner. ol-a. ol-t. p. pet. pol. pru-l. pul. pul-n. rhe. rho. rs. rut. s. s-x. sb-t. sep. si-x. smc. snc. so-d. srr. str. te. teu. thu. trg. trm. tx-b. vr-s. zn.

OBJECTS, APPEARANCE **of.** cl-hx. ery. glo. k-ca. k-o. ner.

Confused. ner.
Large. k-o.
Moving. cl-hx. ery. k-ca. k-o.
Circularly. cl-hx. ery. k-ca. k-o.
Strange. glo.

OBJECTS IMAGINARY. amm-cl. cth. dl-s. dt. ery. euphr. k-o. mrl. na-cl. ner. ol-a. pol.

Black. ol-a.
Blue. dt.
Bright. dl-s. ery. na-cl. ner.
Flashes Bright. dl-s.
Mist. amm-cl. cth. euphr. k-o. mrl.
Serpentine Bodies. ery.
Bright. ery.
Spots. dt. ery. na-cl. ner. ol-a.
Black. ol-a.
Blue. dt.
Bright. na-cl. ner.
White. ery.
Threads. pol.
White. ery.

SIGHT DAZZLED. ner.

SIGHT IMPAIRED. aga. al-o. amm-cl. con. cth. euphr. k-o. men. mll. mrl. n-x. na-cl. thu.

EYEBALL. acon. al-o. anan. bry. ca-ca. ca-o. cb-v. cch. chd. cle. cmc. co. cof. con. cth. cub. dig. euphr. glo. grp.

hg. hg-s. k-bicr. k-ca. k-o. klm'. lpd. n-x. na-cl. na-sa. ol-a. p. pet. pol. pul. pul-n. rhe. rho. rs. rut. s. s-x. sb-t. sep. si-x. snc. te. teu. thu. trm. tx-b. vr-s. zn.

Coldness. acon. al-o. con.

Color Red. hg. na-cl. sb-t. zn.

Contractive. euphr.

Cutting. rs.

Discharge. anan.

Drawing. klm.

Dryness. k-ca.

False Sensations. co. (s-x). sb-t.

Sand. co. s-x). sb-t.

Heat. (co). con. grp. hg. k-ca. (na-sa). ol-a. (rs). s-x. zn.

Itching. (dl-s). (rs).

Lachrymation. al-o. anan. bry. ca-ca. ca-o. cch. chd. cmc. co. cof. cth. cub. dig. euphr. grp. hg. k-bicr. k-o. lpd. lyc. (n-x). na-cl. (na-sa). p. pet. pol. pul. rhe. rho. (rut). s. sb-t. sep. si-x. snc. srr. te. (teu). thu. trm. tx-b. vr-s. zn.

Hot. euphr. (na-sa). teu.

Movements. (grp). (mrl). (so-d).

Convulsions. (so-d).

Paralysis. (rs).

Pressing. (cb-v). euphr. (glo). (rs). (rut). s. s-x.

Shooting. (p). (rs). (sep). thu.

Smarting. euphr. hg. k-bicr. (rs). zn.

Undefined. acon. cle. co. euphr. hg-s. na-cl. pul-n.

EYEBALL SUPERIORLY. cb-v.

Pressing. cb-v.

EYEBALL ANTERIORLY. s-x.

Heat. s-x.

Pressing. s-x.

EYELIDS. co. dl-s. grp. mrl. rs. so-d. thu.

Adhesion of. thu.

Heat. co.

Movements, Closing. grp.

Convulsions. so-d.

Winking. mrl.

Paralysis. rs.

Smarting. rs.

UPPER EYELID. dl-s. rs.

UPPER TARSAL EDGES. dl-s.

Itching. dl-s.
CANTHI. dl-s. p. s-x.
EXTERNAL CANTHUS. s-x.
False Sensations, Sand. s-x.
INTERNAL CANTHUS. dl-s. p.
Itching. dl-s.
Shooting. p.
RIGHT. glo. n-x. na-sa. rs.
Eyeball, Heat. na-sa.
Lachrymation. n-x.
Hot. na-sa.
Pressing. glo. (rs).
Upper Eyelid, Heat. rs.
Itching. rs.
Shooting. rs.
LEFT. rut. sep. teu.
Eyeball, Lachrymation. rut. teu.
Pressing. rut.

ROOM, In.

æth. ag-na. alli. alm. amm-ca. anth. cl-hx. cro. dig. dro. dt. ery. hg. hg-s. jnp-s. k-bicr. k-o. led. na-ca. na-sa. p. pet. pt. pul. rn-b. s. se. sep. si-x. so-d. trg. tx-b. vtx.
OBJECTS, APPEARANCE **of**. dro. pt. si-x.
Moving. dro. si-x.
Circularly. si-x.
Vibrating. dro.
Small. pt.
Strange. pt.
OBJECTS IMAGINARY. dt. ery. na-sa. sep. so-d. trg.
Blue. dt. trg.
Bright. dt. ery. na-sa. so-d.
Flames. so-d.
Flashes, Bright. ery.
Green. dt.
Halo. trg.
Blue. trg.
Red. trg.
Mist. (na-sa). sep.
Moving with Eye. dt.
Near Eye. (na-sa).

Red. trg.
Spots. dt.
Blue. dt.
Bright. dt.
Stars. (na-sa).
Bright. (na-sa).
Near Eye. (na-sa).
Green. (na-sa).
Near Eye. (na-sa).
Near Eye. (na-sa).
Yellow. (na-sa).
Near Eye. (na-sa).
Stripes. dt.
Blue. dt.
Moving with Eye. dt.
Vertical. dt.
Green. dt.
Moving with Eye. dt.
Vertical. dt.
Moving with Eye. dt.
Vertical. dt.
Vertical. dt.
Yellow. (na-sa).

PHOTOPHOBIA. dt.

SIGHT IMPAIRED. alm. dro. hg. na-ca. (na-sa). pul. sep.

EYEBALL. æth. ag-na. alli. anth. cro. dig. hg-s. k-bicr. k-o. p. pt. s. se. tx-b. vtx.

Coldness. hg-s.
Dryness. s.
False Sensations. k-bicr.
Sand. k-bicr.
Heat. æth. dig. k-bicr. pt.
Itching. (alli).
Lachrymation. alli. anth. cro. dig. k-o. p. pt. tx-b. vtx.
Hot. dig.
Pressing. k-bicr. (na-sa). (rn-b).
Sensitive. (na-sa).
Shooting. (na-sa). se.
Smarting. (hg-s).
Softness, Feeling of. (na-sa).

Swelling, Feeling of. (hg-s).
Undefined. ag-na.
EYEBALL EXTERNALLY. rn-b.
Pressing. rn-b.
ORBIT. hg-s. na-sa.
ORBIT INFERIORLY. hg-s. na-sa.
EYELIDS. alli. dig.
Movements, Closing. (dig).
UPPER EYELID. alli.
BACKWARDS. na-sa.
CHANGING CHARACTER **or** PLACE. na-sa.
Objects Imaginary, Mist, then Star Bright Green Yellow Near Eye. na-sa.
Eyeball, Sensitive then Pressing. (na-sa).
„ **Shooting, then** „ (na-sa).
„ **Softness, Feeling of, then** „ (na-sa).
OBJECTS IMAGINARY **then** EYEBALL. na-sa.
SIGHT IMPAIRED **then** OBJECTS IMAGINARY. na-sa.
RIGHT. dig. na-sa.
Objects Imaginary, Bright. na-sa.
Green. na-sa.
Mist. na-sa.
Near Eye. na-sa.
Star. na-sa.
Bright. na-sa.
Near Eye. na-sa.
Green. na-sa.
Near Eye. na-sa.
Near Eye. na-sa.
Yellow. na-sa.
Near Eye. na-sa.
Yellow. na-sa.
Sight Impaired. na-sa.
Eyeball, Pressing. na-sa.
Orbit Inferiorly, Pressing. na-sa.
Sensitive. na-sa.
Shooting. na-sa.
Softness, Feeling of. na-sa.
Eyelids, Movements, Closing. dig.
Backwards. Orbit Inferiorly, Shooting. na-sa.

Changing. Objects Imaginary, Mist, then Star Bright Green Yellow Near Eye. na-sa.
Orbit Inferiorly, Sensitive then Pressing. na-sa.
,, **Shooting, then** ,, na-sa.
,, **Softness, Feeling of, then** ,, na-sa.
Objects Imaginary then Eyeball, Star Bright Green Yellow Near Eye, then Pressing. na-sa.
Sight Impaired, then Object Imaginary, Star Bright Green Yellow Near Eye. na-sa.
LEFT: alli. dt. hg-s.
Objects Imaginary, Blue. dt.
Bright. dt.
Spots Blue. dt.
Bright. dt.
Orbit Inferiorly, Smarting. hg-s.
Swelling. hg-s.
Upper Eyelid, Itching. alli.

UNCOVERING.

thu.
EYEBALL. thu.
Coldness. thu.
Undefined. thu.

WASHING.

al-o. amm-cl. cl-hx. elaps. k-ca. k-na. men. ni-ca. p-x. sa-l. sep.
PHOTOPHOBIA. k-na.
SIGHT IMPAIRED. k-ca.
EYEBALL. amm-cl. cl-hx. elaps. k-na. men. ni-ca. sa-l. sep.
Color Red. ni-ca. sep.
Heat. amm-cl. cl-hx. k-na.
Lacrymation. k-na.
Shooting. sa-l.
Smarting. sa-l.
Tensive. ni-ca.
Undefined. elaps. (men). ni-ca. sep.
LEFT. men.
Eyeball, Undefined. men.

WEATHER DAMP.

crt.
SIGHT IMPAIRED. crt.
EYEBALL. crt.
Lachrymation. crt.

WEATHER DULL.

aga.

WEATHER HOT.

s.
PHOTOPHOBIA. s.
EYEBALL. s.
Shooting. s.

WIND.

anan. asr. chd. euphr. k-bicr. lyc. na-cl. p. pul. sa-l. srr. thu.
EYEBALL. anan. asr. chd. euphr. k-bicr. lyc. na-cl. p. pul. sa-l. srr. thu.
Coldness. sa-l.
Discharge. anan.
Lachrymation. anan. chd. euphr. k-bicr. lyc. na-cl. p. pul. srr. thu.
Hot. euphr.
Shooting. (sa-l). thu.
Cold. sa-l.
Undefined. euphr. na-cl.

KNEELING.

mg-ca.
OBJECTS, FALSE APPEARANCE **of.** mg-ca.
Moving. mg-ca.
Circularly. mg-ca.

LYING.

ag-na. cb-v. cld. cln. dt. f-hx. k-o. led. men. mgs. mtr. sep. zn.

OBJECTS, FALSE APPEARANCE **of**. sep.
Moving. sep.
Circularly. sep.
OBJECTS, IMAGINARY. ag-na. dt. f-hx.
Black. k-o.
Blue. dt.
Bright. dt. f-hx.
Figures. ag-na.
Flashes Bright. f-hx.
Spots. dt. k-o.
Black. k-o.
Blue. dt.
Bright. dt.
SIGHT IMPAIRED. mtr.
EYEBALL. cb-v. cld. cln. f-hx. men. zn.
Color Red. cln.
Lachrymation. zn.
Hot. zn.
Pressing. cb-v. (f-hx).
Shooting. cld.
Tearing. led.
Undefined. (men). zn.
ORBIT. zn.
ORBIT SUPERIORLY. zn.
Undefined. zn.
RIGHT. cld. f-hx.
Eyeball, Pressing. f-hx.
Shooting. cld.
Undefined. f-hx.
LEFT. dt. men.
Objects Imaginary, Blue. dt.
Bright. dt.
Spot Blue. dt.
Bright. dt.
Eyeball, Undefined. men.

LYING on LEFT SIDE.

hg-i.
OBJECTS, IMAGINARY. hg-i.

Black. hg-i.
Mist. hg-i.
Black. hg-i.

LYING on RIGHT SIDE.

dt.
OBJECTS, IMAGINARY. dt.
Blue. (dt).
Bright. dt.
Spots. dt.
Blue. (dt).
Bright. dt.
LEFT. dt.
Objects, Imaginary, Blue. dt.
Bright. dt.
Spots, Blue. dt.
Bright. dt.

REST.

cl-hx. dro.
EYEBALL. cl-hx. dro.
Cutting. (cl-hx).
Itching. (cl-hx).
Shooting. (cl-hx). (dro).
CANTHI. cl-hx.
EXTERNAL CANTHUS. cl-hx.
RIGHT. cl-hx.
Eyeball, Cutting. cl-hx.
Shooting. cl-hx.
External Canthus, Itching. cl-hx.
LEFT. dro.
Eyeball, Shooting. dro.

SITTING.

alm. cic. dt. eug. hg-s. hur. na-ca. na-sa. p. p-x. rut. s-x. sep. smi.
OBJECTS, FALSE APPEARANCE of. cic. eug. rut. s-x. sep.
Inverted. eug.
Moving. cic. rut. s-x. sep.
Circularly. cic. rut. s-x. sep.

OBJECTS IMAGINARY. dt. hur. p-x. smi.
Bright. dt.
Cyphers. p-x.
Far off. dt.
Mist. smi.
Spots. dt.
Bright. dt.
Far off. dt.
Far off. dt.
Zigzags. hur.
SIGHT IMPAIRED. alm.
EYEBALL. na-ca. na-sa. p.
Heat. (hg-s).
Lachrymation. (na-sa).
Shooting. (na-ca). p.
Tearing. p.
Undefined. na-ca.
ORBITAL INTEGUMENTS. hg-s.
ORBITAL INTEGUMENTS INFERIORLY. hg-s.
RIGHT. na-sa.
Eyeball, Lachrymation. na-sa.
Shooting. na-sa.
LEFT. dt. hg-s.
Objects, Imaginary, Bright. dt.
Far off. dt.
Spots. dt.
Bright. dt.
Far off. dt.
Far off. dt.
Orbital Integuments Inferiorly, Heat. hg-s.

STANDING.

bry. ca-ca. dt. euph. hg-s. k-o. mg-ca. pnx. pul.
OBJECTS, FALSE APPEARANCE **of.** bry. ca-ca. euph. mg-ca. pnx.
Moving. bry. ca-ca. euph. mg-ca. pnx.
Circularly. bry. ca-ca. euph. mg-ca.
OBJECTS, IMAGINARY. dt. k-o.
Bright. dt.
Spots. dt.
Bright. dt.

Veil. k-o.
EYEBALL.
Heat. (hg-s).
ORBITAL INTEGUMENTS. hg-s.
ORBITAL INTEGUMENTS INFERIORLY. hg-s.
LEFT. hg-s.
Orbital Integuments Inferiorly, Heat. hg-s.

PRESSURE.

alm. amm-cl. anth. art-v. ba-ca. bry. cit-c. dro. eryn. evo. lac-cg. na-cl. p-x. pet. rs. s. si-x. smi. snp-n. vr-a.
SIGHT IMPAIRED. ba-ca.
EYEBALL. anth. cit-c. eryn. evo. na-cl. pet. rs. s. si-x. smi. snp-n.
Bruised. (alm). s. (smi).
Eruptions. (bry).
Undefined Pain. (bry).
Pressing. (art-v). evo. (p-x).
Shooting. pet. snp-n.
Smarting. (dro).
Tearing. (amm-cl).
Undefined. anth. (bry). (eryn). (lac-cg). (na-cl). rs. si-x. smi.
EYEBALL CENTRE OF. lac-cg.
Undefined. lac-cg.
CORNEA. lac-cg.
Undefined. lac-cg.
ORBIT. alm. amm-cl. art-v. smi.
ORBIT SUPERIORLY. amm-cl.
ORBIT INFERIORLY. alm. art-v. smi.
Bruised. smi.
Pressing. art-v.
EYELIDS. bry. dro. p-x.
UPPER EYELID. dro.
LOWER EYELID. bry. p-x.
Eruptions, Undefined Pain. bry.
BACKWARDS. cit-c.
DOWNWARDS. cit-c.
RIGHT. amm-cl. cit-c. na-cl.
Eyeball, Undefined. na-cl.
Orbit Superiorly, Tearing. amm-cl.

Backwards. Eyeball, Pressing. cit-c.
Downwards. Eyeball, Pressing. cit-c.
LEFT. alm. dro. eryn. p-x.
Eyeball, Undefined. eryn.
Orbit Inferiorly, Bruised. alm.
Upper Eyelid, Smarting. dro.
Lower Eyelid, Pressing. p-x.

RUBBING. (Scratching, Wiping).

aga. anan. cb-a. chd. chi. cit-c. con. frm-s. grc. (k-bicr). k-o. klm. kre. lct. na-ca. nic. p-x. pol. pul. rn-b. rs. rut. sep. smi. spi. sr-ca. trn. zn.

OBJECTS IMAGINARY. k-o. nic. pol. spi. sr-ca.
Blue. sr-ca.
Feathers. spi.
Halo. sr-ca.
Blue. sr-ca.
Red. sr-ca.
Mist. k-o. nic. pol.
Red. sr-ca.
Vibrations. pol.

SIGHT IMPAIRED. k-o. nic. pol. spi.

EYEBALL. aga. anan. chd. cit-c. frm-s. grc. (k-bicr). klm. na-ca. p-x. rn-b. rs. sep. spi. sr-ca. zn.
Color Red. kre.
Eruptions. (smi).
Hot. (smi).
False Sensations. kre. (rs). (sep). (spi). (sr-ca).
Sand. kre. (rs). (sep). (spi). (sr-ca).
Heat. chd. frm-s. (smi).
Itching. (k-o). kre. rn-b. (rut). (sep). (trn). (zn).
Lachrymation. grc. (kre). na-ca. p-x.
Hot. grc. kre.
Salt. kre.
Pressing. aga. (pul). (sep). sr-ca.
Shooting. klm. (pul).
Smarting. anan. (k-o). kre. (rut). (sep). (zn).
Undefined. (k-bicr).
Wrinkled Feeling. anan.

EYEBALL SUPERIORLY. spi.

EYELIDS. kre. smi. trn.

Color Red. kre.
Eruption, Hot. smi.
Itching. kre.
Smarting. kre.
TARSAL EDGES. kre. trn.
Color Red. kre.
Itching. kre.
Smarting. kre.
CANTHI. cb-a. k-o. lct. pul. rs. rut. sep. zn.
EXTERNAL CANTHUS. lct. rs. sep.
Smarting. lct.
INTERNAL CANTHUS. cb-a. k-o. pul. rut. sep. zn.
Itching. rut.
Pressing. pul.
Shooting. pul.
Smarting. rut. sep.
FORWARDS. cit-c.
UPWARDS. cit-c.
RIGHT. cit-c. k-o. sep. spi. sr-ca.
Eyeball, False Sensations, Sand. sep. sr-ca.
Pressing. sep.
Eyeball Superiorly, False Sensations, Sand. spi.
Internal Canthus, Itching. k-o.
Smarting. k-o. zn.
Forwards. Eyeball, Pressing. cit-c.
Upwards. Eyeball, Pressing. cit-c.
LEFT. cb-a. rs. sep. zn.
Eyeball, False Sensations, Sand. rs.
Itching. zn.
Smarting. sep. zn.
External Canthus, Itching. sep.
Smarting. sep.
Internal Canthus, Smarting. cb-a.

TOUCH.

acon. ag-na. aga. alo. atp. atrop. au. ba-ca. bry. buf. buf-s. ca-s. cb-a. cch. chd. chi. chio. chlor. cit-c. cld. cle. cof. cu. cu-asi. dig. dro. elaps. eryn. fe-mgs. gn-l. hg. hg-i. hg-s. hll. hur. k-bicr. k-ca. k-o. lac-cg. ly-b. lyc. mg-cl. mgs-ar. mn-ca. n-x. na-ca. na-cl. na-sa. ni-ca. ner. p. par.

pet. phy. pol. qu-sa. rs-r. rs-v. s. sang. sb-s. sb-t. sep. si-x. sn. spi. spo. spo-f. str. str-i. thu. trn. trx. vtx.

EYEBALL. acon. ag-na. atp. atrop. au. bry. buf-s. ca-s. cch. chi. chio. cit-c. cld. cle. cof. cu-asi. dig. elaps. eryn. gn-l. hg. hg-s. hll. k-bicr. k-ca. ly-b. mg-cl. mgs-ar. na-ca. na-cl. ni-ca. phy. pol. qu-sa. rs-v. sang. sb-s. sb-t. si-x. spi. str-i. thu. trn. vtx.

Bruised. ca-s. (na-cl). sb-t. vtx.

Eruptions. (hg-s). (hur). (sb-s). (sn). (spo).

Undefined Pain. (hg-s). (hur). (sb-s). (sn). (spo).

False Sensations. hg.

Sand. hg.

Heat. (aga). (k-o). (thu).

Itching. (k-o).

Pressing. (au). ca-s. (chd). (chi). (cu). (na-cl). (thu). (trx).

Shooting. (ba-ca). (ni-ca).

Smarting. atrop. (chd). (dro). (hg-s). (ner). (spi). (str).

Softness, Feeling of. (na-sa).

Undefined. (sensitive). acon. ag-na. (aga). (alo). atp. bry. buf-s. ca-s. (cb-a). cch. chi. chio. (chlor). cit-c. cld. cle. cof. cu-asi. dig. elaps. (eryn). (fe-mgs). gn-l. hg. (hg-i). hg-s. hll. (hur). k-bicr. k-ca. (lac-cg). ly-b. (lyc). mg-cl. mgs-ar. (mn-ca). (n-x). na-ca. na-cl. (na-sa). ni-ca. (p). (pet). phy. pol. qu-sa. (rs-r). rs-v. (sang). sb-s. sb-t. si-x. (sn). spi. (spo). spo-f. (str). str-i. (thu). (trn).

EYEBALL SUPERIORLY. acon. thu.

Undefined. acon.

EYEBALL CENTRE OF. lac-cg.

Undefined. lac-cg.

CORNEA. lac-cg.

Undefined. lac-cg.

ORBIT. alo. au. cu-asi. hg. hg-i. hg-s. ly-b. na-cl. na-sa. p. pet. sep. spi. thu.

Undefined. alo. ly-b.

ORBIT CIRCUMFERENCE. ly-b. na-cl. p.

Undefined. ly-b. p.

ORBIT SUPERIORLY. cu-asi. hg. hg-i. hg-s. na-cl. pet. sep.

Smarting. hg-s.

Undefined. hg. sep.

ORBIT INFERIORLY. au. hg-s. na-sa. thu.

ORBIT EXTERNALLY. spi.

Smarting. spi.

ORBITAL INTEGUMENTS. aga. ba-ca. chi. hll. hur. n-x. ner. sb-s. sn. spo. str. thu. trx.

Undefined. n-x.

ORBITAL INTEGUMENTS SUPERIORLY. aga. ba-ca. chi. hll. hur. ner. sb-s. sn. spo. str. thu. trx.

Eruptions, Undefined Pain. hur. sb-s. sn.

Pressing. chi.

Shooting. ba-ca.

Undefined. aga. str.

EYELIDS. atp. atrop. ca-s. cb-a. chd. chlor. cu. dro. hg. k-bicr. k-o. lyc. mgs-ar. mn-ca. ni-ca. spo-f. str.

Eruptions, Undefined Pain. hg-s.

Pressing. cu.

Smarting. atrop. chd.

Undefined. ca-s. cb-a. chlor. hg. k-bicr. lyc. mgs-ar. mn-ca. spo-f.

UPPER EYELID. atp. chd. mn-ca.

Undefined. mn-ca.

LOWER EYELID. dro. k-o.

Heat. k-o.

Itching. k-o.

TARSAL EDGES. ni-ca. str.

Shooting. ni-ca.

Smarting. str.

EYELIDS, INNER SURFACE. s.

Tensive. s.

CANTHI. aga. atp. fe-mgs. rs-r.

EXTERNAL CANTHUS. fe-mgs. rs-r.

Undefined. fe-mgs. rs-r.

INTERNAL CANTHUS. aga. atp.

Heat. aga.

LACHRYMAL GLAND. fe-mgs.

Undefined. fe-mgs.

RIGHT. au. dro. hg-s. na-cl. na-sa. ner. pet. sang. str. thu. trn.

Eyeball, Pressing. au.

  Undefined. sang. thu. trn.

Orbit Superiorly Smarting. hg-s.

  Undefined. na-cl. pet.

Orbit Inferiorly, Softness, Feeling of. na-sa.

  Undefined. au. na-sa. thu.

Orbital Integuments Superiorly, Smarting. ner.

  Undefined. str.

Lower Eyelid, Smarting. dro.
LEFT. atp. chd. cu-asi. eryn. hg-i. hg-s. hll. na-cl. spo. thu. trx.
Eyeball, Undefined. eryn.
Eyeball Superiorly, Heat. thu.
Pressing. thu.
Orbit Circumference, Bruised. na-cl.
Pressing. na-cl.
Orbit Superiorly, Undefined. cu-asi. hg-i.
Orbit Inferiorly, Undefined. hg-s.
Orbital Integuments Superiorly, Eruption, Undefined Pain. spo.
Pressing. trx.
Tensive. hll.
Undefined. thu.
Upper Eyelid, Eruption, Undefined Pain. hg-s.
Pressing. chd.
Undefined. atp.
Internal Canthus, Undefined. atp.

ASCENDING.

cmf. ery. hg-s.
SIGHT IMPAIRED. ery.
EYEBALL. cmf.
Smarting. (hg-s).
Swelling, Feeling of. (hg-s).
Undefined. cmf.
ORBIT. hg-s.
ORBIT SUPERIORLY. hg-s.
Smarting. hg-s.
Swelling, Feeling of. hg-s.

DRIVING.

li-ca. na-cl.
EYEBALL. na-cl.
Dryness. na-cl.
Undefined. (li-ca).
ORBIT. li-ca.
Undefined. li-ca.

ORBITAL INTEGUMENTS. li-ca.
ORBITAL INTEGUMENTS SUPERIORLY. li-ca.
RIGHT. li-ca.
Orbital Integuments Superiorly, Undefined. li-ca.

LIFTING.

ol-a. sb-t.
OBJECTS IMAGINARY. sb-t.
Bright. sb-t.
Spots. sb-t.
Bright. sb-t.
Vibrations. sb-t.

MOVING.

ca-ca. chi. led. na-cl. nic. pb. rn-b. spi.
OBJECTS IMAGINARY. ca-ca.
Black. ca-ca.
Spots. ca-ca.
Black. ca-ca.
EYEBALL. nic. spi.
Boring. nic.
Drawing. nic.
Undefined. spi.

RISING. (Generally, including Varieties).

acon. amb. amm-cl. arn. art-v. as-o. bry. ca-ca. cb-a. cb-v. cmc. cmf. dl-s. dt. glo. hg-i. hg-s. k-bicr. lct. ly-b. lyc. mg-ca. myris. na-cl. ox-x. par. pru-l. pul. rn-b. rs. rs-r. sb-s. sb-t. thr. thu. val. vr-a. vr-s. ziz. zn.
OBJECTS, FALSE APPEARANCE **of.** acon. arn. bry. ca-s. cb-a. k-bicr. ly-b. mg-ca. zn.
Moving. acon. arn. bry. cb-a. k-bicr. ly-b. mg-ca. zn.
Circularly. acon. arn. bry. cb-a. k-bicr. ly-b. mg-ca. zn.
OBJECTS IMAGINARY. mg-cl. sb-t. vr-a.
Black. vr-a.
Bright. sb-t. vr-a.
Flames. vr-a.

High up. mg-cl.
Mist. mg-cl. sb-t.
Rocks. mg-cl.
High up. mg-cl.
Spots. sb-t. vr-a.
Black. vr-a.
Bright. sb-t.
Vibrations. sb-t.
SIGHT IMPAIRED. amb. art-v. ca-s. cmc. dt. glo. myris. na-cl. pul. vr-s.
EYEBALL. hg-s. lyc. ox-x. pul. rn-b. thr. thu. val.
Color Red. pul.
Heat. thu.
Pressing. (lct). (ox-x). rn-b. val.
Smarting. hg-s.
Tearing. lyc.
Throbbing. (thr).
Undefined. (hg-i).
EYEBALL SUPERIORLY. ox-x.
Pressing. ox-x.
ORBIT. hg-i. lct.
Pressing. lct.
ORBIT SUPERIORLY. hg-i.
EYELIDS. (dt).
Movements, Closing. (dt).
RIGHT. hg-i. thr.
Eyeball, Throbbing. thr.
Orbit, Undefined. hg-i.
Orbit Superiorly, Undefined. hg-i.

RISING **from** LYING.

amb. amm-cl. art-v. cb-a. cb-v. cmc. cmf. dt. hg-i. hg-s. lct. ly-b. mg-ca. par. pul. rn-b. rs. rs-r. sb-s. thr. thu. val. zn.
OBJECTS, FALSE APPEARANCE **of.** cb-a. ly-b. mg-ca.
Moving. cb-a. ly-b. mg-sa.
Circularly. ly-b. mg-sa.
SIGHT IMPAIRED. amb. art-v. cmc. dt.
EYEBALL. hg-s. rn-b. thr. thu. val.
Heat. thu.
Pressing. (lct). rn-b. val.

Smarting. hg-s.
Throbbing. (thr).
Undefined. (hg-i).
ORBIT. hg-i. lct.
Pressing. lct.
ORBIT SUPERIORLY. hg-i.
RIGHT. hg-i. thr.
Eyeball, Throbbing. thr.
Orbit, Undefined. hg-i.
Orbit Superiorly, Undefined. hg-i.

RISING **from** SITTING.

acon. bry. k-bicr. mg-cl. sb-t. vr-a. vr-s.
OBJECTS, FALSE APPEARANCE **of**. acon. bry. k-bicr.
Moving. acon. bry. k-bicr.
Circularly. acon. bry. k-bicr.
OBJECTS IMAGINARY. mg-cl. sb-t. vr-a.
Bright. sb-t. vr-a.
Flames. vr-a.
High up. mg-cl.
Mist. mg-cl. sb-t.
Rocks. mg-cl.
High up. mg-cl.
Spots. sb-t.
Bright. sb-t.
SIGHT IMPAIRED. vr-s.

RISING **from** STOOPING. (**Raising Head**).

arn. as-o. ca-s. cb-a. na-cl. pul. zn.
OBJECTS, FALSE APPEARANCE **of**. arn. cb-a. zn.
Moving. arn. cb-a. zn.
Circularly. arn. cb-a. zn.
SIGHT IMPAIRED. ca-s. na-cl.
EYEBALL. pul.
Color Red. pul.

STOOPING. (**Bending Head Down**).

anth. au. br. bry. ca-ca. cch. chi. cit-c. cmc. cof. cph. dl-s. dro. f-hx. grp. hg-i. hg-s. kre. lct. mll. mn-ca. mrl. msc. na-cl. p. pet. pol. s. stach. val. vin. ziz.

OBJECTS, FALSE APPEARANCE **of.** au. dl-s. val.

Moving. au. dl-s. val.

Circularly. au. dl-s. val.

OBJECTS, IMAGINARY. lct. msc. vin.

Black. lct.

Mist. vin.

Moving Circularly. msc.

Spots. lct.

Black. lct.

SIGHT IMPAIRED. cof. hg-s. na-cl. p.

EYEBALL. br. cit-c. cmc. dro. f-hx. kre. mrl. pol. s. stach.

Bursting. stach.

Cutting. (chi). (hg-s).

Drawing. (mn-ca). (val).

Lachrymation. cmc.

Looseness, Feeling of. br.

Pressing. (anth). (bry). cit-c. f-hx. (hg-s). kre. mrl. pol.

Shooting. dro. (s).

Smarting. cit-c.

Swelling, Feeling of. cph.

Throbbing. pol.

Undefined. cmc. (hg-i). mll. (pet). (ziz).

EYEBALL POSTERIORLY. anth.

Pressing. anth.

ORBIT. chi. hg-i. mn-ca. pet. val. ziz.

Cutting. chi.

Drawing. mn-ca.

ORBIT CIRCUMFERENCE. val.

Drawing. val.

ORBIT SUPERIORLY. hg-i. hg-s. pet.

Cutting. hg-s.

FORWARDS. br.

Eyeball, Pressing. br.

BACKWARDS. hg-s.

Eyeball, Pressing. hg-s.

OUTWARDS. hg-s.
Orbit Superiorly, Cutting. hg-s.
TO HEAD. kre.
TO VERTEX. kre.
Eyeball, Pressing. kre.
RIGHT. f-hx. hg-i. ziz.
Eyeball, Pressing. f-hx.
Orbit, Undefined. ziz.
Orbit Superiorly, Undefined. hg-i. pet.
LEFT. bry. s.
Eyeball, Shooting. s.
Downwards Pressing. bry.

TURNING ROUND.

hg.
OBJECTS, FALSE APPEARANCE **of**. hg.
Moving. hg.
Circularly. hg.

WALKING.

acon. aga. arn. as-o. atp. bry. ca-ca. ca-s. can-i. cb-v. chi. cof. con. dl-s. dt. elaps. ery. euphr. fe-a. glo. grp. hg. hur. itu. k-bicr. k-o. led. mgs-ar. na-cl. ner. nic. ol-t. ox-x. p. pb. pet. phy. pul. pul-n. rn-b. s. s-x. sb-t. sep. smc. so-d. spi. spo. str. te. thu. trg. vr-s. vr-v. ziz. zn.
OBJECTS, FALSE APPEARANCE **of**. arn. ery. glo. na-cl. ner. p. sep. spi.
Confused. ner.
Moving. arn. ery. na-cl. p. sep. spi.
Circularly. arn. ery. na-cl. p. sep. spi.
Strange. glo.
OBJECTS, IMAGINARY. acon. atp. can-i. dt. elaps. ery. euphr. hur. k-o. na-cl. ner. nic. ol-t. sb-t. so-d.
Black. (atp). ca-ca. elaps. ol-t.
Blue. dt.
Bright. ery. hur. na-cl. ner. nic. sb-t. so-d.
Circles. elaps.
Black. elaps.
Figures. can-i.
Flames. so-d.
Mist. euphr. k-o.

Serpentine Bodies. ery.
Bright. ery.
Spots. (atp). ca-ca. dt. ery. hur. na-cl. ner. nic. ol-t. sb-t.
Black. (atp). ca-ca. ol-t.
Blue. dt.
Bright. hur. na-cl. ner. nic. sb-t.
White. ery.
Vibrations. acon. sb-t.
White. ery.
Zigzags. hur.
SIGHT DAZZLED. ner.
SIGHT IMPAIRED. aga. euphr. fe-a. k-bicr. k-o. na-cl. pul. sep. so-d. vr-v.
EYEBALL. ca-s. cb-v. cof. con. euphr. glo. grp. hur. itu. nic. ox-x. phy. pul-n. s. smc. spi. spo. te. thu. vr-s.
Boring. nic.
Coldness. con.
Contractive. euphr.
Cutting. (chi).
Drawing. nic.
False Sensations. (s-x).
Sand. (s-x).
Heaviness. itu.
Lachrymation. cof. grp. spo. te. (thu). vr-s.
Movements. (grp). (spo).
Pressing. (cb-v). euphr. (glo). (led). (ox-x). phy. s. (spi).
Shooting. smc.
Swelling, Feeling of. spi.
Tearing. smc.
Throbbing. (trg).
Undefined. ca-s. (chi). hur. (pd). (pet). phy. pul-n. spi. ziz.
EYEBALL SUPERIORLY. cb-v. ox-x.
Pressing. cb-v. ox-x.
ORBIT. chi. hur. led. pet. ziz.
Cutting. chi.
Undefined. hur.
ORBIT SUPERIORLY. chi. pet.
Undefined. chi.
ORBIT EXTERNALLY. led.
Pressing. led.

EYELIDS. cb-v. grp. spo.
Movements, Closing. grp. (spo).
Spasmodically. spo.
UPPER EYELID. cb-v.
Pressing. cb-v.
CANTHI. s-x.
EXTERNAL CANTHUS. s-x.
RIGHT. glo. s-x. spi. trg. ziz.
Eyeball, Pressing. glo. spi.
Throbbing. trg.
Orbit, Undefined. ziz.
Orbit Superiorly, Undefined. pet.
External Canthus, False Sensations, Sand. s-x.
LEFT. atp. pd. thu.
Objects Imaginary, Black. atp.
Spots. atp.
Black. atp.
Eyeball, Lachrymation. thu.
Undefined. pd.

ANGER.

sep.
SIGHT IMPAIRED. sep.

ANXIETY.

chd.
OBJECTS IMAGINARY. chd.
Bright. chd.
Spots. chd.
Bright. chd.

EMOTIONS.

dt.
EYEBALL. dt.
Movements. dt.
Squinting. dt.

FRIGHT.

dt.
EYEBALL. dt.
Movements. dt.
Squinting. dt.

MENTAL EXERTION

ag-na. art-v. au. eryn. lct. men. rn-b. s. stach. str. str-i.
OBJECTS IMAGINARY. au.
Bright. au.
Spots. au.
Bright. au.
EYEBALL. art-v. eryn. lct. s. stach.
Bursting. stach.
Pressing. lct. (rn-b).
Tensive. s.
Undefined. art-v. eryn.
ORBIT. rn-b.
ORBIT SUPERIORLY. rn-b.
Pressing. rn-b.

Being ROUSED.

myris.
EYEBALL.
Movements. (myris).
EYELIDS. myris.
Movements, Winking. myris.

When SCOLDED.

dt.
IRIS. dt.
Pupils, Dilated. dt.

When OTHERS TALK **about it.**

ca-pa.
EYEBALL. ca-pa.
False Sensations. ca-pa.
Sand. ca-pa.

MOVING HEAD.

acon. amm-ca. arn. cmc. dl-s. lac-cg. lch. lyc. msc. mtr. na-cl. pul. spi.

OBJECTS, FALSE APPEARANCE **of.** amm-ca. arn. dl-s.

Moving. amm-ca. arn. dl-s.

Circularly. amm-ca. arn. dl-s.

OBJECTS IMAGINARY. msc.

Moving Up and Down. msc.

SIGHT IMPAIRED. acon. lch. na-cl.

EYEBALL. cmc. lac-cg. lyc. pul. stach.

Bursting. lac-cg. stach.

Pressing. cmc. (mtr).

Shooting. (pul).

Smarting. cmc.

Undefined. (cmc). lyc.

EYELIDS. mtr.

UPPER EYELID. mtr.

Pressing. mtr.

FORWARDS. cmc.

Eyeball, Pressing. cmc.

DOWNWARDS. cmc.

Eyeball Pressing. cmc.

To HEAD. cmc.

To OCCIPUT, cmc.

Eyeball Posteriorly, Undefined. cmc.

LEFT. lyc. pul.

Eyeball, Shooting. pul.

Undefined. lyc.

MOVING HEAD to SHOULDER.

gel.

OBJECTS, FALSE APPEARANCE **of.** gel.

Multiplied. gel.

MOVING HEAD ROUND.

dl-s.

OBJECTS, FALSE APPEARANCE **of.** dl-s.

Moving. dl-s.

Circularly. dl-s.

MOVING HEAD ROUND to LEFT.

dt.
OBJECTS, IMAGINARY. dt.
Bright. dt.
Far off. (dt).
Spots. dt.
  Bright. dt.
    Far off. (dt).
  Far off. (dt).
LEFT. dt.
Bright. dt.
Far off. dt.
Spots. dt.
  Bright. dt.
    Far off. dt.
  Far off. dt.

RESTING HEAD on ARM.

na-cl.
EYEBALL. na-cl.
Pressing. na-cl.

MOVING SCALP.

chi.
EYEBALL.
Pressing. (chi).
ORBITAL INTEGUMENTS. chi.
ORBITAL INTEGUMENTS SUPERIORLY. chi.
Pressing. chi.

Before HEAD Symptoms.

acon. anm. ba-ca. cch. cic. con. cot. cth. dt. ery. hur. hyo. k-bicr. lac-d. na-cl. pod. pso. rhe. sang. (sep). smi. thr. trg.
OBJECTS, FALSE APPEARANCE of. ery. pod. pso. thr.
Confused. ery. pod.
Far too. thr.
Moving. pso.
Multiplied. ery.

OBJECTS IMAGINARY. con. ery. hyo. na-cl. pod. pso. smi. thr. trg.

Black. pso.

Bright. ery. hyo. na-cl. pso. smi. trg.

Circles. pso.

Mist. pod.

Moving. pod.

Moving. pod.

Spots. ery. hyo. pso.

Black. pso.

Bright. ery. hyo.

Veil. thr.

Vibrations. con. ery. pso. smi. thr. trg.

Bright. con. ery.

Zigzags. na-cl. trg.

Bright. na-cl.

SIGHT DAZZLED. na-cl.

SIGHT IMPAIRED. acon. con. cth. dt. (ery). k-bicr. ac-d. na-cl. pod. pso. (sep). smi. thr.

EYEBALL. acon. anm. ba-ca. cch. cic. cot. mrl. rhe. rg.

Appearance Glassy. anm.

Staring. anm. cic.

Drawing. (cch).

Pressing. (trg).

Projecting. anm.

Smarting. cot.

Swelling. rhe.

Tearing. (cch).

Tensive. mrl.

Undefined. acon. (ba-ca). (hur). (k-bicr). (sang).

Same Symptom. (cch). mrl.

ORBIT. hur. k-bicr.

Undefined. hur.

ORBIT SUPERIORLY. k-bicr.

CANTHI. sang.

INTERNAL CANTHUS. sang.

RIGHT. k-bicr. sang. trg.

Eyeball Pressing. trg.

Orbit Superiorly, Undefined. k-bicr.

Internal Canthus, Undefined. sang.

LEFT. ba-ca. cch.
Eyeball, Drawing. cch.
Tearing. cch.
Undefined. ba-ca.
Same Symptoms. cch.

With HEAD **Symptoms.**

ach. acon. æsc. æsc-g. æth. ag. ag-na. aga. al-o. alli. alm. alo. amb. amm-ca. amm-cl. anag. anan. anm. apo. apo-a. aps. ara. arn. art-v. as-o. asc. asr. ast. astac. atp. au. ba-a. ba-ca. ba-cl. bap. bar. ber. bi-na. br. bru. bry. buf. ca-a. ca-ca. ca-o. ca-s. can. cap. cast. cau. cb-a. cb-v. cch. ccs. chd. cic. cis. cit-c. cl-hx. cld. cln. clv. cmc. cmf. cn-sa. co. cof. con. cor. cot. cph. crb-x. cro. crot. crt. cth. cu. cu-ca. cund. cy-hx. cyc. dig. dl-s. dol. dph. dph-i. drm. dro. dt. elaps. erig. ery. eryn. eug. eupat. (eupat-p). euph. euph-c. euphr. evo. f-hx. fe. fe-a. fe-mgs. frm. gel. glo. glp. gn-l. grp. grt. gss. gua. gym. hg. hg-bicl. hg-bini. hg-cl. hg-i. hg-s. hll. hpm. hpp. hum. hur. hydr. hyo. hyp. i. ind. irs. itu. jat. jcr. jnc. jnp-s. jug. k-bicr. k-ca. k-i. k-na. k-o. kd-o. kis. klm. kre. lac-cg. lac-d. lau-c. lch. lct. led. li-ca. lpd. ly-b. lyc. men. menth. mg-ca. mg-cl. mg-sa. mgs. mgs-ar. mgs-au. morph-a. mph. mrl. msc. mtr. myr. myris. n-x. na-ba. na-ca. na-cl. na-sa. narth. ner. ni-ca. nic. ol-t. os. ox-x. p. p-x. pan. par. pb. ped. pet. phl. phy. physo. pip. plb. pnc. pnx. pod. pol. ppv. pru-l. pso. pt. ptv. pul. qu-sa. rhe. rho. rn-b. rs. rs-r. rut. s. s-x. sa-mgs. sang. sb-t. scu. se. sep. si-x. smb. smc. smi. smr. sn. snc. so-d. spi. spo. spo-f. sr-ca. srr. stach. str. str-i. tep. thr. thu. til. trg. trn. tx-b. urt. val. vi-o. vin. vr-a. vr-s. vr-v. vtx. wis. woo. zn. zng.

OBJECTS, FALSE APPEARANCE **of.** acon. ag-na. al-o. (alm). amm-ca. anan. anm. arn. atp. au. ba-ca. ba-cl. ber. bry. ca-a. ca-ca. ca-o. ca-s. can. cb-a. cb-v. chd. cic. cl-hx. con. cy-hx. dl-s. dro. dt. ery. eug. euph. euph-c. fe. frm. gel. glo. grt. gua. hg. hyo. jnc. k-bicr. k-ca. k-o. kis. kre. lct. li-ca. lpd. ly-b. lyc. mg-ca. mg-cl. mrl. msc. mtr. myris. na-cl. ner. nic. p. p-x. par. pb. pnx. ppv. pru-l. pso. rho. rn-b. rs. rut. s. s-x. se. sep. si-x. smc. sn. spi. spo. str. tep. thr. thu. til. val. vin. vr-a. vr-s. vr-v. vtx. wis. zn.

Black. acon. al-o. hg. (na-cl). s-x. vin.

Blue. atp.
Bright. atp.
Confused. anan. ery. lct. ner. pnx.
Far. myris. smc. sn. thr.
Green. dt. hg. mg-cl. tep.
Grey. atp.
Inverted. eug. glo.
Large. ber. dt. k-o.
Moving. acon. ag-na. al-o. amm-ca. anm. arn. atp. au. ba-ca. ba-cl. ber. bry. ca-ca. ca-o. ca-s. can. cb-a. chd. cic. cl-hx. con. cy-hx. dl-s. dro. dt. ery. eug. euph. euph-c. fe. frm. grt. gua. hg. jnc. k-bicr. k-ca. k-o. kre. lct. lpd. ly-b. lyc. mg-ca. mrl. msc. mtr. na-cl. ner. nic. p. p-x. par. pnx. ppv. pru-l. pso. rho. rn-b. rs. rut. s. s-x. se. sep. si-x. smc. spi. spo. str. tep. thu. til. val. vin. vr-a. vr-s. vtx. wis. zn.
Backwards and Forwards. frm.
Circularly. acon. ag-na. al-o. amm-ca. anm. arn. atp. au. ba-ca. ba-cl. ber. bry. ca-ca. ca-o. ca-s. can. cb-a. chd. cic. cl-hx. con. cy-hx. dl-s. dro. ery. euph. euph-c. fe. grt. gua. hg. jnc. k-bicr. k-ca. k-o. kre. lct. lpd. ly-b. lyc. mg-ca. mrl. msc. mtr. na-cl. ner. nic. p. p-x. par. ppv. pru-l. pso. rho. rn-b. rs. rut. s. s-x. se. sep. si-x. spi. str. tep. thu. val. vin. vr-a. vr-s. vtx. zn.
Vertically. dt. msc. spo.
Downward. dt.
Up and Down. msc. spo.
Vibrating. atp. cic. eug. grt. msc. pnx. s-x. smc. til. wis. zn.
Multiplied. (alm). atp. cic. ery. gel. hyo. kis. ner. nic. pb. spo. vr-v.
Part Visible. li-ca. p. vr-v.
Left half Visible. li-ca.
Red. atp. mg-cl.
Small. cb-v. dt.
Strange. ca-a. dt.
White. atp.
Yellow. k-bicr. tep.
OBJECTS, IMAGINARY. acon. ag. ag-na. al-o. amb. amm-ca. ara. arn. as-o. atp. au. ba-cl. bi-na. bry. ca-ca. ca-s. can. cb-a. cb-v. cch. chd. cmf. con. crb-x. cro. cth. cu. cyc. dig. dph. dt. elaps. ery. glo. hg. hyo. k-bicr. k-ca. k-o. kre. mg-ca. mg-cl. mgs-au. msc. myris. na-ca. na-cl. ner. nic. ol-t. p. pet. pnx. ppv. pru-l. pso. pt. pul. qu-sa.

rhe. s. sb-t. sep. si-x. smc. smi. so-d. spo. sr-ca. srr. str. tep. thr. thu. trg. tx-b. vi-o. vin. vr-v. zn.

Black. acon. dt. elaps. (ery). glo. ol-t. str. thu.

Blue. (dt). pso.

Bright. acon. amm-ca. atp. au. ba-cl. ca-ca. ca-s. chd. con. dig. dph. dt. elaps. ery. hyo. k-ca. msc. ner. nic. p. ppv. qu-sa. s. sb-t. sep. spo. sr-ca. srr. str. tep. thr. trg. tx-b. vi-o. vin.

Circles. p. tx-b. vr-v.

Bright. tx-b.

Moving. tx-b.

Green. vr-v.

Moving. tx-b.

Red. vr-v.

Corpses. as-o. atp. ca-s. cth. na-ca. ppv. smc. str.

Figures. ag-na. amb. as-o. atp. bry. ca-ca. cb-a. cch. cmf. (cu). dt. hg. hyo. k-o. mg-ca. mg-cl. mgs-au. myris. na-ca. ppv. pul. rhe. s. sep. si-x. zn.

Flames. atp. ca-ca. ca-s. s. spo. vin.

Flashes, Bright. elaps. ery. hyo.

Moving from Left to Right. elaps.

Green. vr-v. (zn).

Grey. atp. pnx.

Halo. (zn).

Light. qu-sa.

Mist. acon. ag. atp. bi-na. can. cb-a. cro. cyc. (ery). k-ca. k-o. pet. pru-l. pso. (s). sb-t. smi.

Black. (ery).

Grey. atp.

Red. (ery).

Moving. tx-b.

Noving Circularly. ba-cl. msc.

Moving Downwards. ery.

Moving from Left to Right. elaps.

Red. elaps. (ery). vr-v.

Semicircle. vi-o.

Bright. vi-o.

Spirits. as-o. atp. (cu). dt. hyo. ppv. pt. s. so-d. trg.

Spots. acon. atp. au. chd. dig. dt. elaps. ery. glo. k-ca. ner. nic. ol-t. ppv. qu-sa. sb-t. sep. sr-ca. srr. str. tep. thu. trg.

Black. acon. dt. elaps. glo. ol-t. str. thu.

Bright. acon. atp. au. chd. dig. dt. ery. k-ca. ner. nic. ppv. qu-sa. sb-t. sep. sr-ca. srr. str. tep. trg.

Moving Downwards. ery.
Grey. pnx.
Moving Downwards. ery.
Red. elaps.
White. elaps.
Stars. al-o. na-ca. pso.
Blue. pso.
White. al-o. na-ca.
Veil. as-o. cu. dt. k-bicr. kre. mrl. na-cl. pru-l. thr. vin.
Crooked. (na-cl).
Yellow. k-bicr.
Vibrations. acon. amm-ca. ara. arn. atp. ba-cl. chd. con. crb-x. dph. dt. msc. ner. p. pt. sb-t. sep. thr. trg. vin.
Bright. acon. amm-ca. atp. ba-cl. chd. con. dph. msc. ner. p. sb-t. sep. thr. trg.
Visions. ag-na. as-o. atp. cb-v. dt. ppv. pul. spo. str.
Beautiful. ppv.
Horrible. atp. cb-v. (dt). ppv. pul.
Water. ca-s. hg. sb-t.
Waves. ca-ca.
Light of. ca-ca.
White. al-o. elaps. na-ca.
Yellow. k-bicr.
Zigzags. p. trg.
Bright. p.

PHOTOMANIA. acon. amm-ca. atp. ca-a. ca-ca. dt.

PHOTOPHOBIA. acon. amm-ca. aps. arn. as-o. atp. ba-ca. ca-ca. ca-s. chd. chi. cic. con. crb-x. cro. dig. (dt). euphr. glo. grp. hg. hll. hyo. k-bicr. k-ca. lac-d. lau-c. lyc. mgs-ar. mtr. na-ba. na-ca. p. p-x. pul. qu-sa. rs. s. scu. sep. si-x. str. str-i. thu. trn. zn. zng.

Artificial Light, to. lac-d.

SIGHT DAZZLED. buf. cic. dig. euphr. (na-cl).

SIGHT IMPAIRED. acon. æsc-g. æth. ag. ag-na. aga. al-o. alm. apo. apo-a. art-v. as-o. asc. ast. atp. bi-na. bry. buf. ca-ca. ca-s. can. cap. cau. cb-a. cb-v. chd. chi. cic. cit-c. cl-hx. clv. cof. con. cot. cro. crot. crt. cth. cu. cy-hx. cyc. dig. dl-s. dph. drm. dt. (ery). eryn. evo. fe. fe-a. gel. glo. grp. grt. gym. hg. hg-s. hydr. hyo. ind. irs. jnp-s. k-bicr. k-ca. k-na. k-o. kre. lct. ly-b. lyc. mg-cl. mph. mrl. msc. mtr. myris. n-x. na-ca. na-cl. na-sa. narth. ner. nic. ol-a. ol-t. ox-x. p. p-x. par. pb. pet. phl. phy. pip. pnc. pnx. pol. ppv. pru-l. pt. pul. qu-sa. rph. rs. rs-r. s. s-x.

sa-mgs. sang. sb-t. se. sep. si-x. smc. smi. sn. so-d. spo. srr. str. str-i. tep. til. thr. thu. trg. trn. trx. tx-b. urg. vin. (vr-a). vr-s. vr-v. zn.

Hemeralopia (Night-blindness). vr-a.

Myopia (Short-sightedness). ca-ca. chi. na-cl.

EYEBALL. acon. æsc. æth. ag. ag-na. aga. al-o. alli. (alm). alo. amb. amm-ca. anag. anan. anm. aps. ara. arn. art-v. as-o. asr. ast. atp. ba-a. ba-ca. bap. ber. bi-na. br. bru. bry. buf. c-bis. ca-a. ca-ca. ca-s. cast. cb-a. cb-v. cch. ccs. chi. cic. cis. cit-c. cld. cln. clv. cmc. cmf. cn-sa. co. cof. con. cot. cph. cro. crot. crt. cth. cu. cu-ca. cund. dig. dol. dph. dph-i. dt. elaps. erig. ery. eug. eupat. eupat-p. euph. euphr. evo. f-hx. fe-mgs. gel. glo. gn-l. gss. gym. hg. hg-bicl. hg-bini. hg-i. hg-s. hll. hpm. hum. hur. hyo. hyp. irs. itu. jat. jcr. jnp-s. jug. k-bicr. k-ca. k-i. k-na. k-o. kd-o. kre. lac-cg. lac-d. lau-c. lch. lct. led. li-ca. ly-b. lyc. men. menth. mg-ca. mg-cl. mgs. mgs-ar. morph-a. mrl. msc. mtr. myr. myris. n-x. na-ba. na-ca. na-cl. nic. os. ox-x. p. p-x. pan. pb. phy. physo. pnc. pnx. pod. pol. ppv. pru-l. pso. pt. ptv. pul. rhe. rho. rn-b. rs. rs-r. s. s-x. sa-l. sang. scu. se. sep. si-x. smb. sn. snc. spi. spo. spo-f. sr-ca. stach. str. str-i. thr. thu. trg. trn. tx-b. val. vi-o. vp-t. vr-a. vr-s. woo. zn.

Appearance Astonished. lau-c.

Bright. acon. (ag-na). (alm). atp. bry. cch. cth. dt. eupat. hyo. jat. lch. lyc. morph-a. ppv. trg. trn.

Dim. ara. as-o. bry. buf. (cu). dt. ery. gym. k-ca. ppv. trg.

Glassy. anm. atp. bry. (dt). glo. ppv. rs.

Impudent. (dt).

Spiteful. (dt).

Staring. acon. æth. al-o. amm-ca. anm. arn. as-o. atp. ca-s. chi. cic. cit-c. clv. cof. con. cth. cu. dol. dt. ery. glo. hg. hg-bicl. hyo. hyp. k-ca. k-o. lau-c. lyc. mgs. mgs-ar. msc. mtr. p-x. ppv. pru-l. rs. s. sep. si-x. spi. (spo). str. str-i. vr-a. zn.

Downwards. dt. ery.

Sideways. (dt).

Suspicious. dt.

Upward-looking. jat.

Wild. (alm). cu. cu-ca. dt. hyo. hyp. pb. vp-t.

Boring. bi-na. ca-ca. nic. s.

Bruised. (crt). (cu). (ly-b).

Bursting. acon. hg-s. lac-cg. sep. si-x. stach.

Coldness. (cro). s.

Color Dark. (anm). (as-o). (ca-s). (chi). (clv). (cu). (dl-s). (dt). (ery). (grp). (hg). (k-ca). (lyc). (mtr). (myris). (p). (p-x). (rs). (s). (s-x). (sep). (smc). (sn). (str). (str-i). (trg). (vr-a).

Red. acon. ag. (ag-na). al-o. arn. as-o. atp. bi-na. bry. buf. ca-ca. ca-s. cch. chi. cln. clv. cmf. (con). crot cu. cu-ca. dt. (eupat). (eupat-p). euphr. glo. gym. hg. hg-bini. hg-s. hum. hyo. (ind). k-bicr. kre. led. morph-a. myris. n-x. na-cl. p. (par). pnx. pol. ppv. pul. s. sep. si-x. (spi). (spo-f). str. str-i. trg. vr-a. (vr-s). (zn).

Contractive. (ag). ag-na. (anan). atp. bi-na. elaps. evo. (jnp-s). k-na. na-ba. physo. trg.

Crampy. buf. na-ca. sr-ca.

Creeping. crot.

Cutting. (cund). s.

Discharge. ag-na. (cch). (hg-bicl). (k-i). led. (na-cl).

Fetid. led.

Mucus. ag-na.

Pus. (cch). (hg-bicl). (na-cl).

Thin. (k-i).

Drawing. (acon). aga. (as-o). (atp). (cch). (ccs). (crt). (dph). k-o. kre. (ly-b). nic. p. pod. rho. (s). sr-ca. tx-b (val). (vr-s).

Dryness. myris. ppv.

Eruptions. (ca-ca). euphr. (hg-bicl). (rs). (zn).

Pimples. (rs).

Pterygium. (ca-ca). zn.

Rhagades. (zn).

Ulcers. (ca-ca). euphr. (hg-bicl).

Vesicles. (rs).

False Sensations. ca-s. cmf. (cro). k-na.

Sand. ca-s. cmf.

Stones. k-na.

Wind Cold. (cro).

Gnawing. ox-x. s.

Hæmorrhage. cb-v. (ery).

Hairs, Inverted. (zn).

Heat. (acon). æsc. (alm). amb. ara. asr. bi-na. br. c-bis. ca-ca. (cit-c). cro. crot. ery. eug. gym. hg-bini. hg-s. (hpm). jug. k-bicr. k-ca. k-na. (lau-c). lct. ly-b. mg-cl.

myris. n-x. na-ba. na-ca. (na-cl). (par). ppv. rho. s. s-x. sep. sn. spi. str-i. thu. trn. vr-a. zn.

Heaviness. alli. alo. anan. ast. chi. (cit-c). cmf. cph. (crot). ery. (euph). (frm). hg-s. (hur). jcr. k-bicr. (lac-d). lyc. (physo). pol. ptv. rs-r. s. str-i. thu. (trn). woo.

Itching. ca-ca. cot. (cu). (ly-b). s. sep. trg. (trn). vtx. zn.

Lachrymation. ag-na. alli. aps. asr. atp. ber. br. bru. bry. ca-ca. cb-a. cb-v. ccs. (chi). (con). cro. dt. eug. euph. euphr. fe-mgs. hg. k-bicr. k-ca. k-i. kd-o. kre. lac-d. lct. ly-b. (menth). myris. na-cl. os. p. pnx. ppv. pt. pul. rs-r. s. (sep). si-x. (smi). (spi). spo. str. str-i. trg. trn. tx-b. vr-a. zn.

Hot. bry. euphr. kre. (pul). (spi).

Feeling of. cro. (na-cl).

Movements. (ach). (acon). æth. (ag). (aga). (alm). (alo). (amm-ca). anm. aps. as-o. atp. (bar). (br). bry. buf. (ca-a). ca-ca. (ca-s). (can). (cb-a). (cb-v). (chd). (chi). cic. (cit-c). (cmf). (cof). (cor). (crb-x). cth. cu. (cyc). dig. (dol). dt. (dt-t). (euph). gel. glo. (glp). (hg-bicl). (hg-s). hll. hyo. (hyp). (jnp-s). (k-na). (k-o). kre. (lac-cg). lau-c. (li-ca). (ly-b). (lyc). (mg-ca). (mg-cl). (mg-sa). (msc). (mtr). (myris). (n-x). (na-cl). (na-sa). (ox-x). (p). (p-x). pb. (pet). (phl). (plb). (pnx). (pod). (ppv). (pru-l). (pt). (ptv). (qu-sa). (rs-r). s. (sb-t). (sep). si-x. (smr). (spi). (spo). (srr). (str). (thu). trg. vi-o. (vr-a). (vr-s).

Convulsions. (ach). æth. anm. as-o. atp. (br). bry. buf. (chi). cic. (cit-c). (cmf). cth. cu. dt. (hyo). kre. lau-c. (sep). si-x. trg. vi-o.

Feeling of. ara. glo. trn.

Squinting. æth. (alm). aps. atp. (ca-ca). dig. dt. gel. hll. hyo. (pb). s.

Feeling, of. ca-ca. pod.

Downwards. æth. cb-a.

Upwards. aps. buf. cic. cu. glo. hll.

Inwards. (alm). (ca-ca). (pb).

To the Left. buf.

Motion, in. eug.

Rolling. eug.

Numbness. hur.

Paralysis. (bap). (dt). (gel). (k-o). mg-ca. msc. (ped). (ptv). spi. (trg). (trn).

Pressing. acon. (æth). ag-na. aga. amb. anag. (as-o). asr. ast. atp. bap. ber. br. bry. buf. ca-a. ca-ca. cb-v. (ccs).

cis. (cit-c). cld. cmc. cmf. cn-sa. (con). cph. cro. crot. (crt). ery. (f-hx). glo. gn-l. gym. hg-bini. (hg-s). itu. jcr. (jnp-s). k-bicr. k-ca. (k-na). (k-o). kre. (lch). lct. (ly-b). lyc. men. menth. mg-ca. mgs-ar. mrl. msc. (mtr). (myris). n-x. na-ba. na-ca. na-cl. nic. (p). p-x. (pan). (ped). phy. pol. (pru-l). ppv. (pso). ptv. (pul). (qu-sa). rn-b. rs. s. s-x. (sang). (scu). se. sep. si-x. smb. (smc). spi. (spo). (spo-f). (sr-ca). (str). str-i. thu. trg. val. (zn). (zng).

Like a Plug. asr. (smc).

Projecting. æth. anm. atp. (chi). glo. hyo. myris. ppv. spi. (spo). str-i.

Sensitive. atp. (lac-cg). na-ba. (na-cl). (sep).

Shooting. (acon) anag. (anan). (as-o). (ba-ca). buf. ca-ca. (chd). (cis). cit-c. (cld). cmf. gss. (hg-bini). hpp. (k-bicr). k-ca. (lau-c). na-ca. ox-x. (pan). pnx. (pso). s. (sa-l). se. sep. si-x. snc. (spi). trg. zn.

Cold. sa-l.

Hot. as-o.

Small Feeling. (kre) s.

Smarting. (acon). art-v. (as-o). asr. bap. bry. cast. cit-c. cmc. (co). cro. hg-s. k-bicr. (lac-cg). li-ca. mg-cl. na-ba. ox-x. pso. trn. zn.

Sticky Feeling. elaps.

Strained. dph.

Sunken. as-o. clv. (cu). dt. ery. k-ca. morph-a. rs. spo. vp-t.

Feeling. amb. hg-s. lyc.

Swelling. anm. as-o. (bry). (cch). (clv). (dt). (eupat-p). (hg-bicl). (hyo). (k-ca). (k-i). led. mg-ca. pb. rhe. sep. str-i. trg. (u-na).

Chemosis. euphr.

Œdematous. (bry). (u-na).

Feeling of. ag-na. (cit-c). cro. mg-ca. p-x. pru-l.

Tearing. (ag-na). (anm). (as-o). bi-na. ca-ca. (cb-a). cb-v. (cch). (chd). (con). (cro). (k-ca). (kd-o). led. lyc. na-ba. na-ca. (ni-ca). (os). p. (pnc). pul. (s). sep. smb. (smc). str. zn.

Tensive. ba-a. ba-ca. ber. jnp-s. k-ca. (k-o). mrl. n-x. ox-x. par. s. sep. si-x. trg.

Throbbing. (atp). (ba-a). bry. (cb-a). crb-x. (glo). (myris). (na-cl). p. se. (sn). (thr). (thu). trg.

Tingling. crot.

Undefined. (alo). art-v. atp. (br). bry. cb-v. cit-c. cmf. (co). con. cro. (cu). dph-i. dt. (erig). f-hx. fe-mgs. (frm). (gym). hg-bini. hg-i. hpp. hur. irs. jug. k-i. lac-cg. lac-d.

(li-ca). (men). mg-ca. mgs-ar. myr. n-x. ox-x. pb. pod. (ppv). pul. rs. (s). (sang). sep. si-x. (spi). spo-f. str-i. thr. thu. trg. zn.

Wrinkled. (zn).

Same Symptom. (ach). acon. æsc. ag. ag-na. aga. alli. alo. anag. ara. (as-o). asr. (atp). (ba-a). ba-ca. (ber). bi-na. br. bry. buf. (ca-a). ca-ca. ca-o. cb-a. cb-v. (cch). (ccs). (chd). (cic). cis. cit-c. (cld). cmf. (co). con. crb-x. cro. (crt). (cu). (cund). dt. elaps. eug. fe-mgs. (glo). gn-l. gym. hg-bini. hg-s. hur. irs. itu. jcr. jnp-s. jug. k-bicr. k-ca. k-na. (k-o). kre. lac-d. (lau-c). lct. led. (ly-b). lyc. (men). mg-ca. mrl. msc. myr. n-x. na-ba. na-ca. na-cl. (ni-ca). nic. ox-x. p. phy. physo. (pnc). pnx. pod. ppv. (pso). (pul). (qu-sa). rn-b. s. s-x. (sang). se. sep. si-x. (smc). snc. (spi). sr-ca. stach. str. (str-i). thu. trg. urt. val. (vr-s). woo. zn. (zng).

EYEBALL SUPERIORLY. phy.

Pressing. phy.

EYEBALL EXTERNALLY. rn-b. spo.

Pressing. rn-b.

EYEBALL INTERNALLY. zn.

Color, Red. zn.

EYEBALL POSTERIORLY. co. menth. spo-f.

Pressing. menth. spo-f.

Undefined. co.

Same Symptom. co.

SCLEROTIC. as-o. eupat.

Color, Red. eupat.

Yellow. as-o. eupat.

CORNEA. ca-ca. hg-bicl. lac-cg. rs. s.

Color, Red. s.

White. hg-bicl. s.

Eruptions, Pimples. rs.

Ulcers. ca-ca. hg-bicl.

Vesicles. rs.

Sensitive. lac-cg.

Smarting. lac-cg.

CHAMBERS **of** EYE. hg-bicl.

Discharge, Pus. hg-bicl.

IRIS. æth. (alm). anm. aps. arn. ast. astac. atp. ba-ca. (br). (buf). ca-ca. cap. chi. cic. clv. cmf. crb-x. cro. crt. cu. cy-hx. dph. dt. ery. glo. hll. hyo. hyp. lau-c. lyc. morph. morph-a. msc. mtr. myris. n-x. na-cl. nic. p. pb. pnx. ppv. pru-l. pul. rhe. s. sep. si-x. smc. str. str-i. thu. trg. vr-v. zn.

Color, Discoloured. na-cl.

Pupils Contracted. anm. arn. ast. atp. cap. chi. cic. crb-x. cu. dph. dt. glo. lau-c. morph. msc. mtr. na-cl. p. pul. rhe. s. sep. si-x. smc. str-i. thu. zn.

Dilated. æth. (alm). anm. aps. astac. atp. br. buf. ca-ca. chi. cic. clv. cmf. cro. crt. cy-hx. dt. ery. hll. hyo. hyp. lyc. mgs. morph-a. myris. nic. pb. pnx. ppv. pru-l. rhe. str. vr-v.

Insensible. atp. ba-ca. buf. (cu). dt. hyo. mtr. myris. n-x. ppv. pru-l. trg.

Mobile. atp. mtr.

ORBIT. acon. alo. atp. ba-a. ba-ca. cb-a. cis. cit-c. con. crot. crt. cu. frm. glo. hg-i. hur. kd-o. lau-c. li-ca. lyc. msc. myris. na-cl. nic. os. ped. pol. ppv. pru-l. pul. qu-sa. sep. smc. sn. sr-ca. trg. val. zn.

Bruised. crt. cu.

Drawing. val.

Heaviness. crot. hur.

Pressing. acon. cit-c. crt. msc. na-cl. nic. ped. pol. pru-l. qu-sa. sr-ca.

Shooting. lau-c.

Tearing. cb-a. con. lyc.

Throbbing. cb-a.

Undefined. alo. con. hur. li-ca. trg.

Same Symptom. acon. alo. con. cu. hur. qu-sa. sr-ca.

ORBIT SUPERIORLY. cis. frm. hg-i. kd-o. myris. na-cl. os. sep. smc.

Tearing. kd-o. os.

Pressing. na-cl.

Sensitive. sep.

ORBITAL INTEGUMENTS. anm. as-o. ca-s. cb-a. chi. clv. cu. dl-s. dt. ery. grp. hg. lyc. mtr. myris. ox-x. p. p-x. par. rs. s. s-x. sep. smc. sn. spi. str. str-i. trg. vr-a. vtx.

Color Dark. anm. arn. ca-s. chi. clv. cu. dl-s. dt. ery. grp. hg. lyc. mtr. p. p-x. rs. s. sep. smc. sn. str. str-i. trg. vr-a.

Red. par.

Yellow. spi.

Shooting. as-o.

Hot. as-o.

Smarting. as-o.

Same Symptom. as-o.

ORBITAL, INTEGUMENTS SUPERIORLY. cb-a. ox-x. par. sep. vtx.

Gnawing. ox-x.

Itching. vtx.

Movements, Convulsions. sep.
Downwards-Pressing. cb-a.
Smarting. ox-x.
Tensive. ox-x. par.
ORBITAL INTEGUMENTS INFERIORLY. dt. myris. s-x.
Color, Dark. dt. myris.
EYELIDS. ach. acon. æth. ag. ag-na. alm. alo. amm-ca. anm. aps. atp. bap. bar. br. bry. buf. ca-a. ca-ca. ca-s. can. cb-v. cch. chd. chi. cit-c. clv. cmf. cof. con. cor. cph. crb-x. crot. cu. cyc. dig. dol. dt. dt-t. ery. euph. euphr. frm. glo. glp. grp. hg-bicl. hg-s. hll. hpm. hyo. hyp. ind. jnp-s. k-bicr. k-ca. k-na. k-o. kre. lac-cg. lac-d. lau-c. led. li-ca. ly-b. lyc. mg-ca. mg-cl. mg-sa. msc. mtr. myris. n-x. na-cl. na-sa. ox-x. p. p-x. par. pb. pet. phl. physo. plb. pnx. pod. ppv. pru-l. pt. ptv. qu-sa. rs-r. s. sb-t. sep. smr. spi. spo. srr. str. thu. trg. trn. u-na. vr-a. vr-s. zn.
Adhesion. ca-ca. (con). k-ca. led.
Color, Dark. clv. k-ca.
Red. par.
Discharge Fetid. led.
Drawing. acon.
Hæmorrhage. (ery).
Hairs, Inverted. zn.
Heat. lau-c. par.
Itching. (cu). trn.
Movements, Closing. acon. æth. ag. aga. alm. alo. amm-ca. anm. aps. atp. bar. (br). bry. (buf). ca-a. (ca-ca). ca-s. can. cb-v. chd. cor. crb-x. cu. cyc. (dig). (dt). euph. glo. glp. (hg-bicl). hg-s. hll. hyo. (hyp). jnp-s. k-na. k-o. kre. lac-cg. lau-c. li-ca. ly-b. lyc. mg-ca. mg-cl. mg-sa. msc. myris. n-x. na-cl. (na-sa). ox-x. p. p-x. pb. pet. phl. plb. pnx. pod. ppv. pt. ptv. qu-sa. rs-r. s. sb-t. sep. smr. spi. spo. srr. str. thu. vr-a. vr-s.
Spasmodically. br. ca-ca. cyc. hg-bicl. (hyp). myris. spo.
Convulsions. ach. (chi). cmf. cu. hyo. kre.
Opening Wide. (alm). buf. cit-c. cof. dol. dt. dt-t. lyc. mtr. pb. ppv. pru-l. vr-a.
Upwards Drawn. acon. lyc.
Winking. aga. myris.
Paralysis. Opening Difficult. bap. gel. mg-ca. ped. ptv. trg. trn.
Pressing. æth. msc.
Shooting. acon. k-bicr.

Small Feeling. kre.
Smarting. acon. trn.
Swelling. clv. hg-bicl. hyo. k-i.
Tensive. n-x.
Same Symptom. ach.
UPPER EYELID. cit-c. cph. crot. ery. euph. frm. hg-s. jnp-s. k-ca. lac-d. p. ptv. trn. zn.
Heaviness. cit-c. cph. crot. ery. euph. frm. hg-s. lac-d. ptv. trn.
Pressing. p.
Swelling. k-ca.
LOWER EYELID. bry. cch. grp. u-na.
Swelling. bry. u-na.
Œdematous. bry.
TARSAL EDGES. euphr. hpm. vr-s.
Color Red. euphr. vr-s.
Eruptions, Ulcers. euphr.
Heat. hpm.
EYELIDS, INNER SURFACE. cch. ind. k-bicr. zn.
Color Red. ind. k-bicr.
Wrinkled. zn.
CANTHI. anan. co. k-i. na-cl. ppv. zn.
Discharge. na-cl.
Pus. na-cl.
EXTERNAL CANTHUS. co. zn.
Eruptions, Rhagades. zn.
Smarting. zn.
INTERNAL CANTHUS. anan. k-i. ppv.
Contractive. anan.
Discharge. k-i.
Thin. k-i.
Shooting. anan.
Swelling. k-i.
Undefined. k-i.
CARUNCULA LACHRYMALIS. ca-ca.
LEFT **then** RIGHT. zn.
Eyeball, Eruption, Pterygium. zn.
FORWARDS. acon. anm. atp. br. cb-v. glo. gym. k-na. lch. mgs-ar. mtr. na-ca. na-cl. p. pan. pso. pul. rn-b. rs. sang. scu. sep. si-x. snc. str. str-i. val. zng.
Eyeball, Pressing. acon. atp. br. glo. gym. k-na. lch. mgs-ar. mtr. na-cl. p. pso. pul. rn-b. rs. sang. scu. sep. si-x. str. val.

Like a Plug. asr.
Shooting. na-ca. snc.
Tearing. anm. cb-v.
Orbit Superiorly, Pressing. na-cl.
BACKWARDS. acon. dph. hg-s. ly-b. s.
Eyeball, Drawing. dph. ly-b. s.
Pressing. acon. hg-s.
UPWARDS, vr-s.
DOWNWARDS. atp. s.
Eyeball, Pressing. s.
To BACK. trg.
To NAPE. trg.
Eyeball, Tensive like a Thread. trg.
RIGHT. (alm). as-o. atp. ber. buf. ca-a. ca-ca. ccs. cis. cit-c. cld. cmf. con. cro. crt. dig. dt. erig. f-hx. hyp. k-bicr. k-o. ly-b. menth. mg-cl. na-cl. ner. pb. pnc. ppv. pso. pul. s-x. smc. sn. spi. spo-f. str-i. thr. thu. trg. vr-s. zn. zng.
Objects Imaginary, Veil Crooked. na-cl.
Photophobia. str-i.
Sight Impaired. cro. k-bicr. ner.
Eyeball Bruised. ly-b.
Coldness. cro.
Color Red. as-o. con. spo-f.
Drawing. as-o. ccs. crt. vr-s.
False Sensations, Wind Cold. cro.
Heat. ly-b. thu.
Itching. ly-b. trg.
Lachrymation. con. menth.
Hot. pul.
Feeling of. na-cl.
Movements, Squinting. (alm). pb.
Inwards. (alm). pb.
Paralysis. (k-o).
Pressing. as-o. atp. ber. ca-a. ccs. cmf. con. f-hx. k-o. pul. spi. str-i. thu. trg. zn.
Shooting. ca-ca. cld. pso.
Tearing. as-o. cro. pnc.
Tensive. k-o.
Throbbing. atp. thr. thu. trg.
Undefined. erig. f-hx. str-i.
Same Symptom. as-o. atp. ber. ca-a. ca-ca. ccs. cld. cro. k-o. ly-b. pnc. pso. pul. spi. str-i. vr-s.

Eyeball Internally, Color Red. zn.
Swelling. zn.
Eyeball Posteriorly, Undefined. spo-f.
Orbit, Drawing. atp.
Pressing. pul.
Tearing. zn.
Throbbing. sn. trg.
Same Symptom. atp. ppv. trg.
Orbit Superiorly, Heat. na-cl.
Pressing like a Plug. smc.
Sensitive. na-cl.
Shooting. cis.
Throbbing. na-cl.
Orbital Integuments, Color Red. dt.
Swelling. dt.
Orbital Integuments Inferiorly, Color Dark. s-x.
Eyelids, Adhesion of. con.
Movements, Closing. ca-a. dig. mg-cl.
Spasmodically. hyp.
Open Wide. buf.
Upper Eyelid, Heat. na-cl.
Movements, Convulsions. cit-c.
Hangs Down. na-cl.
Tearing. zn.
Internal Canthus, Pressing. ppv.
Same Symptom. ppv.
Caruncula Lachymalis, Swelling. ca-ca.
Forwards. Eyeball, Pressing. str-i. zng.
Upwards. Eyeball, Drawing. vr-s.
Downwards. Orbit, Drawing. atp.
LEFT. acon. ag-na. ba-a. ba-ca. br. buf. ca-ca. cch. ccs. chd. cit-c. co. cund. euph. frm. glo. grp. gym. hg-bini. hg-i. jnp-s. k-ca. lac-cg. ly-b. men. myris. na-cl. na-sa. ni-ca. nic. pan. ppv. s. sang. sep. smc. spi. spo. str-i. thu. trg. zn. zng.
Objects, False Appearance of, Dark. na-cl.
Objects Imaginary, Green. zn.
Halo. zn.
Green. zn.
Mist. s.
Sight Dazzled. na-cl.
Sight Impaired. ca-ca. ly-b. na-cl.
Eyeball Appears Bright. ag-na.
Boring. s.

Color Red. ag-na. glo. spi.
Contractive. ag. jnp-s.
Cutting. cund. s.
Drawing. cch. nic.
Eruptions, Pterygium. ca-ca.
Gnawing. s.
Heat. acon. k-ca. s.
Lachrymation. ag-na. euph. k-ca. ly-b. (sep). spi. trg.
Hot. spi.
Movements, Convulsions. trg.
Squinting. ca-ca.
Inwards. ca-ca.
Pressing. acon. ccs. cit-c. hg-bini. ly-b. pan. s. spi. str-i. zng.
Shooting. hg-bini. s. spi.
Tearing. ag-na. cch. chd. k-ca. ni-ca. s. smc.
Throbbing. na-cl.
Undefined. br. cit-c. hg-bini. gym. lac-cg. men. ppv. sang. spi.
Same Symptom. acon. ag-na. ba-a. br. cch. ccs. chd. cit-c. cund. glo. gym. hg-bini. ly-b. men. na-cl. ni-ca. nic. ppv. s. sang. smc. spi. str-i. zng.
Eyeball Externally, Pressing. spo.
Orbit, Heat. cit-c.
Pressing. cit-c.
Shooting. ba-ca.
Swelling, Feeling of. cit-c.
Throbbing. ba-a. glo.
Same Symptom. ba-ca. glo.
Orbit Superiorly, Pressing. myris.
Throbbing. myris.
Undefined. frm. hg-i.
Eyelids, Movements, Closing. buf. euph. na-sa. thu.
Convulsions. trg.
Upper Eyelid, Pressing. jnp-s.
Lower Eyelid, Movements, Hangs Down. grp.
Swelling. cch.
Eyelids Inner Surface, Discharge. cch.
Pus. cch.
External Canthus, Smarting. co.
Forwards. Eyeball, Shooting. pan.

After HEAD Symptoms.

anag. anm. ba-ca. ber. bry. cb-v. con. (cu). dt. frm-s. gel. hyp. k-bicr. k-o. mg-ca. p. rhe. si-x. str-i. thu. trg.

OBJECTS IMAGINARY. p. trg.
Vibrations. p. trg.
Zigzags. trg.
PHOTOMANIA. gel.
SIGHT IMPAIRED. con. dt. frm-s. gel. k-bicr. k-o. p. si-x.
EYEBALL. anag. anm. ba-ca. ber. bry. cb-v. con. hyp. str-i.
Appearance Staring. hyp.
Wild, hyp.
Heat. str-i.
Heaviness. str-i.
Itching. (p).
Lacrymation. (ba-ca). cb-v.
Movements. (ba-ca). cb-v.
Paralysis. (cu).
Pressing. anag. (ba-ca). ber. bry.
Shooting. anag.
Swelling. anm.
Tensive. ber.
Throbbing. (thu).
Undefined. con.
LENS. mg-ca.
Cataract. mg-ca.
IRIS. dt. hyp. rhe.
Pupils Dilated. dt. hyp. rhe.
EYELIDS. ba-ca. cb-v. (cu). hyp. p.
Itching. p.
Movements Closing. (ba-ca). cb-v. (hyp.)
Spasmodically. (hyp).
Paralysis. (cu).
RIGHT. hyp. thu.
Eyeball, Throbbing. thu.
Eyelids, Movements, Closing Spasmodically. hyp.
LEFT. ba-ca.
Eyeball, Lacrymation. ba-ca.
Pressing. ba-ca.
Eyelids, Movements, Closing. ba-ca.

DARKNESS or DUSK.

acon. ag-na. al-o. amm-cl. atp. ba-ca. ca-ca. cb-v. cd-sa. chd. cund. dig. dl-s. dt. ery. fe-mgs. hg. hyo. lyc. myris. na-cl. p. pul. rut. s-x. sr-ca. thu. val. vr-a.

OBJECTS, FALSE APPEARANCE **of**. myris.

Closer Together. myris.

Far, Too. myris.

Oblique. myris.

OBJECTS IMAGINARY. acon. ag-na. al-o. ba-ca. ca-ca. cb-v. cund. dig. dl-s. dt. ery. fe-mgs. lyc. p. sr-ca. thu. val.

Blue. (cund). dt. fe-mgs.

Bright. ag-na. al-o. ba-ca. ca-ca. dl-s. dt. ery. fe-mgs. lyc. p. thu. val.

Circles. fe-mgs.

  Blue. fe-mgs.

  Bright. fe-mgs.

  Red. fe-mgs.

  Zigzags. fe-mgs.

Flames. ag-na. dl-s.

Flashes, Bright. ag-na. dt. ery. thu.

Green. dt. sr-ca.

Light. al-o. val.

Mist. (ag-na).

Moving with Eye. dt.

Pyriform Body. (cund).

  Blue. (cund).

Red. fe-mgs.

Spots. ba-ca. ca-ca. dt. lyc. p. sr-ca. thu.

  Blue. dt.

  Bright. ba-ca. ca-ca. dt. lyc. p. thu.

  Green. sr-ca.

  White. sr-ca.

Stripes. dt.

  Blue. dt.

    Moving with Eye. dt.

    Vertical. dt.

  Green. dt.

    Moving with Eye. dt.

    Vertical. dt.

  Moving with Eye. dt.

  Vertical. dt.

Vertical. dt.
Vibrations. dig.
  Bright. dig.
Visions. cb-v. p.
  Horrible. cb-v.
White. sr-ca.
Zigzags. fe-mgs.
SIGHT IMPAIRED. ag-na. amm-cl. atp. cd-sa. chd. dig. (dt). fe-mgs. grp. hg. hyo. rut. srr. vr-a.
EYEBALL. al-o. amm-cl. na-cl. s-x.
Heat. amm-cl. s-x.
Lachrymation. s-x.
Movements. (ba-ca). (na-cl).
Paralysis. (na-cl).
Pressing. al-o. na-cl.
Smarting. (lyc).
EYELIDS. ba-ca. na-cl.
Closing. ba-ca. na-cl.
  Spasmodically. ba-ca. na-cl.
Paralysis. na-cl.
CANTHI. lyc.
EXTERNAL CANTHUS. lyc.
Smarting. lyc.
RIGHT. cund.
Objects Imaginary, Blue. cund.
  Pyriform Body. cund.
    Blue. cund.
LEFT. ag-na. dt.
Objects Imaginary, Blue. dt.
  Bright. dt.
  Mist. ag-na.
  Spots. dt.
    Blue. dt.
    Bright. dt.

LIGHT, **Artificial**.

(alm) alo. amph. art-v. as-o. asc. ber. ca-ca. ca-o. ca-pa. ca-s. cb-v. chd. chi. cmc. con. cor. cph. cro. dl-s. dph. dro. dt. ele. gel. grp. hg. i. k-ca. krm. lac-d. lo-c. lyc. mg-cl. mg-sa. mn-ca. mrl. myris. n-x. na-ba. na-sa. ni-ca. ol-a. p. p-**x**. pb. pet. phy. pol. pru-l. pt. pul. rs-r. rut. s. sb-t. sep. si-**x**. smi. srr. stach. str-i. thu. til. trg.

OBJECTS, FALSE APPEARANCE **of.** ele. hg. lyc. mrl. smi. til.

Confused. ele. hg. mrl. til.

Moving. lyc.

Vibrating. lyc.

Red. smi.

OBJECTS, IMAGINARY. ber. cb-a. chi. cro. dt. krm. mn-ca. n-x. na-sa. p-x. sep. srr. til.

Black. cb-a. dt. mn-ca.

Blue. dt.

Bright. chi. dt. (na-sa). p-x. srr. til.

Circles. mn-ca.

Black. mn-ca.

Cobwebs. n-x.

Light. chi.

Red. chi.

Yellow. chi.

Mist. (na-sa). sep.

Moving with Eye. dt.

Near Eye. (na-sa).

Red. chi.

Spots. cb-a. dt. krm. srr.

Black. cb-a. dt.

Moving with Eye. dt.

Symmetrical, Lines in. cb-a.

Blue. dt.

Bright. dt. srr.

Moving with Eye. dt.

Symmetrical Lines in. cb-a.

White. krm.

Yellow. cb-a.

Symmetrical Lines in. cb-a.

Stars. (na-sa).

Bright. (na-sa).

Near Eye. (na-sa).

Green. (na-sa).

Near Eye. (na-sa).

Near Eye. (na-sa).

Yellow. (na-sa).

Near Eye. (na-sa).

Veil. ber. cro.

Vibrations. (dt). p-x. til.

Bright. (dt). p-x. til.

White. krm.
Yellow. cb-a.
SIGHT DAZZLED. cph. hg. p.
SIGHT IMPAIRED. ber. cro. myris. na-sa. rs-r. sep.
EYEBALL. alo. amph. art-v. asc. ca-ca. ca-o. ca-pa. cb-a. chd. cmc. con. cor. cph. cro. dro. dt. gel. grp. hg. i. lac-d. lo-c. lyc. mg-cl. mg-sa. mn-ca. mrl. na-ba. na-sa. ni-ca. ol-a. p. p-x. pet. pol. pru-l. pt. pul. rut. s. sb-t. sep. smi. stach. str-i. thu.
Appearance Dim. lyc.
Bursting. pol. stach.
Color Red. sb-t.
Contractive. sep.
Cutting. ca-ca.
Dryness. (art-v). cro. mg-cl. pru-l.
Eruptions. sb-t.
Blisters. sb-t.
False Sensations. art-v.
Sand. art-v.
Heat. (art-v). ca-o. cor. cro. grp. mg-cl. mg-sa. ni-ca. ol-a. p-x. pru-l. rut. thu.
Heaviness. (na-sa).
Lachrymation. cmc.
Movements. (ber). (cro). (mrl).
Convulsions. (ber).
Pressing. (alo). (art-v). cb-a. cro. mn-ca. na-sa. pet. pol. smi. str-i.
Sensitive. (na-sa).
Shooting. amph. ca-ca. lyc. (na-sa). pul. s. sep.
Smarting. (cro). lyc. p-x. (phy).
Softness, Feeling of. (na-sa).
Undefined. amph. art-v. asc. ca-ca. ca-pa. chd. cmc. con. cph. dro. dt. gel. hg. i. lac-d. lo-c. lyc. mrl. na-ba. p. pt. s.
IRIS. (alm). pb.
Pupils Dilated. (alm). pb.
ORBIT. na-sa.
ORBIT INFERIORLY. na-sa.
ORBITAL INTEGUMENTS. chd.
EYELIDS. art-v. as-o. ber. ca-ca. cro. mrl. na-sa. p-x. srr.
Cutting. ca-ca.
Dryness. art-v. as-o.
Heat. art-v. p-x.

Movements, Closing. srr.
Convulsions. ber.
Winking. cro. mrl.
Pressing. art-v.
Smarting. cro.
UPPER EYELID. na-sa.
Heaviness. na-sa.
CANTHI. art-v. p-x. phy.
Heat. p-x.
INTERNAL CANTHUS. art-v. phy.
Heat. art-v.
Smarting. phy.
FORWARDS. cmc. pol.
Eyeball, Pressing. cmc. pol.
BACKWARDS. na-sa.
DOWNWARDS. cmc.
Eyeball, Pressing. cmc.
To HEAD. cmc.
To OCCIPUT. cmc.
Eyeball Posteriorly, Undefined. cmc.
CHANGING CHARACTER **or** PLACE. na-sa.
Objects Imaginary, Mist, then Star Bright Green Yellow Near Eye. (na-sa).
Eyeball, Sensitive then Pressing. (na-sa).
,, **Shooting then** ,, (na-sa).
,, **Softness, Feeling of, then** ,, (na-sa).
OBJECTS IMAGINARY, **then** EYEBALL. na-sa.
SIGHT IMPAIRED **then** OBJECTS IMAGINARY. na-sa.
RIGHT. alo. chd. na-sa.
Objects Imaginary, Bright. na-sa.
Green. na-sa.
Mist. na-sa.
Near Eye. na-sa.
Star. na-sa.
Bright. na-sa.
Near Eye. na-sa.
Green. na-sa.
Near Eye. na-sa.
Near Eye. na-sa.
Yellow. na-sa.
Near Eye. na-sa.
Yellow. na-sa.

Sight Impaired. na-sa.
Eyeball, Pressing. alo. na-sa.
Orbit Inferiorly, Pressing. na-sa.
Sensitive. na-sa.
Shooting. na-sa.
Softness, Feeling of. na-sa.
Backwards. Orbit Inferiorly, Shooting. na-sa.
Changing. Objects Imaginary, Mist, then Star Bright Green Yellow Near Eye. na-sa.
Orbit Inferiorly, Sensitive then Pressing. na-sa.
„ **Shooting then** „ na-sa.
„ **Softness, Feeling of then** „ na-sa.
Objects Imaginary then Eyeball, Star Bright Green Yellow Near Eye then Pressing. na-sa.
Sight Impaired then Objects Imaginary, Star Bright Green Yellow Near Eye. na-sa.
LEFT. dt.
Objects Imaginary, Blue. dt.
Bright. dt.
Spots. dt.
Blue. dt.
Vibrations. dt.
Bright. dt.

LIGHT, Natural.

acon. æth. ag-na. aga. al-o. alli. alo. amm-ca. amm-cl. amph. anan. aps. arn. art-v. arum-t. as-o. ast. atp. ba-ca. ber. br. bry. buf. ca-ca. (ca-i). ca-o. ca-pa. ca-s. cast. cb-a. cch. chd. chi. chio. cic. cl-hx. cle. cmc. co. cof. con. cop. crb-x. cro. crv. cu-a. cund. dig. dl-s. drm. dro. dt. elaps. ery. eryn. eug. eupat. euphr. fe-mgs. gel. grc. grp. hg. hg-bicl. hg-bini. hll. hyo. irs-f. k-bicr. k-ca. k-i. k-na. k-o. kre. lac-d. lac-f. lau-c. lct. li-ca. lo-c. lyc. mg-ca. mg-cl. mg-sa. mgs-ar. mgs-au. mn-ca. mrl. mtr. myris. n-x. na-ba. na-ca. na-cl. na-sa. nic. ol-a. p. p-x. pb. pet. phl. phy. pnx. pol. pru-l. pso. pul. qu-sa. rho. rs. rs-r. rs-v. s. s-x. sa-l. sb-s. sb-t. scu. sep. si-x. smb. smc. smi. sn. so-d. spi. srr. str. str-i. thr. thu. trn. trx. u-na. vr-a. vr-s. vtx. woo. ziz. zn. zng.
OBJECTS, FALSE APPEARANCE **of.** thr.
Multiplied. thr.
OBJECTS IMAGINARY. alo. con. cund. dt. (ery). fe-mgs. k-ca. qu-sa. s. sb-t. sep. so-d. thr. thu.

Black. dt. k-ca. (s). thu.
Blue. dt. fe-mgs.
Bright. dt. fe-mgs. (qu-sa). sb-t. sep. so-d. thr.
Circle. fe-mgs.
  Blue. fe-mgs.
  Bright. fe-mgs.
  Red. fe-mgs.
  Zigzags. fe-mgs.
Flames. so-d.
Flashes Bright. sb-t.
Halo. con.
  Variegated. con.
High up. dt.
Pyriform Body. (cund).
  Red. (cund).
Rain. thu.
Red. (cund). fe-mgs.
Semicircle. dt.
  Bright. dt.
    High Up. dt.
  High Up. dt.
Spots. amm-cl. dt. k-ca. (qu-sa). s. thu.
  Black. dt. k-ca. (s). thu.
  Blue. dt.
  Bright. dt. (qu-sa).
  White. s. thu.
  Yellow. amm-cl.
Stripes. dt.
  Bright. dt.
    Upwards to Right. dt.
    Vertical. dt.
  Upwards to Right. dt.
  Vertical. dt.
Threads. (ery).
Upwards to Right. dt.
Variegated. con.
Vertical. dt.
Veil. k-ca.
Vibrations. alo. (dt). sep. thr.
  Bright. (dt). sep. thr.
White. s. thu.
Yellow. amm-cl.
Zigzags. fe-mgs.
SIGHT DAZZLED. dt. euph. mrl. p. sa-l. sep.

SIGHT IMPAIRED. atp. con. dt. eug. fe-mgs. grp. k-ca. k-o. myris. p. s. sb-s. si-x. trn. vr-a.

EYEBALL. acon. æth. ag-na. aga. al-o. (alli). amm-ca. amm-cl. anan. aps. arn. art-v. arum-t. as-o. ast. atp. au. ba-ca. ber. br. bry. buf. ca-ca. (ca-i). ca-o. ca-pa. ca-s. cast. cb-a. cch. (chd). chi. chio. cic. cl-hx. cle. clv. cmc. co. cof. con. cop. cro. crv. cu-a. dig. dl-s. drm. dro. dt. elaps. ery. eryn. eug. eupat. euphr. gel. grc. grp. hg. hg-bicl. hg-bini. hll. hyo. irs-f. k-bicr. k-ca. k-i. k-na. k-o. kre. lac-d. lac-f. lau-c. (led). li-ca. lo-c. lyc. mg-ca. mg-cl. mg-sa. mgs-ar. mgs-au. mn-ca. mrl. mtr. myris. n-x. na-ba. na-ca. na-cl. na-sa. nic. ol-a. p. p-x. pb. pet. phl. phy. pnx. pol. pru-l. pso. pul. qu-sa. rho. rs. rs-r. rs-v. s. s-x. sa-l. sb-s. sb-t. scu. sep. si-x. smc. smi. spi. srr. str. str-i. thr. thu. trn. trx. (u-na). vr-s. vtx. woo. ziz. zn. zng.

Color Red. eryn. sb-t.

Dryness. (mn-ca). rho.

Eruptions. sb-t.

Blisters. sb-t.

Heat. (chd). dl-s. eryn. (k-bicr). kre. mg-ca. mg-cl. rho.

Heaviness. (lyc).

Itching. anan.

Lachrymation. al-o. bry. dig. dl-s. dt. eug. grp. k-bicr. kre. lyc. mg-cl. qu-sa. s-x. (str-i). vr-s. zn.

Hot. al-o. dig. dl-s. str-i.

Movements. (as-o). eryn. (k-bicr). (mrl).

Convulsions. (k-bicr).

Squinting. eryn.

Paralysis. ast. lyc.

Pressing. mg-cl. phy. (pul). s. sep. (str).

Shooting. co. euphr. grp. pul. s. thu.

Smarting. as-o. (chd). co. dl-s. eryn. grp.

Undefined. (Photophobia). as-o. æth. ag-na. aga. al-o. (alli). amm-ca. amm-cl. anan. aps. arn. art-v. arum-t. as-o. ast. atp. au. ba-ca. ber. br. bry. buf. ca-ca. (ca-i). ca-o. ca-pa. ca-s. cast. cb-a. cch. chi. chio. cic. cl-hx. cle. clv. cmc. co. cof. con. cop. cro. crv. cu-a. dig. dl-s. drm. dro. dt. elaps. ery. eupat. euphr. gel. grc. grp. hg. hg-bicl. hg-bini. hll. hyo. irs-f. k-bicr. k-ca. k-i. k-na. k-o. kre. lac-d. lac-f. lau-c. (led). li-ca. lo-c. lyc. mg-ca. mg-cl. mg-sa. mgs-ar. mgs-au. mn-ca. mrl. mtr. myris. n-x. na-ba. na-ca. na-cl. na-sa. nic. ol-a. p. p-x. pb. pet. phl. phy. pnx. pol. pru-l. pso. pul. rs. rs-r. rs-v. s. s-x. sa-l. sb-s. scu. sep. si-x. smc. smi. spi. srr. str. str-i. thr. thu. trn. trx. (u-na). vtx. woo. ziz. zn. zng.

EYELIDS. as-o. k-bicr. lyc. mn-ca. mrl. (myris). s. sa-l.
Dryness. mn-ca.
Heat. k-bicr.
Movements, Closing. (as-o). sa-l.
Spasmodically. as-o.
Convulsions. k-bicr.
Winking. mrl. (myris).
Pressing. s.
UPPER EYELID. lyc.
Heaviness. lyc.
RIGHT. aps. atp. cund. (hg-bini). lac-f. str-i.
Objects Imaginary, Pyriform Body. cund.
Red. cund.
Red. cund.
Eyeball Undefined. aps. atp. (hg-bini). lac-f. str-i.
LEFT. al-o. alli. as-o. atp. dt. led. s. u-na.
Objects Imaginary, Black. s.
Blue. dt.
Bright. dt.
Spots. dt. s.
Black. s.
Blue. dt.
Bright. dt.
Vibrations. dt.
Bright. dt.
Sight Impaired. atp.
Eyeball, Lacrymation. alo.
Undefined. alli. as-o. led. u-na.

CHANGE of LIGHT.

dt.
EYEBALL. dt.
Pressing. (dt).
EYEBALL INTERIORLY. dt.
Pressing. dt.

During LIGHTNING Flash.

rn-b.
OBJECTS IMAGINARY. rn-b.
Rope across Sky. rn-b.

READING.

ach. ag-na. aga. al-o. amm-ca. anan. anm. aps. ara. art-v. as. as-o. asr. atp. atrop. bar. ber. br. bry. c-bis. ca-ca. ca-o. ca-pa. ca-s. cb-v. cd-sa. chd. chi. cic. cmc. co. cof. con. cot. cro. crt. cth. cund. cyc. dl-s. dph. drm. dro. dt. ery. glo. glp. gn-c. grp. grt. hæm. hg. hrc. hur. hyo. i. jnp-s. k-ca. k-i. k-o. klm. kre. lac-c. lac-d. lac-f. lch. li-ca. lpd. lyc. men. mg-ca. mg-cl. mgs-ar. mn-ca. mph. mrl. myris. n-x. na-ca. na-cl. na-sa. narth. ner. nic. p. p-x. pet. phy. pnx. pol. pul. rho. rmx. rs-v. rut. s. s-x. sb-t. sep. si-x. smi. so-d. sr-ca. stach. str-i. thu. trg. val. vi-o. vin. vtx. zn.

OBJECTS, FALSE APPEARANCE **of**. aga. anm. atp. atrop. bry. chd. chi. co. cro. cund. dro. dt. ery. glo. gn-c. grp. hg. hyo. jnp-s. lac-c. li-ca. lyc. na-cl. pb. pnx. pol. sb-t. si-x. smi. thu. trg. vi-o.

Black. hg. thu.

Blue. atp.

Confused. anm. atp. atrop. bry. chd. chi. co. (cund). dro. dt. ery. glo. grp. hæm. hg. hyo. jnp-s. k-o. lyc. na-cl. pnx. pol. si-x. trg. vi-o.

Green. lac-c.

Grey. dt.

Large. atp.

Moving. aga. atp. cic. con. dt. hg. hyo. k-o.

Vertically. con.

Vibrating. atp. k-o.

Multiplied. dt. sb-t.

Horizontally. sb-t.

Part Visible. lac-c. li-ca. pb.

Vertical. pb.

Red. cro. lac-c. smi.

Small. glo.

Variegated. atp. cic. lac-c.

White. chi. dro. ery. si-x.

Yellow. atp. lac-c.

OBJECTS, IMAGINARY. ag-na. ca-ca. ca-pa. cd-sa. chi. cic. cot. cro. dl-s. dro. dt. ery. gn-c. grt. hæm. k-ca. k-o. lac-c. lch. mg-cl. mph. n-x. na-ca. p-x. pet. pol. rmx. sb-t. sr-ca. trg. vin.

Black. ca-ca. ca-pa. ery. k-ca. sb-t. trg.

Bright. dl-s. dt. sb-t.

Circles. k-ca.
Cobweb. k-ca.
Figures. ca-pa.
Moving from Right to Left. ca-pa.
Flashes, Bright. dl-s. sb-t.
Green. lac-c. n-x. sr-ca.
Grey. (ca-pa). lch.
Halo. chi. cic.
Variegated. cic.
White. chi.
High up. mg-cl.
Mist. (ag-na). cd-sa. cro. dro. gn-c. grt. hæm. k-ca. k-o. mg-cl. mph. na-ca. p-x. pet. pol. rmx. vin.
Moving from Right to Left. ca-pa.
Red. cot. lac-c.
Rocks, High up. mg-cl.
Spots. ca-ca. ca-pa. cot. dt. ery. k-ca. lac-c. lch. n-x.
Black. ca-ca. ca-pa. ery. k-ca.
Bright. dt.
Green. lac-c. n-x.
Grey. ca-pa. (lch).
Red. cot. lac-c.
White. ery.
Yellow. cot. lac-c. lch.
Variegated. cic.
Veil. dro. gn-c.
Vibrations. dt. p-x. pol. trg.
Black. trg.
Bright. dt.
Waves. sr-ca.
Green. sr-ca.
White. chi. ery.
Yellow. cot. lac-c. lch.
PHOTOPHOBIA. (lac-f).
SIGHT DAZZLED. pol.
SIGHT IMPAIRED. ag-na. aga. art-v. asr. br. bry. ca-ca. ca-s. cd-sa. chd. cro. crt. dph. dro. dt. glo. gn-c. grt. hæm. hur. i. k-ca. k-i. k-o. lac-f. lch. li-ca. men. mg-ca. mph. myris. n-x. na-ca. na-cl. p. p-x. pet. pol. rho. rmx. rs-v. s. sep. smi. str-i. thu. vin.
Myopia. p-x.
Presbyopia. rmx.
EYEBALL. ach. aga. al-o. amm-ca. aps. ara. art-v. as.

asr. bar. c-bis. ca-ca. ca-o. cmc. con. cro. cyc. dph. ery. grp. grt. hrc. k-ca. k-i. lac-c. lac-f. li-ca. lpd. mn-ca. mrl. n-x. na-ca. na-sa. ner. nic. p. pet. phy. pol. pul. rho. rs-v. rut. s. s-x. sep. smi. so-d. stach. thu. vtx.

Bursting. asr. stach.

Color, Red. (lac-f).

Contractive. sep.

Cutting. ca-ca. pet.

Drawing. art-v.

Dryness. art-v. (as-o). bar. (grp). li-ca. na-ca. p.

False Sensations. pul.

Sand. pul.

Gnawing. (str-i).

Heat. bar. ca-ca. ca-o. cro. cyc. (grp). na-ca. ner. nic. pol. rho. rut. s. s-x. thu. vtx. (zn).

Heaviness. (na-sa).

Lachrymation. amm-ca. c-bis. cro. grt. hrc. (lac-f). lpd. n-x. ner. p. s-x..

Movements. (aga). (ber). (ca-ca). (cro). (lac-d). (mrl).

Convulsions. (aga). (ber). (lac-d).

Feeling of. ara.

Paralysis. asr. k-i.

Pressing. ach. (aga). (al-o). con. cro. mn-ca. na-sa. pul. smi. zn.

Shooting. ach. aps. k-ca.

Smarting. (ca-ca). cro. (li-ca). p. (s-x). (sep). (str-i).

Stiffness. ca-ca.

Tensive. ca-ca. ner.

Throbbing. (lac-f).

Undefined. art-v. as-o. (chd). dph. ery. lac-c. (lac-d). li-ca. phy. rs-v. rut.

ORBITAL INTEGUMENTS. chd.

EYELIDS. as-o. ber. ca-ca. cro. grp. mrl. na-sa. ner. str-i. zn.

Cutting. ca-ca.

Dryness. as-o. grp.

Heat. ca-ca. grp.

Movements, Convulsions. ber.

Winking. ca-ca. cro. mrl.

Smarting. ca-ca.

UPPER EYELID. na-sa. zn.

Heaviness. na-sa.

TARSAL EDGES. li-ca. str.

Gnawing. str-i.
Smarting. li-ca. str-i.
CANTHI. lac-d. sep.
INTERNAL CANTHUS. li-ca. sep.
Smarting. sep.
FORWARDS. cmc.
Eyeball, Pressing. cmc.
BACKWARDS. lac-f.
DOWNWARDS. cmc.
Eyeball, Pressing. cmc.
To HEAD. lac-f.
To FOREHEAD. lac-f.
To TEMPLE. lac-f.
RIGHT. al-o. lac-f. mg-ca. rho.
Photophobia. lac-f.
Sight Impaired. mg-ca.
Eyeball, Color Red. lac-f.
Heat. rho.
Lachrymation. lac-f.
Pressing. al-o.
Shooting. lac-f.
Backwards, Eyeball Shooting. lac-f.
To Forehead. Eyeball, Shooting. lac-f.
Throbbing. lac-f.
To Temple. Eyeball, Shooting. lac-f.
Throbbing. lac-f.
LEFT. ag-na. aga. cund. dt. lac-d. lch. ner. s-**x**. zn.
Objects, False Appearance of, Confused. cund.
Objects, Imaginary, Bright. dt.
Grey. lch.
Mist. ag-na.
Spots, Bright. dt.
Grey. lch.
Eyeball, Heat. s-x.
Lachrymation. s-x.
Movements, Convulsions. aga.
Pressing. aga.
Smarting. s-x.
Eyelids, Tensive. ner.
Upper Eyelid, Heat. zn.
Pressing. zn.
Internal Canthus, Movements, Convulsions. lac-d.
Undefined. lac-d.

READING WRITING.

con. dt. lch.
OBJECTS, FALSE APPEARANCE **of**. con. dt.
Moving. con.
  Vertically. con.
Multiplied. dt.
OBJECTS, IMAGINARY. lch.
Grey. (lch.)
Spots. (lch).
  Grey. (lch).
LEFT. lch.
Objects, Imaginary, Grey. lch.
  Spots. lch.
  Grey. lch.

SEWING.

ag-na. amm-ca. amm-cl. ca-ca. eupat. k-ca. lac-d. lct. mrl.
OBJECTS, FALSE APPEARANCE **of**. lct. mrl.
Confused. lct. mrl.
OBJECTS IMAGINARY. ag-na. amm-ca. amm-cl.
Black. amm-ca.
Mist. (ag-na).
Spots. amm-ca. amm-cl.
  Black. amm-ca.
  Yellow. amm-cl.
Yellow. amm-cl.
SIGHT IMPAIRED. ca-ca. eupat.
EYEBALL. k-ca. rmx.
Movements. (lac-d).
  Convulsions. (lac-d).
Shooting. k-ca.
Smarting. rmx.
Undefined. (lac-d).
CANTHI. lac-d.
INTERNAL CANTHUS. lac-d.
LEFT. ag-na. lac-d.
Objects Imaginary, Mist. ag-na.
Internal Canthus, Movements, Convulsions. lac-d.
  Undefined. lac-d.

SPINNING.

dt. mg-sa.
OBJECTS IMAGINARY. mg-sa.
Figures. mg-sa.
SIGHT IMPAIRED. dt.

WRITING.

ag-na. al-o. alo. ara. ca-ca. ca-s. cb-v. chd. cle. co. crb-x. cth. dl-s. dph. ele. ery. fe. grp. grt. k-bicr. k-ca. lac-f. lch. lct. lyc. mrl. na-ca. na-cl. narth. ol-a. p-x. pet. physo. pol. ppv. rho. rs-v. sep. sr-ca. thu. val. vin. zn.

OBJECTS, FALSE APPEARANCE **of**. chd. cle. crb-x. ery. grp. k-ca. lyc. ppv.

Confused. chd. cle. crb-x. ery. k-ca. lyc. ppv.
Moving. k-ca. thu.
Circularly. k-ca.
Vibrating. thu.
Multiplied. cle. ery. grp.

OBJECTS IMAGINARY. cle. ery. grt. k-ca. na-ca. ol-a. p-x. sr-ca. vin.

Black. na-ca.
Bright. cle. ery. ol-a.
Green. sr-ca.
Mist. vin.
Spots. ery. na-ca. ol-a.
Black. na-ca.
Bright. ery. ol-a.
Stars. k-ca.
Veil. grt. ol-a. p-x.
Vibrations. cle.
Bright. cle.
Waves. sr-ca.
Green. sr-ca.

PHOTOPHOBIA. (lac-f).

SIGHT IMPAIRED. ag-na. alo. chd. co. cth. ele. grt. k-ca. lct. na-cl. ol-a. p-x. physo. rho. sep. zn.

Myopia. p-x.

EYEBALL. al-o. ara. ca-ca. co. dl-s. fe. lac-f. na-ca. na-cl. ol-a. pol. rho. rs-v. sep. thu. zn.

Color Red. (lac-f).

Contractive. sep.
Creeping. ol-a.
Dryness. na-ca. na-cl.
Heat. dl-s. (k-bicr). (lct). na-ca. na-cl. pol. rho. thu. zn.
Lachrymation. ca-ca. fe. (lac-f). ol-a. zn.
Movements. (ca-s). (dph). (ery).
Convulsions, Feeling of. ara.
Paralysis. (fe).
Pressing. co.
Shooting. co. (lac-f).
Smarting. co. dl-s.
Throbbing. (lac-f).
Undefined. rs-v.
IRIS. lct.
Pupils Dilated. lct.
EYELIDS. ca-s. dph. ery. fe. lct. pol.
Heat. lct. pol.
Movements, Closing. dph. ery.
Winking. ca-s.
Paralysis. fe.
CANTHI. k-bicr.
INTERNAL CANTHUS. k-bicr.
Heat. k-bicr.
BACKWARDS. lac-f.
To HEAD. lac-f.
To FOREHEAD. lac-f.
To TEMPLE. lac-f.
RIGHT. al-o. lac-f.
Photophobia. lac-f.
Eyeball, Color Red. lac-f.
Lachrymation. lac-f.
Pressing. al-o.
Shooting. lac-f.
Backwards. Eyeball Shooting. lac-f.
To Forehead. Eyeball, Shooting. lac-f.
Throbbing. lac-f.
To Temple. Eyeball, Shooting. lac-f.
Throbbing. lac-f.

LOOKING FIXEDLY. (**Long, Exerting Eyes**).

ac-s. aga. al-o. amm-ca. amm-cl. aps. art-v. au. ba-a. ba-ca. ca-ca. cast. cb-v. chd. cic. cl-hx. cmc. co. con. (cph). cro. cth. dl-s. dro. eug. gel. grp. hæm. hg. hg-s. k-bicr. (k-ca). k-o. kre. lac-c. lch. led. lyc. mg-ca. mn-ca. mtr. n-x. na-cl. na-sa. ni-ca. nic. p. p-x. pet. pnx. pol. pru-l. pt. qu-sa. rhe. rho. rn-b. rs. rs-v. rut. s. s-x. smc. smi. spi. spo. sr-ca. thu. trn. tx-b. val.

OBJECTS, FALSE APPEARANCE **of.** aga. amm-ca. cic. cl-hx. con. eug. k-o. lac-c. n-x. pnx. pol.

Black. n-x.
Confused. cic. cl-hx. eug. (k-bicr). k-o.
  Outlines. k-bicr.
Moving. eug. k-o. pol.
  Vibrating. eug. k-o. pol.
Multiplied. amm-ca. con. pnx.
Red. lac-c.
White. aga.

OBJECTS, IMAGINARY. ac-s. aga. al-o. amm-ca. amm-cl. art-v. ca-ca. lac-c. lch. na-sa. nic. p-x. pet. rut.

Black. ac-s. amm-ca.
Bright. (na-sa). nic. p-x.
Circles. lch.
  Grey. lch.
Green. sr-ca.
Grey. lch.
Mist. (na-sa).
Near Eye (na-sa).
Red. lac-c.
Spots. ac-s. amm-ca. amm-cl. lac-c.
  Black. ac-s. amm-ca.
  Red. lac-c.
  Yellow. amm-cl.
Stars. (na-sa).
  Bright. (na-sa).
    Near Eye. (na-sa).
  Green. (na-sa).
    Near Eye. (na-sa).
  Near Eye. (na-sa).
  Yellow. (na-sa).
    Near Eye. (na-sa).

Veil. aga. al-o. art-v. ca-ca. lch. pet. rut.
Vibrations. nic. p-x.
Bright. nic. p-x
Waves. sr-ca.
Green. sr-ca.
Yellow. amm-cl.
SIGHT DAZZLED. s.
SIGHT IMPAIRED. aga. al-o. art-v. ca-ca. cast. cb-v. hæm. k-bicr. lch. mg-ca. mn-ca. n-x. (na-sa). nic. pet. qu-sa. rs-v. rut. spi. thu. trn.
Myopia. cb-v.
EYEBALL. aps. au. ba-ca. cb-v. cmc. dl-s. dro. hg. hg-s. k-bicr. kre. mn-ca. na-cl. na-sa. ni-ca. nic. p. pet. pol. pru-l. pt. rhe. rho. rs. s. s-x. smc. smi. spo. sr-ca. tx-b. val.
Color Red. au. sr-ca.
Drawing. (pru-l).
Dryness. rho.
False Sensations. hg.
Sand. hg.
Heat. ba-ca. k-bicr. ni-ca. pet. rho. s-x. sr-ca.
Lachrymation. (cph). (hg-s). (k-ca). kre. nic. pol. (s). spo. sr-ca. tx-b.
Hot. (k-ca).
Movements. (gel).
Pressing. ba-ca. cmc. mn-ca. na-cl. (na-sa). p. pet. rhe. rs. s-x. smc. val.
Shooting. dl-s.
Smarting. cmc. (co). dro.
Tensive. au.
Undefined. aps. (cb-v). (cmc). (co). nic. pt. rhe. (rut). smi.
EYEBALL SUPERIORLY. pru-l.
Drawing. pru-l.
EYEBALL ANTERIORLY. s-x.
Heat. s-x.
Pressing. s-x.
IRIS. p-x.
Pupils, Dilated. (p-x).
EYELIDS. co. gel. pru-l.
Movements, Closing. gel.
Smarting. co.
Undefined. co.
UPPER EYELID. co. pru-l.

Smarting. co.
TARSAL EDGES. pru-l.
UPPER TARSAL EDGE. pru-l.
Drawing. pru-l.
CANTHI. p-x.
INTERNAL CANTHUS. p-x.
Pressing. p-x.
CHANGING CHARACTER **or** PLACE **in** EYES. na-sa.
Objects Imaginary Mist, then Star Bright Green Yellow Near Eye. (na-sa).
OBJECTS IMAGINARY **then** EYEBALL. na-sa.
SIGHT IMPAIRED **then** OBJECTS IMAGINARY. na-sa.
RIGHT. hg-s. mg-ca. na-sa. p-x. s. trn.
Objects Imaginary, Bright. na-sa.
Green. na-sa.
Mist. na-sa.
Near Eye. na-sa.
Star. na-sa.
Bright. na-sa.
Near Eye. na-sa.
Green. na-sa.
Near Eye. na-sa.
Near Eye. na-sa.
Yellow. na-sa.
Near Eye. na-sa.
Yellow. na-sa.
Sight Impaired. mg-ca. na-sa. trn.
Eyeball, Lachrymation. hg-s. s.
Pressing. na-sa.
Iris, Pupil Dilated. p-x.
Changing. Objects Imaginary Mist, then Star Bright Green Yellow Near Eye. na-sa.
Objects Imaginary, then Eyeball, Star Bright Green Yellow Near Eye, then Pressing. na-sa.
Sight Impaired, then Star Bright Green Yellow Near Eye. na-sa.
LEFT. cb-v.
Eyeball Undefined. cb-v.

LOOKING UP.

al-o. as-o. atp. ba-ca. cb-v. chd. crot. cu. dt. hg-s. jnp-s. k-ca. lac-c. mn-ca. p. pul. s. vr-s. zn.

OBJECTS IMAGINARY. atp. cu. dt. p. zn.

Black. p. (zn).
Bright. dt. zn.
High up. dt.
Mist. atp. p.
  Black. p.
  White. atp.
Semicircle. dt.
  Bright. dt.
    High up. dt.
  High up. dt.
Spots. dt. zn.
  Bright dt.
    High up. dt.
  High up. dt.
Stars. atp.
  White. atp.
Stripes. dt. (zn).
  Black. (zn).
    Upwards to Left. zn.
  Bright. dt.
    High up. dt.
    Upwards to Right. dt.
    Vertical. dt.
  High up. dt.
  Upwards to Right, dt.
  Upwards to Left. (zn).
  Vertical. dt.
Upwards to Right. dt.
Upwards to Left. (zn).
Veil. cu.
Vertical. dt.
White. atp.

SIGHT IMPAIRED. cu.

EYEBALL. al-o. as-o. atp. ba-ca. cb-v. chd. crot. hg-s. k-ca. lac-c. mn-ca. p. s. vr-s.

Heat. al-o.
Movements. (al-o).
    Convulsions. (al-o).

Paralysis. (dt).
Pressing. (as-o). atp. ba-ca. crot. mn-ca. vr-s.
Shooting. (as-o).
Swelling, Feeling of. (hg-s).
Tensive. (hg-s). p. s. vr-a.
Undefined. (as-o). cb-v. chd. (k-ca). lac-c.
EYEBALL SUPERIORLY. as-o.
Pressing. as-o.
Undefined. as-o.
EYELIDS. as-o. hg-s.
Swelling, Feeling of. hg-s.
UPPER EYELID. as-o.
Undefined. as-o.
LEFT. al-o. as-o. k-ca. zn.
Objects Imaginary, Black. zn.
Stripe. zn.
Black. zn.
Upwards to Left. zn.
Upwards to Left. zn.
Eyeball, Movements, Convulsions. al-o.
Undefined. k-ca.
Eyeball Superiorly, Shooting. as-o.

LOOKING DOWN.

acon. al-o. dt. klm. mll. ner. p. pnx. s. tep.
OBJECTS, FALSE APPEARANCE **of.** mll. ner. pnx. tep.
Large. mll.
Moving. pnx. tep.
Multiplied. ner.
OBJECTS, IMAGINARY. dt. klm. p.
Black. p.
Blue. dt.
Bright. klm.
Mist. p.
Black. p.
Spots. dt.
Blue. dt.
Vibrations. klm.
Bright. klm.
SIGHT IMPAIRED. klm.

EYEBALL. acon. al-o.
Heat. acon.
Movements. (al-o).
Convulsions. (al-o).
Pressing. acon. (s).
EYELIDS. s.
UPPER EYELID. s.
Pressing. s.
LEFT. alo.
Eyeball, Movements, Convulsions. alo.

LOOKING SIDEWAYS. (**Around**).

acon. ba-a. gel. mg-ca. mg-sa. ner. pol. sr-ca.
OBJECTS, FALSE APPEARANCE **of.** ca-ca. gel.
Moving. ca-ca.
Circularly. ca-ca.
Multiplied. gel.
OBJECTS IMAGINARY. pol. sr-ca.
Bright. pol.
Green. sr-ca.
Spots. pol. sr-ca.
Bright. pol.
Green. sr-ca.
SIGHT IMPAIRED. ner.
EYEBALL. acon. ba-a. mg-sa. si x.
Heat. acon.
Pressing. acon. ba-a. mg-sa.
Undefined. si-x.
FORWARDS. mg-sa.
Eyeball, Pressing. mg-sa.

LOOKING INWARDS.

mn-ca.
EYEBALL. mn-ca.
Pressing. mn-ca.

LOOKING **to** RIGHT.

dig. sep.
OBJECTS, FALSE APPEARANCE **of.** dig.
Multiplied. dig.
EYEBALL. dig. sep.
Pressing. sep.
Undefined. dig.

LOOKING to LEFT.

na-sa. smi.
OBJECTS, IMAGINARY. na-sa.
Bright. (na-sa).
Green. (na-sa).
Mist. (na-sa).
Near Eye. (na-sa).
Star. (na-sa).
  Bright. (na-sa).
    Near Eye. (na-sa).
  Green. (na-sa).
    Near Eye. (na-sa).
  Near Eye. (na-sa).
  Yellow. (na-sa).
    Near Eye. (na-sa).
Yellow. (na-sa).
SIGHT IMPAIRED. (na-sa).
EYEBALL. smi.
Bruised. (smi).
RIGHT. na-sa. smi.
Objects, Imaginary, Bright. na-sa.
  Green. na-sa.
  Mist. na-sa.
  Near Eye. na-sa.
  Star. na-sa.
    Bright. na-sa.
      Near Eye. na-sa.
    Green. na-sa.
      Near Eye. na-sa.
    Near Eye. na-sa.
    Yellow. na-sa.
      Near Eye. na-sa.
  Yellow. na-sa.
Sight Impaired. na-sa.
Eyeball, Bruised. smi.

LOOKING into the AIR.

amm-cl. dt. k-ca. s. thu.
OBJECTS, IMAGINARY. amm-cl. dt. k-ca. s. thu.
Black. k-ca.

Bright. dt.
Far off. dt.
Spots. amm-cl. dt. k-ca. s. thu.
Black. k-ca.
Bright. dt.
Far off. dt.
Far off. dt.
White. s. thu.
Yellow. amm-cl.
Veil. k-ca.
White. s. thu.
Yellow. amm-cl.
LEFT. dt.
Objects Imaginary, Bright. dt.
Far off. dt.
Spots. dt.
Bright. dt.
Far off. dt.
Far off. dt.

LOOKING at NEAR **Objects**.

ag-na. al-o. amm-ca. atp. bry. buf. ca-a. ca-ca. cb-a. chd. con. cub. dph. dro. dt. f-hx. glp. grt. hyo. k-o. lyc. mg-cl. mn-ca. na-cl. p-x. pet. phy. pul. s. sep. si-x. spi. srr. str. trg. val.

OBJECTS, FALSE APPEARANCE **of**. amm-ca.
Multiplied. amm-ca.
OBJECTS, IMAGINARY. (dt).
Figures. (dt).
SIGHT DAZZLED. p-x.
SIGHT IMPAIRED. (**Presbyopia**). ag-na. al-o. amm-ca. atp. bry. buf. ca-a. ca-ca. cb-a. con. dph. dro. dt. f-hx. glp. grt. hyo. k-o. lyc. mg-cl. na-cl. p-x. pet. phy. pul. rmx. s. sep. si-x. spi. srr. str. trg. val.
EYEBALL. mn-ca. p-x.
Pressing. mn-ca. p-x.
LEFT. cb-a.
Sight Impaired. cb-a.

LOOKING at DISTANT Objects.

ach. aga. amm-ca. as-o. atp. ber. buf. ca-ca. ca-s. cac. cb-v. chi. cmf. con. cyc. dig. dph. dt. eupat-p. euph. euphr. gel. glp. grp. grt. hyo. i. krm. lyc. mn-ca. n-x. na-ca. na-cl. ni-ca. nic. ol-a. p-x. pb. pet. physo. pul. rut. s. s-x. sb-t. se. si-x. smc. spo. srr. thu. trg. val. vi-o. vi-t. vrb. woo.

OBJECTS, FALSE APPEARANCE **of.** atp. chi. gel. i. n-x. ni-ca. nic.

Blue. i.

Confused. chi. gel.

Large. ni-ca.

Multiplied. amm-ca. atp. n-x. nic.

Horizontally. n-x.

OBJECTS, IMAGINARY. dig.

Black. dig.

Spots. dig.

Black. dig.

SIGHT IMPAIRED. (**Myopia**). ach. aga. amm-ca. (as-o). ber. buf. ca-ca. ca-s. cac. cb-v. chi. cmf. con. cyc. dph. dt. eupat-p. euph. gel. glp. grp. grt. hyo. krm. lyc. mn-ca. n-x. na-ca. na-cl. ol-a. p. p-x. pb. pet. physo. pul. rut. s. s-x. sb-t. se. si-x. smc. spo. srr. thu. trg. val. vi-o. vi-t. vrb. woo.

LEFT. as-o. ca-ca.

Sight Impaired. as-o. ca-ca.

CHANGING AXIS of VISION.

lac-c.

SIGHT IMPAIRED. lac-c.

LOOKING at SMALL Objects.

atp. cd-sa. cof. cyc. dro. dt. elc. eupat. i. mph. na-ca. pet. s.

OBJECTS, FALSE APPEARANCE **of.** dt.

Multiplied. dt.

OBJECTS, IMAGINARY. dro.
Bright. dro.
Vibrations. dro.
Bright. dro.
SIGHT IMPAIRED. (atp). cd-sa. cyc. dt. ele. eupat. i. mph. na-ca. pet. s.
Presbyopia. atp.

LOOKING at LINEAR **Objects**.

ox-x.
OBJECTS, FALSE APPEARANCE **of**. ox-x.
Far. ox-x.
Large. ox-x.

LOOKING at FIXED **Objects**.

pb.
OBJECTS, FALSE APPEARANCE **of**. pb.
White. pb.

LOOKING at DIFFERENT **Objects**.

lac-c.
EYEBALL. lac-c.
Pressing. lac-c.

LOOKING at FLOWING WATER.

fe.
OBJECTS, FALSE APPEARANCE **of**. fe.
Moving. fe.
Circularly. fe.

LOOKING at BLACK **Objects**.

dt. (str). trn.
OBJECTS, FALSE APPEARANCE **of**. dt. (str).
Grey. dt. (str).
OBJECTS, IMAGINARY. trn.
Mist. trn.

N

LOOKING at BLUE **Objects**.

art-v. lpd. snt.
OBJECTS, FALSE APPEARANCE **of**. art-v.
Green. art-v.
Grey. lpd.

LOOKING at GREEN **Objects**.

trn.
OBJECTS, IMAGINARY. trn.
Mist. trn.

LOOKING at GREY **Objects**.

snt.
OBJECTS, FALSE APPEARANCE **of**. snt.
Blue. snt.
Yellow. snt.

LOOKING at RED **Objects**.

art-v. grp. trn.
OBJECTS, FALSE APPEARANCE **of**. art-v.
Yellow. art-v.
OBJECTS, IMAGINARY. trn.
Mist. trn.
EYEBALL. grp.
Shooting. grp.
INWARDS. grp.
Eyeball, Shooting. grp.

LOOKING at WHITE **Objects**.

acon. as-o. cro. dt. (ery). grp. hyo. k-ca. mtr. na-cl. nic. (p). smi. sr-ca.
OBJECTS, FALSE APPEARANCE **of**. art-v. cro. smi.
Red. cro. smi.
Yellow. art-v.
OBJECTS, IMAGINARY. acon. dt. (ery). hyo. k-ca. (p). sr-ca.
Black. acon. (p).

Blue. dt.
Bright. acon. dt.
Figures. hyo. (p).
Green. sr-ca.
Grey. dt.
Halo. dt. hyo.
  Grey. dt.
  Red. dt.
  Yellow. hyo.
Red. dt.
Spots. acon. dt. k-ca. (p).
  Black. acon. (p).
  Blue. dt.
  Bright. acon. dt.
  White. k-ca.
Threads. (ery).
Waves. sr-ca.
  Green. sr-ca.
White. k-ca.
Yellow. hyo.
SIGHT DAZZLED. as-o. grp.
SIGHT IMPAIRED. mtr. nic.
EYEBALL. grp.
Lachrymation. grp.
Shooting. grp.
INWARDS. grp.
Eyeball, Shooting. grp.

LOOKING at YELLOW Objects.

snt. trn.
OBJECTS, FALSE APPEARANCE of. snt.
Red. snt.
OBJECTS, IMAGINARY. trn.
Mist. trn.

LOOKING at BRIGHT OBJECTS.

amm-cl. buf. cch. cmc. dt. grp. grt. mg-cl. p-x. sep. str-i. vr-s.
SIGHT DAZZLED. p-x.
SIGHT IMPAIRED. dt. grt.
EYEBALL. buf. cmc. grp. p-x.
Pressing. cmc. p-x.

Shooting. grp.
Undefined. buf. (cmc).
EYEBALL POSTERIORLY. cmc.
FORWARDS. cmc.
Eyeball, Pressing. cmc.
DOWNWARDS. cmc.
Eyeball, Pressing. cmc.
INWARDS. grp.
Eyeball, Shooting. grp.
To HEAD. cmc.
To OCCIPUT. cmc.
Eyeball Posteriorly, Undefined. cmc.

LOOKING at ARTIFICIAL LIGHT.

acon. ag-na. al-o. anan. atp. ba-ca. ca-ca. (chd). cic. cmc. cph. dig. dl-s. dt. euph. euphr. fe-mgs. hpp. i. k-ca. k-na. k-o. kre. lyc. mg-cl. mim. mtr. n-x. ni-ca. os. os-x. p. p-x. pb. ptv. pul. rut. s. sep. smc. smi. sn. sr-ca. srr. til. trg. vr-v. zn.

OBJECTS, FALSE APPEARANCE **of**. (**Appearance of Flame**). acon. ag-na. anan. atp. ba-ca. (chd) dig. euphr. fe-mgs. hpp. i. k-na. k-o. kre. lyc. n-x. ni-ca. os. pb. ptv. smc. sn. til.
Black. euphr. k-o. smc.
Blue. dig. hpp. kre.
Bright. dig.
Confused. ag-na. euphr. i. n-x. os. os-x. til.
Large. anan. dig. os. os-x.
Moving. acon. euphr. lyc. smc.
Vibrating. acon. euphr. lyc. smc.
Multiplied. ni-ca. pb.
Small. (chd).
Variegated. ag-na. atp. ba-ca. fe-mgs. k-na. ni-ca. sn.
Yellow. ptv.

OBJECTS IMAGINARY. al-o. atp. ba-ca. ca-ca. cic. cmc. cph. dig. dl-s. dt. euph. k-ca. k-na. k-o. mg-cl. mim. mtr. n-x. os. p. p-x. ptv. pul. rut. s. sep. smc. smi. sn. sr-ca. srr. trg. vr-v. zn.
Black. k-o. p.
Blue. cph. trg.
Bright. ca-ca. dt. pul. trg.
Green. k-o. mg-cl. p. rut. sep. vr-v. zn.

Grey. p. sep.
Halo. al-o. atp. ba-ca. ca-ca. cic. cmc. cph. dig. dl-s. euph. k-ca. k-na. k-o. mg-cl. mim. n-x. os. p. p-x. ptv. pul. rut. s. sep. smc. smi. sn. sr-ca. trg. vr-v. zn.
  Black. k-o. p.
  Blue. cph. trg.
  Bright. ca-ca. dt. pul. trg.
  Green. k-o. mg-cl. p. rut. sep. vr-v. zn.
  Grey. p. sep.
  Red. atp. (cmc). cph. ptv. rut. s. trg. vr-v.
  Star-like. pul.
  Variegated. atp. ba-ca. cic. k-na. k-o. os.
Rays. atp. k-ca. mtr. srr. trg.
Red. atp. (cmc). cph. ptv. rut. s. trg. vr-v.
Spots. dt.
  Bright. dt.
Stars. pul.
Variegated. atp. ba-ca. cic. k-na. k-o. os.
RIGHT. cmc.
Objects Imaginary, Halo. cmc.
  Red. cmc.
 Red. cmc.
LEFT. atp. zn.
Objects Imaginary. **Green**. zn.
 Halo. atp.
  Green. zn.
  Variegated. atp.
 Rays. atp.
 Variegated. atp.

LOOKING SUDDENLY in the DARK.

p-x.
EYEBALL. p-x.
Pressing. p-x.

LOOKING through SPECTACLES.

na-ba.
EYEBALL. na-ba.
Heat. na-ba.

Movements. (na-ba).
EYELIDS. na-ba.
Movements, Closing. na-ba.
Spasmodically. na-ba.

LOOKING **with** RIGHT EYE.

lyc.
OBJECTS, FALSE APPEARANCE **of**. lyc.
Part Visible. lyc.
Vertical. lyc.
Left Side Visible. lyc.

LOOKING **into** IMAGINARY BRIGHT SPOT.

chd.
EYEBALL. chd.
Lachrymation. chd.

LACHRYMATION.

(ca-s). mgs.
EYEBALL. ca-s. mgs.
Eruptions. (ca-s).
Blisters. (ca-s).
Undefined. mgs.
EYEBALL ROUND CORNEA. (ca-s).
Eruptions, Blisters. (ca-s).

MOVING EYES.

acon. ag-na. arn. as-o. atp. bry. ca-a. ca-ca. ca-o. ca-s. cb-v. chd. chi. cit-c. cle. cmc. con. cor. cph. crt. cu. dig. eryn. gel. hg. hpp. k-bicr. k-ca. k-o. klm. lau-c. lo-cœ. lyc. mg-ca. mn-ca. mph. mtr. n-x. na-cl. nic. ox-x. p. pb. pul. rn-b. rn-s. rs. s. sa-l. sep. si-x. sn. spi. spo. spo-f. sr-ca. stc. str-i. trg. val. vi-t. vtx. ziz. zn.
OBJECTS, FALSE APPEARANCE **of**. gel.
Confused. gel.
OBJECTS IMAGINARY. atp. p.
Black. p.
Bright. atp.

Mist. p.
Black. p.
Spots. atp.
Bright. atp.
PHOTOPHOBIA. ca-s.
SIGHT IMPAIRED. con.
EYEBALL. acon. ag-na. as-o. atp. bry. ca-ca. ca-s. cb-v. chd. chi. cmc. cor. cph. crt. eryn. hg. hpp. k-bicr. k-ca. klm. lau-c. lo-cœ. lyc. mph. n-x. nic. ox-x. pb. pul. rn-b. rn-s. rs. s. sa-l. sep. sn. spi. spo-f. sr-ca. stc. str-i. trg. val. vi-t. vtx.
Bruised. (cu). (vtx).
Bursting. acon. (lau-c).
Drawing. pb.
Dryness. (arn). (as-o). atp. crt.
False Sensations. chi. hg. (rs).
Sand. chi. hg. (rs).
Heat. acon.
Heaviness. chi. pb.
Motion, in. (rs).
Passing Round, like Something. (rs).
Movements. gel.
Convulsions. gel.
Pressing. acon. atp. ca-s. cph. crt. hg. mn-ca. (mtr). nic. sep. spi. trg. (val).
Shooting. acon. (as-o). (sn). (spi). (spo). sr-ca. (vi-t).
Smarting. (arn). (chd). (cmc). cor. lo-cœ. stc.
Stiffness. atp. ca-ca.
Swelling, Feeling of. spi.
Tensive. ca-ca. n-x. s. (sn). (spo). (vi-t).
Undefined. acon. ag-na. (as-o). bry. (ca-o). cb-v. chd. eryn. hpp. k-bicr. k-ca. klm. lyc. mph. ox-x. pul. rn-b. rn-s. rs. s. (sa-l). si-x. spi. spo-f. str-i. (ziz).
EYEBALL SUPERIORLY. acon.
Bursting. acon.
Undefined. acon.
EYEBALL EXTERNALLY. vtx.
Bruised. vtx.
EYEBALL INTERIORLY. as-o.
ORBIT. chd. cu. ziz.
Bruised. cu.
Smarting. chd.
EYELIDS. arn. as-o. ca-a. ca-o. mtr.
Adhesion of. ca-a.

UPPER EYELID. ca-o. mtr.
Pressing. mtr.
Undefined. ca-o.
TARSAL EDGES. arn. as-o.
Dryness. arn. as-o.
Smarting. arn.
Undefined. as-o.
CANTHI. spo.
EXTERNAL CANTHUS. spo.
FORWARDS. val.
Eyeball, Pressing. val.
To HEAD. spo-f.
To TEMPLE. spo-f.
Eyeball, Undefined. spo-f.
RIGHT. as-o. cmc. lau-c. rs. spi. vi-t. ziz.
Eyeball, Bursting. lau-c.
Motion in, Passing Round like Something. rs.
Shooting. as-o. spi. vi-t.
Smarting. cmc.
Tensive. vi-t.
Orbit, Undefined. ziz.
LEFT. as-o. sa-l. sn. spi. spo.
Eyeball, Pressing. spi.
Shooting. as-o. sn.
Tensive. sn.
Undefined. sa-l.
Eyeball Interiorly, Shooting. as-o.
External Canthus, Shooting. spo.
Tensive. spo.

MOVING EYELIDS.

alm. arn. as-o. atp. ber. c-bis. chd. chi. cor. euphr. k-bicr. mgs-au. mn-ca. str-i. thu. trg.
OBJECTS, IMAGINARY. atp.
Bright. atp.
Spots. atp.
Bright. atp.
EYEBALL. arn. chd. chi. k-bicr. str-i. trg.
Bruised. (alm). trg.
Dryness. (as-o). chi.

False Sensations. chi. (thu).
Sand. chi. (thu).
Heaviness. (ber).
Scraping. chd. k-bicr.
Smarting. arn. (c-bis).
Undefined. euphr. (mn-ca). str-i.
ORBIT. alm. trg.
Bruised. trg.
ORBIT INFERIORLY. alm.
EYELIDS. as-o. ber. c-bis. mn-ca.
Dryness. as-o.
Undefined. mn-ca.
UPPER EYELID. ber. c-bis.
Heaviness. ber.
CANTHI. thu.
INTERNAL CANTHUS. thu.
RIGHT. thu.
Internal Canthus, False Sensations, Sand. thu.
LEFT. alm. c-bis.
Orbit Inferiorly, Bruised. alm.
Upper Eyelid, Smarting. c-bis.

When EYELID is STILL.

asr.
EYEBALL. asr.
Movements. (asr).
Convulsions. (asr).
EYELIDS. asr.
UPPER EYELID. asr.
LEFT. asr.
Upper Eyelid, Movements, Convulsions. asr.

OPENING EYELIDS.

acon. ag-na. al-o. asr. atp. au. (ca-i). chd. co. con. cph. cro. cth. euph. grp. hg. k-bicr. mg-cl. na-ba. p. p-x. physo. rs-r. s-x. spi. str. str-i. zn.
OBJECTS, IMAGINARY. (spi).
Black. (spi).
Bright. (spi).

Spots. (spi).
Black. (spi).
Bright. (spi).
EYEBALL. acon. al-o. au. (ca-i). cph. grp. mg-cl. p-x. s-x. str-i. zn.
Bursting. acon.
Discharge. hg.
False Sensations. chd. s-x. str-i.
Sand. chd. s-x. str-i.
Hæmorrhage. (atp).
Heat. al-o. mg-cl.
Lachrymation. au. (ca-i). con. cph. physo. (spi). zn.
Hot. au. (ca-i). (spi).
Movements. (chd). (k-bicr).
Convulsions. (k-bicr).
Pressing. acon. (na-ba). str-i.
Shooting. str-i.
Smarting. chd. (cth).
Undefined. al-o. (cth). grp. p-x.
EYELIDS. atp. chd. co. cth. k-bicr. na-ba.
Hæmorrhage. atp.
Movements, Closing. (chd).
Spasmodically. chd.
Convulsions. k-bicr.
As if connecting Strings Snapped. co.
UPPER EYELID. cth. na-ba.
Pressing. na-ba.
Undefined. cth.
TARSAL EDGES. cth.
Smarting. cth.
CANTHI. s-x.
EXTERNAL CANTHUS. s-x.
FORWARDS. acon.
Eyeball, Pressing. acon.
OUTWARDS. s-x.
RIGHT. s-x.
External Canthus, False Sensation, Sand. s-x.
Outwards. Eyeball, False Sensation, Sand. s-x.
LEFT. (spi).
Objects Imaginary, Black. (spi).
Bright. (spi).
Spots, Black. (spi).
Bright. (spi).
Eyeball, Lachrymation. (spi).

CLOSING EYELIDS.

ag-na. aga. al-o. am-ni. as-o. atp. atrop. ba-ca. ber. ca-ca. ca-s. cb-v. chd. cle. cmf. con. cor. cro. cu. dig. dl-s. dt. elaps. f-hx. grt. hll. hpm. hur. jnp-s. k-o. lac-d. lau-c. lch. led. lo-c. lyc. mn-ca. na-ca. os. p. p-x. phy. pod. ptv. pul. rs-r. s. s-x. sep. si-x. smi. smr. spo. stc. str. thr. thu. vr-v.

OBJECTS, FALSE APPEARANCE **of.** ca-s. grt. si-x.

Moving. ca-s. grt. si-x.

Circularly. ca-s. grt. si-x.

OBJECTS, IMAGINARY. ag-na. al-o. am-ni. as-o. atp. atrop. ba-ca. ca-ca. con. dig. dt. elaps. f-hx. k-o. lau-c. led. mn-ca. na-ca. p. pod. ptv. pul. s. sep. spo. thr. thu. vr-v.

Black. thu.

Bright. al-o. as-o. atp. dig. f-hx. k-o. mn-ca. na-ca. p. sep. spo. thr.

Circles. am-ni. elaps. f-hx. mn-ca.

Bright. mn-ca.

Red. elaps.

Yellow. am-ni.

Figures. ag-na. k-o.

Flames. spo.

Flashes, Bright. as-o. atp. na-ca. sep.

Green. dt.

Halo. vr-v.

Red. vr-v.

Increasing and Decreasing in Size. lau-c.

Light. al-o. p.

Low Down. dt.

Mist. ba-ca. pod.

Moving. pod.

Moving. dt. pod.

Red. elaps. vr-v.

Spots. dig. dt. k-o. thu.

Black. thu.

Bright. dig. k-o.

Green. dt.

Low Down. dt.

Moving. dt.

Low Down. dt.

Moving. dt.

Stars. p.
Vibrations. f-hx. thr.
Bright. f-hx. thr.
Visions. atp. ca-ca. k-o. led. ptv. pul. s. sep. thu.
Horrible. atp. ca-ca. k-o.
Waves. (p).
Concentric. (p).
Yellow. am-ni.
Zigzags. con.
SIGHT IMPAIRED. ba-ca. (os).
Sensation as if Axis of Vision was Moved Backwards and Forwards. os.
EYEBALL. aga. al-o. atp. ber. ca-ca. cle. con. cor. cro. (cu). hll. k-o. lac-d. lo-c. lyc. p-x. s. sep. si-x. smi. smr. spo. stc.
Broken. si-x.
Bruised. s.
Coldness. (hur). (p-x).
Contractive. lac-d.
Like a Band. lac-d.
Dryness. (ber).
False Sensations. (s-x). (sep).
Sand. (s-x). (sep).
Heat. (aga). ca-ca. (cb-v). cle. cor. cro. (hpm). lyc. (ptv). si-x.
Lachrymation. ber. spo.
Movements. (al-o). (cu). (lch). (na-cl).
Convulsions. (al-o). (cu). (lch).
Pressing. aga. atp. (chd). con. (dl-s). (hll). (jnp-s). lac-d. (sep).
Shooting. hll. smi.
Smarting. (dig). lo-c. smr. stc. (str-i).
Stiffness. k-o.
Undefined. (cmf). lac-d. lyc. (rs-r). si-x. (thu).
EYEBALL SUPERIORLY. aga.
Pressing. aga.
ORBIT. p-x. thu.
ORBIT INTERNALLY. p-x.
Coldness. p-x.
ORBIT INFERIORLY. thu.
EYELIDS. ber. cb-v. chd. cro. dig. dl-s. hpm. hur. jnp-s. lac-d. lch. na-cl. ptv.
Coldness. hur.

Dryness. ber.
Heat. cb-v. cro.
Movements, Closing. na-cl.
Spasmodically. na-cl.
UPPER EYELID. chd. cmf. dl-s. jnp-s. lch.
Movements, Convulsions. lch.
Pressing. dl-s.
TARSAL EDGES. dig. hpm. lac-d. p-x. ptv.
Coldness. p-x.
Heat. hpm. ptv.
Small Feeling. lac-d.
Smarting. dig.
CANTHI. aga. hll. rs-r. s-x. str-i.
EXTERNAL CANTHUS. rs-r. str-i.
Smarting. str-i.
Undefined. rs-r.
INTERNAL CANTHUS. aga. hll. s-x.
Heat. aga.
INWARDS. s-x.
RIGHT. cmf. hll. s-x. sep. thu.
Eyeball, False Sensations, Sand. sep.
Pressing. sep.
Orbit Inferiorly, Undefined. thu.
Upper Eyelid, Undefined. cmf.
Internal Canthus, False Sensations, Sand. s-x.
Pressing. hll.
Inwards. **Eyeball, False Sensations, Sand**. s-x.
LEFT. al-o. chd. jnp-s.
Eyeball, Movements, Convulsions. al-o.
Upper Eyelid, Pressing. chd. jnp-s.

NOISE.

hg-i.
EYEBALL.
Undefined. (hg-i).
ORBIT. hg-i.
ORBIT SUPERIORLY. hg-i.
LEFT. hg-i.
Orbit Superiorly, Undefined. hg-i.

Before EAR **Symptoms.**

anag. ery. frm. pet.
OBJECTS, FALSE APPEARANCE **of.** ery.
Confused. ery.
Multiplied. ery.
OBJECTS, IMAGINARY. ery.
Bright. ery.
Spots. ery.
  Bright. ery.
Vibrations. ery.
EYEBALL. anag. pet.
Boring. (frm).
Pressing. anag.
Undefined. (pet).
ORBIT. frm.
RIGHT. frm.
Orbit, Boring. frm.
LEFT. pet.
Eyeball, Undefined. pet.

With EAR **Symptoms.**

acon. al-o. as-o. atp. ba-cl. buf. ca-ca. can. cb-v. chi. cic. cle. clv. cmf. crot. cy-hx. dig. dro. dt. ery. fe-a. frm-s. glo. ind. k-bicr. k-ca. k-i. kre. ly-b. men. mgs. mph. n-x. na-cl. na-sa. ni-ca. p. pb. ppv. pul. qu-sa. s. sa-l. sep. si-x. spo. srr. thu. trg. trn. vr-a.

OBJECTS, FALSE APPEARANCE **of.** al-o. cic. ery. si-x.
Black. al-o.
Confused. ery.
Moving. si-x.
  Vertically. si-x.
    Up and Down. si-x.
Multiplied. cic. ery.

OBJECTS IMAGINARY. as-o. atp. can. (dt). ery. k-ca. p. qu-sa. spo. trg. vr-a.
Bright. ery. k-ca. p. qu-sa. spo. vr-a.
Flames. spo. vr-a.
Light. qu-sa.
Mist. can.

Spots. ery. k-ca. qu-sa.
Bright. ery. k-ca. qu-sa.
Vibrations. atp. ery. p. trg.
Bright. p.
Visions. as-o. spo.
PHOTOPHOBIA. ca-ca. cle. k-na.
SIGHT IMPAIRED. acon. al-o. as-o. can. cb-v. chi. clv. cy-hx. dt. (ery). fe-a. k-bicr. mph. pb. ppv. pul. qu-sa. sep. srr. trn.
EYEBALL. ba-cl. bi-na. buf. ca-ca. cle. crot. dro. dt. frm-s. glo. k-ca. ly-b. men. n-x. na-sa. ppv. s. sa-l. thu. vr-a.
Appearance Bright. dt.
Dim. k-ca. vr-a.
Staring. k-ca.
Bursting. frm-s.
Coldness. (ni-ca). (sa-l).
Color Dark. (k-ca).
Red. bi-na. (ca-ca). crot. glo. (ind). n-x. ppv. s.
Discharge. ba-cl.
Dryness. (thu).
Eruptions. ca-ca. (p).
Pterygium. (ca-ca).
Styes. (p).
Ulcers. ca-ca.
False Sensations. (ni-ca). (thu).
Sand. (thu).
Water, Cold. (ni-ca).
Heat. crot. (dro). (k-ca). s. thu.
Itching. ly-b. na-sa. s.
Lachrymation. (dt). k-ca. vr-a.
Movements. (ca-ca). (dt). (kre). (ppv).
Pressing. k-ca. (na-cl).
Projecting. dt.
Shooting. ca-ca. k-ca. n-x. (sa-l). (thu).
Cold. sa-l.
Swelling. (ca-ca). (k-i).
Tearing. (k-ca).
Undefined. buf. cle. (men).
Same Symptom. ba-cl. buf. cmf. crot. frm-s. ly-b. (men). na-sa. thu.
EYEBALL INTERNALLY. ca-ca.
CORNEA. ca-ca.
Eruptions, Ulcers. ca-ca.

IRIS. cic. dt. mgs. ppv.
Pupils Dilated. cic. dt. mgs. ppv.
Insensible. dt. ppv.
ORBIT. na-cl.
Pressing. na-cl.
EYELIDS. ca-ca. dig. dt. ind. k-ca. k-i. kre. p. ppv. thu.
Color Dark. k-ca.
Movements, Closing. (ca-ca). (dig). dt. kre. p. ppv.
Spasmodically. ca-ca.
Swelling. k-i.
UPPER EYELID. k-ca. thu.
Heaviness. thu.
Swelling. k-ca.
LOWER EYELID. p. thu.
TARSAL EDGES. thu.
LOWER TARSAL EDGE. thu.
EYELIDS, INNER SURFACE. ind.
Color Red. ind.
CANTHI. ca-ca. ni-ca. thu.
EXTERNAL CANTHUS. ni-ca. thu.
INTERNAL CANTHUS. ca-ca.
CARUNCULA. ca-ca.
RIGHT. ca-ca. dig. dro. na-sa. ni-ca. thu.
Eyeball, Dryness. thu.
Heat. dro.
Itching. na-sa.
Same Symptom. na-sa.
Eyeball Internally, Color Red. ca-ca.
Swelling. ca-ca.
Eyelids, Movements, Closing. dig.
Lower Tarsal Edge, Heat. thu.
External Canthus, Coldness. ni-ca.
Dryness. thu.
False Sensations, Sand. thu.
Water Cold. ni-ca.
Shooting. thu.
Caruncula, Swelling. ca-ca.
LEFT. ca-ca. cle. (dt). glo. k-ca. men. na-sa. p.
Eyeball, Color Red. glo.
Eruptions Pterygium. ca-ca.
Heat. k-ca.
Itching. na-sa.

Lachrymation. (dt). k-ca.
Tearing. k-ca.
Undefined. cle. men.
Same Symptom. men. na-sa.
Lower Eyelid, Eruptions Stye. p.

After EAR **Symptoms.**

arn. hur. thu.
EYEBALL. arn. thu.
Drawing. arn.
Shooting. arn.
Tearing. thu.
Undefined. (hur).
Same Symptom. thu.
ORBIT. hur.
OUTWARDS. arn.
Eyeball, Drawing. arn.
LEFT. hur.
Orbit, Undefined. hur.

BLOWING NOSE.

al-o. k-o. n-x. na-cl. na-sa..
OBJECTS, IMAGINARY. al-o. na-sa.
Bright. na-sa.
Spots. na-sa.
Bright. na-sa.
Yellow. na-sa.
Stars. al-o.
Yellow. na-sa.
SIGHT IMPAIRED. k-o.
EYEBALL. k-o. n-x.
False Sensations. (k-o).
Pellicle. (k-o).
Swelling. (na-cl).
Tensive. (k-o).
Undefined. n-x.
EYEBALL INTERNALLY. k-o.
False Sensations, Pellicle. k-o.
LACHRYMAL SAC. na-cl.
Swelling. na-cl.

RIGHT. k-o.
Sight Impaired. k-o.
Eyeball, False Sensations, Pellicle. k-o.
Tensive. k-o.

HÆMORRHAGE **from** NOSE.

cb-v.
SIGHT IMPAIRED. cb-v.

SNEEZING.

amm-ca. (hydr). k-cla.
OBJECTS, IMAGINARY. amm-ca. (hydr). k-cla.
Bright. k-cla.
Spots. k-cla.
Bright. k-cla.
Stars. amm-ca.
Vibrations. (hydr).
Bright. (hydr).

Before NOSE **Symptoms.**

br. ca-ca. cic. k-bicr. k-i. mgs. sang.
SIGHT IMPAIRED. k-i.
EYEBALL. br. ca-ca. cic. k-bicr. k-i. sang.
Dryness. (mgs).
Heat. k-bicr. (sang).
Lachrymation. (sang).
Sensitive. (sang).
Shooting. ca-ca. cic.
Smarting. k-i.
Throbbing. ca-ca.
Undefined. br.
EYELIDS. mgs.
Dryness. mgs.
CANTHI. ca-ca.
INTERNAL CANTHUS. ca-ca.
Shooting. ca-ca.
To HEAD. cic.
To OCCIPUT. cic.

Eyeball, Shooting. cic.
RIGHT. sang.
Eyeball, Heat. sang.
Lachrymation. sang.
Sensitive. sang.

With NOSE **Symptoms**.

ag-na. aga. al-o. alli. amm-ca. anan. anm. arn. art-v. arum. as-o. atp. au. ba-cl. ber. bi-na. br. bru. bry. ca-ca. (ca-i). ca-pa. ca-s. cau. cb-v. ccs. chi. cit-c. clv. co. con. cr-o. crb-x. cro. crt. (cu). cu-asi. dl-s. dt. eug. (eupat-p). euphr. fe. fe-a. fe-mgs. frm. frm-o. gel. grc. hg. hg-bini. hg-s. hll. hydr. ind. jcr. k-bicr. k-ca. k-cla. k-i. k-o. lyc. mg-ca. mg-cl. mrl. na-ca. na-cl. ox-x. p. pb. pet. pnx. ppv. pt. qu-sa. rho. rn-b. rph. rs. rs-r. s. s-x. sep. smc. smi. so-d. spi. (spo). str. te. teu. thu. trg. trn. urg. vr-a. vr-s. vr-v. woo. ziz.

OBJECTS, FALSE APPEARANCE **of**. gel.
Multiplied. gel.
OBJECTS, IMAGINARY. amm-ca. atp. (hydr). k-cla. na-ca. smi.
Bright. atp. (hydr). k-cla.
Mist. smi.
Spots. atp. k-cla.
Bright. atp. k-cla.
Stars. amm-ca. na-ca.
White. na-ca.
Vibrations. (hydr).
Bright. (hydr).
White. na-ca.
PHOTOPHOBIA. alli. atp. ca-ca. con. euphr. k-bicr.
SIGHT IMPAIRED. atp. br. dt. fe-a. gel. (grc). ind. ox-x. pb. qu-sa. sep. smi.
EYEBALL. ag-na. aga. al-o. alli. anan. anm. arn. art-v. as-o. atp. au. ba-cl. ber. bi-na. br. bru. bry. ca-ca. ca-pa. ca-s. cb-v. ccs. chi. cit-c. clv. co. con. cr-o. crb-x. crot. dt. (eupat-p). euphr. fe-mgs. frm. frm-o. grc. hg. hg-s. hll. hydr. jcr. k-bicr. k-ca. k-i. lyc. mg-ca. mg-cl. mrl. na-cl. pnx. pt. rho. rn-b. rph. s. s-x. sep. smc. so-d. spi. str. te. teu. thu. trg. trn. urg. vr-a. vr-v. woo. ziz.
Appearance, Bright. trg.
Dim. alli. as-o. (con). (cu). k-ca. urg.
Staring. (cu). (spo).

Boring. bi-na.
Bursting. (mg-ca).
Coldness. pnx.
Color, Dark. (art-v). (chi). (clv). (cu). (rs).
Red. al-o. (alli). arn. atp. (ca-i). clv. con. (eupat-p). euphr. (hg-s). k-i. rn-b. teu. (vr-s). vr-v.
Yellow. as-o.
Creeping. frm-o.
Discharge. ba-cl.
Drawing. ca-s.
Dryness. atp. (cr-o). grc. spi.
Eruptions. (ca-ca). (p).
Styes. (p).
Ulcers. (ca-ca).
False Sensations. ca-pa. (grc).
Sand. ca-pa. (grc).
Heat. aga. al-o. as-o. (bry). (cit-c). hg. lyc. na-cl. rho. (s). thu. ziz.
Heaviness. jcr. thu. woo.
Itching. arum. eug. (hg-s). (s). sep. (smi).
Lachrymation. ag-na. aga. al-o. alli. anan. atp. au. ber. br. bru. bry. cb-v. ccs. chi. co. con. (crb-x). crot. dl-s. (eupat-p). euphr. hg. hg-bini. (hg-s). hydr. k-bicr. k-i. mg-ca. mg-cl. mrl. pt. rn-b. s. smc. so-d. spi. str. te. (teu). trg. urg. vr-a..
Cold. (trg).
Hot. atp. bry. euphr.
Movements. (aga). art-v. (ca-ca). dt. (k-o). (lyc). spi.
Convulsions. (aga). art-v. dt.
Squinting. art-v. hll. spi.
Paralysis. (ppv).
Pressing. al-o. (atp). br. (cit-c). (crt). (fe). (grc). (hg-s). lyc. (na-cl). (rs-r). thu.
Projecting. spi. (spo).
Sensitive. thu.
Shooting. (aga). ca-ca. cit-c. (hg-s). s. sep.
Smarting. alli. bry. ca-s. (cb-v). (cu-asi). k-bicr. rn-b. s-x. ziz.
Sunken. ag-na. as-o. chi. rph.
Swelling. anm. (clv). (con). (euphr). (hg). (k-i). (pet).
Chemosis. euphr.
Feeling of. cit-c.
Throbbing. (atp). trn.

Undefined. co. fe-mgs. sep.
Same Symptom. aga. al-o. anm. arum. as-o. ba-cl. br. ca-pa. ca-s. (cit-c). co. (cr-o). (cu-asi). eug. k-i. lyc. rn-b. (rs-r). s. sep. (smi). spi. ziz.
SCLEROTIC. con.
Color Red. con.
CORNEA. ca-ca. con.
Eruptions, Ulcers. ca-ca.
Opacity. con.
IRIS. art-v. as-o. atp. hll. spi.
Pupils, Dilated. art-v. as-o. atp. hll. spi.
Insensible. as-o.
ORBIT. cit-c. crt. cu-asi. na-cl. trn.
Pressing. crt. na-cl.
Throbbing. trn.
ORBITAL INTEGUMENTS. art-v. bry. chi. (cu). fe. rs. s. smi.
Color Dark. art-v. chi. (cu).
Itching. smi.
Same Symptom. s. smi.
ORBITAL INTEGUMENTS SUPERIORLY. bry. fe. s.
Heat. bry.
Itching. s.
Pressing. fe.
ORBITAL INTEGUMENTS INFERIORLY. rs.
Color Dark. rs.
EYELIDS. aga. alli. clv. con. hg. hg-s. k-ca. k-i. k-o. lyc. p. ppv. vr-s.
Adhesion of. k-ca. k-o.
Color Dark. clv.
Red. k-o. lyc.
Movements, Closing. (ca-ca). k-o. lyc.
Spasmodically. ca-ca.
Convulsions. aga.
Paralysis, Opening Difficult. ppv.
Swelling. clv. con. k-i.
Same Symptom. aga.
LOWER EYELID. aga. hg. hg-s. p.
Swelling. hg.
TARSAL EDGES. vr-s.
Color Red. vr-s.
CANTHI. cb-v. grc. hg-s. pet. rs-r.

Smarting. cb-v.
INTERNAL CANTHUS. grc. hg-s. pet.
Swelling. pet.
FORWARDS. mg-ca.
RIGHT. aga. atp. br. cr-o. frm. grc. hg-s. na-cl. s.
Sight Impaired. grc.
Eyeball, Color Red. hg-s.
Dryness. cr-o.
Heat. s.
Lachrymation. br. hg-s. teu.
Pressing. atp. na-cl.
Shooting. aga. s.
Throbbing. atp.
Same Symptom. aga. cr-o. s.
Lower Eyelid, Itching. hg-s.
Movements, Convulsions. aga.
Pressing. hg-s.
Shooting. hg-s.
Internal Canthus, False Sensations, Sand. grc.
Itching. hg-s.
Pressing. grc. hg-s.
Shooting. hg-s.
LEFT. alli. cit-c. crb-x. cu-asi. mg-ca. p. rs-r. s. trg.
Photophobia. alli.
Eyeball, Bursting. mg-ca.
Color Red. alli.
Lachrymation. alli. crb-x.
Cold. trg.
Shooting. s.
Same Symptom. s.
Orbit, Heat. cit-c.
Pressing. cit-c.
Smarting. cu-asi.
Swelling, Feeling of. cit-c.
Same Symptom. cit-c. cu-asi.
Lower Eyelid, Eruptions, Styes. p.
Internal Canthus, Pressing. rs-r.
Same Symptom. rs-r.
Forwards. **Eyeball Pressing**. mg-ca.

After NOSE, **Symptoms.**

ca-s. cb-v. hg.
SIGHT IMPAIRED. cb-v.
EYEBALL. ca-s. hg.
Heat. (hg).
Lachrymation. hg.
Smarting. ca-s.
Swelling. (hg).
EYELIDS. hg.
LOWER EYELID. hg.
LEFT. hg.
Lower Eyelid, Heat. hg.
  Swelling. hg.

Moving FACE **Muscles.**

pul. (spi).
EYEBALL. (spi).
Drawing. (pul).
Eruptions. (pul).
  Styes. (pul).
Tensive. (pul).
Undefined. (spi).
CANTHI. pul.
Drawing. pul.
Eruptions, Stye. pul.
Tensive. pul.

Moving JAWS.

ca-a.
EYEBALL.
Boring. (ca-a).
Shooting. (ca-a).
ORBITAL INTEGUMENTS. ca-a.
ORBITAL INTEGUMENTS SUPERIORLY. ca-a.
LEFT. ca-a.
Orbital Integuments Superiorly, Boring. ca-a.
  Shooting. ca-a.

YAWNING.

(arn). atp. ba-ca. ca-pa. dl-s. drm. fe. hg-bicl. k-ca. mph. p-x. sb-t. smi. str. str-i. vi-o. vr-s.

OBJECTS, FALSE APPEARANCE **of**. hg-bicl.

Far. hg-bicl.

Small. hg-bicl.

EYEBALL. (arn). atp. ba-ca. ca-pa. dl-s. drm. fe. hg-bicl. k-ca. mph. p-x. sb-t. smi. str. str-i. vi-o. vr-s.

Heat. hg-bicl.

Lachrymation. (arn). atp. ba-ca. ca-pa. dl-s. drm. fe k-ca. mph. p-x. sb-t. smi. vi-o. vr-s.

PRESSING **on** CHEEK.

atp.

OBJECTS, IMAGINARY. atp.

Flames. atp.

Mist. atp.

Before FACE **Symptoms**.

anm.

EYEBALL. anm.

Appearance, Glassy. anm.

Staring. anm.

Projecting. anm.

With FACE **Symptoms**.

acon. æth. ag-na. al-o. alo. amb. anm. ara. (arn). art-v. as-o. ast. atp. au. ba-ca. ber. bi-na. bry. buf. ca-ca. ca-pa. cap. cast. chi. cic. cit-c. clv. cmf. cn-sa. con. cop. cph. cr-o. crb-x. cro. crot. crt. cth. cu. cu-ca. cub. cyc. dig. dl-s. dor. dph. drm. dt. ery. eupat. (eupat-p). f-hx. fe. glo. glp. grp. grt. gym. hg. hg-bicl. hg-bini. hg-i. hg-s. hll. hyo. hyp. jat. jnp-s. k-bicr. k-ca. k-i. k-na. kre. lau-c. lch. lct. led. ly-b. lyc. men. mg-cl. mgs-ar. morph-a. mph. mrl. msc. mtr. myris. n-x. na-ba. na-ca. na-cl. na-sa. ner. (nic). ox-x. p. p-x. pb. pet. pnx. ppv. pso. pt. pul. qu-sa. rhe. rph. rs. rs-v. rut. s. s-x. sb-t. sep. si-x. smb. smi. sn. spi. spo. str. str-i. teu. trg. trn. urg. urt-u. val. vi-o. vp-r. vp-t. vr-a. vr-s. woo. zn.

OBJECTS, FALSE APPEARANCE **of**. atp. cic. hg-bicl. mg-cl. myris. s-x.

Black. s-x.

Blue. atp.
Bright. atp.
Far. hg-bicl. myris.
Green. mg-cl.
Grey. atp.
Moving. s-x.
Vibrating. s-x.
Multiplied. atp. cic.
Red. atp. mg-cl.
Small. hg-bicl.
White. atp.

OBJECTS, IMAGINARY. alo. atp. au. dt. (ery). (hg). k-ca. pet. pt. qu-sa. trg. (vr-a). zn.

Black. (ery).
Bright. au. k-ca. qu-sa. (vr-a).
Circles. zn.
Variegated. zn.
Figures. dt.
Green. (zn).
Grey. atp.
Halo. (zn).
Green. (zn).
Mist. atp. (ery).
Black. (ery).
Grey. atp.
Red. (ery).
Red. (ery).
Spots. au. k-ca. qu-sa. (vr-a).
Bright. au. k-ca. qu-sa. (vr-a).
Veil. pet.
Vibrations. alo. (hg). pt. trg.
Visions. dt.
Horrid. (dt).

PHOTOMANIA. dt.

PHOTOPHOBIA. acon. au. ca-ca. con. k-ca. str.

SIGHT IMPAIRED. ag-na. as-o. ast. atp. cap. chi. cro. dt. grp. grt. msc. pet. pul. s-x. str-i. trn.

Myopia. chi. grt.

EYEBALL. acon. æth. ag-na. al-o. amb. anm. ara. arn. art-v. as-o. atp. au. ba-ca. ber. bry. buf. ca-ca. ca-pa. cap. cast. chi. cit-c. clv. cmf. cn-sa. con. crot. crt. cth. cu. cu-ca. cyc. dl-s. dor. dph. drm. dro. dt. ery. eupat. f-hx. fe. glo. gym. hg. hg-bicl. hg-bini. hg-i. hg-s. hll. hyo. hyp. jnp-s.

k-bicr. k-ca. k-na. lau-c. lch. lct. led. ly-b. lyc. mg-cl. morph-a. mph. mrl. msc. mtr. myris. n-x. na-ba. na-ca. na-cl. na-sa. ox-x. p. p-x. pb. pet. pnx. ppv. pt. pul. qu-sa. rph. rs. rs-v. rut. s. sb-t. sep. si-x. smc. smi. sn. spi. spo. str. str-i. teu. trg. trn. urg. urt-u. vi-o. vp-r. vp-t. vr-a. vr-s. zn.

Appearance Bright. atp. crot. cth. dt. eupat. hg-bicl. hyo. jnp-s. lch. lyc. mtr. pb. trg. trn.

Dim. acon. ara. as-o. bry. buf. cit-c. (con). cu. dt. ery. hg. jnp-s. k-ca. lch. mtr. p-x. ppv. qu-sa. sep. trg. **vr-a.**

Glassy. anm. atp. (dt). glo. ppv.

Impudent. (dt).

Spiteful. (dt).

Staring. acon. æth. anm. atp. chi. crot. cth. cu. dor. dt. glo. hyp. k-ca. lau-c. lyc. msc. p-x. ppv. si-x. (spo). urg.

Wild. dt. hyp. ppv.

Coldness. lch.

Color Dark. (art-v). (as-o). (ber). (bi-na). (buf). (chi). (clv). (cn-sa). (cph). (cu). (cub). (dig). (dl-s). (dt). (ery). (jat). (jnp-s). (lyc). (myris). (na-ca). (ner). (p). (p-x). (rs). (s-x). (sep). (str-i). (woo).

Red. acon. (as-o). atp. buf. (ca-ca). clv. cmf. con. crot. (cu). cu-ca. dt. (eupat). (eupat-p). hg-s. hyo. led. morph-a. myris. na-cl. (pet). pnx. ppv. qu-sa. rs-v. rut. s. sep. str. (zn).

White. (hg-bicl).

Yellow. as-o. cth. (eupat). mg-cl. (n-x). s. sep. (spi) (str). vr-a.

Contractive. k-na.

Cutting. au.

Discharge. lyc. s.

Drawing. (as-o). (dph). (f-hx). (nic). p. val.

Eruptions. (ca-ca). (hg-bicl). (kre). (rs). zn.

Dry. (kre).

Herpetic. (kre).

Dry. (kre).

Pimples. (rs).

Pterygium. (ca-ca). zn.

Rhagades. (zn).

Scales. (kre).

Dry. (kre).

Ulcers. (ca-ca). (hg-bicl).
Vesicles. (rs).
Gnawing. (s).
Heat. amb. (aps) ara. hg-bicl. k-bicr. lct. ly-b. lyc. mrl. mtr. n-x. na-ca. pet. pt. s. spi. trn. vr-a. zn.
Itching. (cr-o). pet. s. zn.
Lachrymation. ag-na. al-o. (arn). atp. (au). ba-ca. (br). bry. ca-pa. con. crt. dl-s. drm. dt. (eupat). (eupat-p). fe. gym. k-ca. lct. lyc. mph. (na-sa). p-x. pnx. ppv. pt. (pul). qu-sa. sb-t. smi. spi. (spo). str. str-i. (trg). vi-o. vr-a. vr-s. zn.
Hot. au. bry. (pul). spo.
Movements. acon. æth. anm. art-v. atp. (ba-ca). buf. (ca-ca). (chi). cth. cu. (dig). dt. (glp). (grp). hg-bicl. hll. lau-c. (lyc). (men). mtr. ppv. (rhe). si-x. (smb). spi. (spo). trg.
Convulsions. acon. anm. art-v. atp. buf. cth. cu. dt. hg-bicl. (hll). lau-c. (men). mtr. (rhe). si-x. trg.
Squinting. æth. art-v. atp. dt. hll. spi.
Downwards. æth. (grp).
Upwards. acon. buf. (cu). lau-c.
To Left. buf.
Paralysis. (ppv).
Pressing. (as-o). cit-c. dph. (dt). (hg-bini). k-ca. lyc. (myris). na-ba. (na-cl). (ner). p. (pul). s.
Projecting. æth. anm. atp. au. cap. cu. dt. myris. pb. ppv. qu-sa. spo. vp-r. vp-t.
Shooting. ca-ca. (hg-bini). k-ca. (mgs-ar). pnx. (spo).
Smarting. (aps). bry. cast. na-ba. zn.
Small Feeling. al-o.
Strained. dph.
Sunken. ag-na. as-o. ber. buf. ca-ca. chi. cit-c. clv. cn-sa. cu. cyc. dl-s. dro. (dt). ery. hg. k-bicr. k-ca. lyc. n-x. ox-x. p. p-x. pb. ppv. pul. qu-sa. rph. s. smc. sn. spo. teu. vp-t.
Swelling. (as-o). au. (bry). buf. (ca-ca). (con). (cu). dt. (hg-s). (k-i). na-ca. (p). (pb). (pso). rs. s. urt-u.
Feeling of. lch.
Tearing. ca-ca. lyc. p. pul. (spo).
Tensive. jnp-s. k-ca. (nic). spi.
Throbbing. (myris).
Undefined. hg-i. str. trg.
Wrinkled. (zn).

Same Symptom. ara. as-o. (bry). buf. cmf. (cr-o). crot. cth. (cu). (dig). dph. dt. (hg-bini). hg-i. (hg-s). k-bicr. lau-c. ly-b. lyc. mg-cl. (mgs-ar). morph-a. mtr. n-x. (na-cl). pet. ppv. (rhe). s. sep. si-x. sn. spi. (spo). trg. trn. vr-a.

EYEBALL INTERNALLY. zn.

Color Red. zn.

SCLEROTIC. con. eupat.

Color Red. eupat.

Yellow. eupat.

CORNEA. au. ca-ca. con. hg-bicl. rs.

Color Red. au.

White. hg-bicl.

Eruptions, Pimples. rs.

Ulcers. ca-ca. hg-bicl.

Vesicles. rs.

Opacity. con.

CHAMBERS **of** EYE. hg-bicl.

Discharge, Pus. hg-bicl.

IRIS. acon. æth. anm. art-v. as-o. ast. atp. buf. chi. cic. crb-x. crt. cu. dt. glo. hg-bicl. hll. hyo. hyp. lyc. msc. mtr. na-ca. pnx. ppv. spi. str. trg.

Pupils Contracted. acon. ast. atp. crb-x. dt. glo. hg-bicl. msc. pnx.

Dilated. æth. anm. art-v. as-o. atp. buf. chi. cic. crt. cu. dt. hll. hyo. hyp. lyc. msc. mtr. na-ca. ppv. spi. str. trg.

Insensible. acon. æth. as-o. buf. (crb-x.) cu. dt. ppv.

Irregular. trg.

ORBIT. hg-i. lyc. myris. na-cl. pul. sn. val.

Drawing. sn. val.

Pressing. na-cl.

Tearing. lyc.

Same Symptom. na-cl. sn.

ORBIT SUPERIORLY. myris.

ORBITAL INTEGUMENTS. art-v. as-o. ber. bi-na. buf. chi. clv. cn-sa. cph. cr-o. crt. cu. cub. dl-s. dt. ery. hg-s. hll. jat. jnp-s. k-i. lyc. myris. n-x. na-ca. ner. p. p-x. pb. rs. sep. smc. spi. str. str-i. woo.

Color Dark. art-v. ber. bi-na. buf. chi. clv. cn-sa. cph. crt. cu. cub. dl-s. ery. jat. jnp-s. lyc. na-ca. ner. p. p-x. sep. smc. str-i. woo.

Yellow. n-x. spi. str.

Itching. cr-o.
Swelling. as-o. hg-s. k-i. p. pb. rs.
Same Symptom. cr-o. hg-s.
ORBITAL INTEGUMENTS SUPERIORLY. hll.
Movements, Convulsions. hll.
ORBITAL INTEGUMENTS INFERIORLY. dt. jat. myris. p. rs. s-x.
Color Dark. dt. jat. myris. p. rs.
Swelling. dt. p.
Same Symptom. dt.
EYELIDS. acon. anm. aps. as-o. atp. au. ba-ca. bry. buf. ca-ca. chi. clv. con. cu. dig. dt. (cry). glp. grp. hg-bicl. hll. k-ca. kre. lau-c. lyc. men. mtr. pnx. ppv. rhe. spo. zn.
Adhesion of. au. k-ca.
Color Dark. as-o. clv. dig.
Red. con. cu.
Eruptions, Dry. kre.
Herpes. kre.
Dry. kre.
Scales. kre.
Dry. kre.
Hæmorrhage. (ery).
Hairs Inverted. zn.
Heat. aps.
Movements, Closing. acon. anm. (atp). ba-ca. (buf). (ca-ca). chi. cu. dt. glp. (hg-bicl). lau-c. mtr. pnx. ppv. smb. spo.
Spasmodically. ca-ca. hg-bicl. spo.
Convulsions. hll. men. rhe.
Opening Wide. acon. (cu). lau-c. lyc. mtr. ppv.
Paralysis, Opening Difficult. ppv.
Smarting. aps.
Swelling. bry. clv. con. cop. cu. hg-bicl, na-ca. pso.
Same Symptom. as-o. bry. cop. cu. dig. hll. men. rhe.
UPPER. EYELID. k-ca.
Swelling. k-ca.
LOWER EYELID. bry.
Swelling. bry.
EYELIDS, INNER SURFACE. zn.
Wrinkled. zn.
CANTHI. ca-ca. mgs-ar. zn.
EXTERNAL CANTHUS. zn.

Eruptions, Rhagades. zn.
Smarting. zn.
INTERNAL CANTHUS. ca-ca. mgs-ar.
Shooting. mgs-ar.
Same Symptom. mgs-ar.
CARUNCULA. ca-ca.
LACHRYMAL SAC. pet.
FORWARDS. (dt). p.
Eyeball, Pressing. p.
BACKWARDS. dph.
Eyeball, Drawing. dph.
DOWNWARDS. ner.
LEFT **then** RIGHT. zn.
Eyeball, Eruptions, Pterygium. zn.
RIGHT. as-o. br. ca-ca. cit-c. dig. grp. na-sa. pul. s-x.
Objects Imaginary, Vibrations. hg.
Eyeball, Color Red. as-o.
Drawing. as-o.
Lachrymation. br. na-sa.
Hot. pul.
Pressing. as-o. cit-c. pul.
Same Symptom. cit-c.
Eyeball Internally, Color Red. ca-ca.
Swelling. ca-ca.
Orbit, Pressing. pul.
Orbital Integuments Inferiorly, Color Dark. s-x.
Eyelids, Movements, Closing. dig.
Opening Wide. grp.
Caruncula, Swelling. ca-ca.
LEFT. atp. buf. ca-ca. (dt). f-hx. grp. hg-bini. k-ca. myris. ner. s. spo. trg. vr-a. zn.
Objects Imaginary, Bright. vr-a.
Green. zn.
Halo Green. zn.
Spots Bright. vr-a.
Eyeball, Drawing. f-hx.
Eruptions, Pterygium. ca-ca.
Gnawing. s.
Heat. k-ca.
Lachrymation. k-ca. trg.
Movements, Convulsions. trg.
Pressing. hg-bini. ner.
Shooting. hg-bini. spo.

Tearing. k-ca. spo.
Undefined. s.
Same Symptom. hg-bini. ner. s. spo.
Orbit Superiorly, Pressing. myris.
Throbbing. myris.
Eyelids, Movements, Closing. atp. buf. grp.
Convulsions. trg.
Forwards. Eyeball, Pressing. (dt).
Downwards. Eyeball, Pressing. ner.

After FACE Symptoms.

rho.
EYEBALL. rho.
Pressing. rho.
LEFT. rho.
Eyeball, Pressing. rho.

Before TEETH Symptoms.

anm. hur.
EYEBALL. anm. hur.
Appearance Glassy. anm.
Staring. anm.
Projecting. anm.
Undefined. hur.

With TEETH Symptoms.

aps. art-v. as-o. atp. bry. ca-ca. cast. chi. cit-c. cle. cmc. cro. cth. dt. hg. hur. ind. k-ca. k-i. k-o. lyc. mn-ca. myris. na-ba. s. sep. spi. trg. trn.
OBJECTS, FALSE APPEARANCE **of**. dt.
Large. dt.
OBJECTS IMAGINARY. (hg).
Vibrations. (hg).
PHOTOPHOBIA. cle. k-ca.
SIGHT IMPAIRED. as-o. (cro). sep.
EYEBALL. aps. art-v. as-o. atp. bry. ca-ca. cast. chi. cle. cmc. cro. cth. dt. hur. k-ca. k-o. lyc. myris. na-ba. s. trg. trn.

Appearance Bright. cth. trg.
Dim. dt.
Staring. cth. k-o.
Boring. s.
Color Dark. (dt).
Coldness. (cro).
Drawing. (s).
Heat. atp. (cit-c). (myris).
Lachrymation. bry. chi. dt.
Hot. bry.
Movements. aps. art-v. cth. dt. (k-o).
Convulsions. cth. dt.
Squinting. aps. art-v.
Numbness. hur.
Pressing. (cit-c). na-ba.
Shooting. ca-ca. (myris).
Smarting. bry. cast. cmc.
Tearing. (cro). lyc.
Throbbing. trn.
Undefined. cle. hur. s.
Same Symptom. (cro). hur. lyc. (myris).
IRIS. aps. dt. mn-ca.
Pupils Dilated. aps. dt. mn-ca.
ORBIT. cit-c. hg-i. hur. k-i. myris.
Pressing. cit-c.
Throbbing. trn.
ORBIT SUPERIORLY. hg-i.
ORBITAL INTEGUMENTS. dt. spi.
Color Yellow. spi.
ORBITAL INTEGUMENTS INFERIORLY. dt.
Color Dark. dt.
EYELIDS. ind. k-o.
Movements, Closing. k-o.
EYELIDS, INNER SURFACE. ind.
Color Red. ind.
RIGHT. as-o. cro. hg. k-i.
Objects Imaginary, Vibrations. hg.
Sight Impaired. cro.
Eyeball, Coldness. cro.
Color Red. as-o.
Drawing. as-o.
Pressing. as-o.

Tearing. cro.
Same Symptom. cro.
Orbit, Tearing. k-i.
Same Symptom. k-i.
LEFT. cit-c. (dt). hg-i. hur. k-ca. myris. s.
Eyeball, Drawing. s.
Heat. k-ca. myris.
Lachrymation. (dt). k-ca.
Shooting. hur. myris.
Tearing. k-ca.
Undefined. cle. s.
Same Symptom. hur. myris. s.
Orbit, Heat. cit-c.
Pressing. cit-c.
Orbit Superiorly, Undefined. hg-i.
Same Symptom. hg-i.

After TEETH **Symptoms.**

ccs.
EYEBALL. ccs.
Pressing. (ccs).
LEFT. ccs.
Eyeball, Pressing. ccs.

PRESSING **on** THROAT.

trg.
EYEBALL. trg.
Pressing. trg.
FORWARDS. trg.
Eyeball, Pressing. trg.

Before THROAT **Symptoms.**

hyp. na-cl.
SIGHT DAZZLED. (na-cl).
SIGHT IMPAIRED. (na-cl).
EYEBALL. hyp.
Appearance, Staring. hyp.
Wild. hyp.

IRIS. hyp.
Pupils, Dilated. hyp.
LEFT. na-cl.
Sight Dazzled. na-cl.
Sight Impaired. na-cl.

With THROAT **Symptoms.**

acon. æth. ag-na. (alm). anm. aps. as-o. atp. br. bru. bry. buf. ca-ca. cast. cb-v. ccs. cic. cld. clv. con. cop. cth. cu. dt. dt-t. ery. eug. eupat. (eupat-p). gel. glo. hg. hg-bini. hll. hyo. jnp-s. k-bicr. k-ca. k-i. k-na. k-o. klm. lau-c. lyc. mgs. morph-a. msc. myris. na-ba. na-cl. nic. p. par. pb. ppv. pru-l. pt. pul. rn-b. rs. s. sb-t. si-x. smb. spi. spo. str. thu. trg. trn. vr-a.

OBJECTS, FALSE APPEARANCE **of.** (alm). atp. cic. dt. gel. myris. pb.
Blue. atp.
Bright. atp.
Far. gel. myris.
Grey. atp.
Inverted. gel.
Large. dt.
Multiplied. (alm). atp. cic. gel. pb.
Red. atp.
White. atp.
OBJECTS, IMAGINARY. atp. dt. pt.
Black. dt.
Bright. atp.
Grey. atp.
Mist. atp.
  Grey. atp.
Spots. atp. dt.
  Black. dt.
  Bright. atp.
Vibrations. pt.
PHOTOPHOBIA. acon. aps. con. hg. na-ba.
SIGHT IMPAIRED. (alm). as-o. atp. cb-v. dt. gel. klm. par. pb. pru-l.

EYEBALL. acon. æth. ag-na. (alm). anm. aps. as-o. atp. br. bru. bry. buf. ca-ca. cast. cb-v. ccs. cic. cld. clv. cth. cu. dt. ery. eug. eupat. (eupat-p). glo. hg. hg-bini. hll. hyo. jnp-s.

k-ca. k-na. klm. lau-c. lyc. mgs. msc. myris. na-ba. nic. p. pb. ppv. pul. rn-b. rs. s. sb-t. si-x. spi. spo. str. thu. trg. trn. vr-a.

Appearance, Bright. (alm). atp. bry. cth. dt. eupat. lyc. pb.

Dim. as-o. bry. buf. (cu). dt. ery. k-ca. trg. vr-a.

Glassy. anm. atp. bry. (dt). glo. rs.

Impudent. (dt).

Spiteful. (dt).

Staring. æth. anm. atp. cth. (cu). dt. glo. lyc. msc. si-x. spo.

Wild. dt.

Color Dark. (ery). (p).

Red. acon. atp. bry. cld. clv. cu. dt. (eupat). hg. myris. ppv. s. sb-t. str.

White. (s).

Yellow. as-o. (eupat). (eupat-p). s. str. vr-a.

Discharge. (str).

Hard. (str).

Yellow. (str).

Dryness. atp. (mgs). spi.

Eruptions. (k-bicr).

Granulations. (k-bicr).

Pustules. (k-bicr.)

Heat. as-o. eug. k-na. na-ba. myris. s.

Heaviness. ppv. thu.

Itching. s.

Lachrymation. ag-na. aps. br. bru. bry. cb-v. ccs. dt. nic. ppv. pt. rn-b. str. (trg). vr-a.

Movements. æth. (alm). buf. cic. cth. cu. dt. dt-t. hll. (k-o). lau-c. lyc. pb. ppv. pul. si-x. spi. trg.

Convulsions. buf. cic. cth. cu. dt. lau-c. ppv. pul. si-x. trg.

Squinting. æth. (alm). dt. hll. (pb). spi.

Upwards. buf. cic. cu. ppv.

Downwards. æth.

Inwards. (alm). (pb).

To Left. buf.

Paralysis. (trg).

Pressing. atp. (hg-bini). (myris). (na-cl). p. thu.

Projecting. acon. anm. atp. cu. ~~hyo~~. myris. pb. (spo).

Shooting. (cth). (hg-bini). k-ca. klm. (myris). (trn).

Smarting. ca-ca. cast. rn-b.

Sunken. as-o. (cu). (dt). ery. k-ca. p. rs.

Swelling. (cu). dt. (k-i).
Feeling of. cld.
Tearing. pul.
Tensive. jnp-s. k-ca.
Throbbing. (myris).
Undefined. (hg-bini). (s). trg.
Same Symptom. as-o. atp. buf. dt. (hg-bini). lau-c. pul. spi. trg.
EYEBALL ROUND CORNEA. k-bicr.
Color Red. k-bicr.
SCLEROTIC. eupat.
Color Red. eupat.
Yellow. eupat.
CORNEA. k-bicr. s.
Color Red. s.
White. s.
Eruptions, Pustules. k-bicr.
IRIS. æth. (alm). anm. as-o. atp. buf. cic. dt. glo. hll. lyc. morph-a. msc. pb. ppv. pul. spi. str. trg.
Pupils Contracted. atp. dt. glo.
Dilated. æth. (alm). anm. as-o. atp. buf. cic. dt. hll. lyc. morph-a. msc. pb. ppv. pul. spi. str.
Insensible. æth. as-o. buf. dt. ppv.
Irregular. trg.
ORBIT. myris. na-cl.
Pressing. na-cl.
ORBIT SUPERIORLY. myris.
ORBITAL INTEGUMENTS. cth. cu. ery. p.
ORBITAL INTEGUMENTS SUPERIORLY. cth.
Color Dark. cu. ery. p.
EYELIDS. (alm). buf. clv. cop. cu. dt. dt-t. k-bicr. k-ca. k-i. k-o. lyc. mgs. p. pb. ppv. smb. trg.
Adhesion of. k-ca.
Color Dark. clv. k-ca.
Red. cu.
Dryness. mgs.
Eruptions, Granulations. k-bicr.
Movements, Closing. (buf). cu. dt. k-o. ppv. smb.
Convulsions. cu.
Opening Wide. (alm). dt-t. lyc. pb. ppv.
Paralysis, Opening Difficult. trg.
Swelling. clv. cop. cu. k-i.
UPPER EYELID. k-o,

Heaviness. k-o.
CANTHI. str.
Discharge, Hard. str.
Yellow. str.
FORWARDS. atp. p. trg.
Eyeball, Pressing. atp. p. trg.
To HEAD. cth.
To FOREHEAD. cth.
Orbital Integuments Superiorly, Shooting. cth.
RIGHT. (alm). as-o. pb.
Eyeball, Color Red. as-o.
Drawing. as-o.
Movements, Squinting. (alm). pb.
Inwards. (alm). pb.
Pressing. as-o.
LEFT. buf. hg-bini. k-ca. myris. s. trg. trn.
Eyeball, Heat. myris.
Lachrymation. trg.
Movements, Convulsions. trg.
Pressing. hg-bini.
Shooting. hg-bini. myris. trn.
Undefined. hg-bini. s.
Same Symptom. hg-bini. s.
Orbit Superiorly, Pressing. myris.
Throbbing. myris.
Eyelids, Adhesion of. k-ca.
Movements, Closing. buf.
Convulsions. trg.

DRINKING.

crot.
SIGHT IMPAIRED. crot.

EATING.

aga. al-o. amb. arum. atp. ba-ca. ca-ca. cb-v. cro. dig. dph. dt. ery. grt. hg. i. irs-f. k-bicr. k-o. lct. li-ca. lyc. mg-ca. mg-cl. n-x. na-ca. na-sa. ner. ol-a. p. pb. phl. pol. ppv. ptv. rut. s. si-x. str. str-i. thu. val. vr-a. zn.
OBJECTS, FALSE APPEARANCE **of**. dt. hg. p.
Black. hg.

Green. hg.
Moving. hg.
Circularly. hg.
Multiplied. dt.
Part Visible. p.
OBJECTS, IMAGINARY. ba-ca. dig. dph. ery. lct. p. si-x. str-i. zn.
Black. lct. lyc. p.
Bright. dig. dph. ery. p.
Circles. p.
Mist. si-x.
Serpentine Bodies. ery. str-i.
Bright. ery.
Spots. dig. ery. lct. lyc. p.
Black. lct. lyc. p.
Bright. dig.
White. ery.
Veil. ba-ca. zn.
Vibrations. dph. p.
Bright. dph. p.
White. ery.
Zigzags. p.
Bright. p.
PHOTOPHOBIA. str.
SIGHT DAZZLED. dig. si-x.
SIGHT IMPAIRED. atp. ba-ca. ca-ca. cb-v. k-bicr. na-sa. (ner). p. ppv. ptv. str. zn.
EYEBALL. aga. al-o. amb. dph. k-o. lyc. mg-ca. mg-cl. na-ca. na-sa. ol-a. s. thu. zn.
Color Red. s.
Drawing. aga.
Dryness. (vr-a).
Heat. (cb-v). k-o. mg-cl. na-ca. thu. zn.
Heaviness. (cro).
Itching. (mg-ca).
Lachrymation. dph. (na-sa). (ol-a). zn.
Movements. (arum). (dph). (grt). (n-x).
Convulsions. (dph). (grt). (n-x).
Presssing. aga. pol. s. (val).
Shooting. (irs-f). (na-ca). ol-a.
Small Feeling. al-o.
Smarting. mg-cl.
Swelling, Feeling of. (cro).

Tearing. amb. (ol-a). (phl).
Undefined. lyc.
IRIS. s. str.
PUPILS, **Dilated.** s. str.
ORBIT. pol.
Pressing. pol.
ORBITAL INTEGUMENTS. amb. n-x. phl.
Tearing. amb.
ORBITAL INTEGUMENTS SUPERIORLY. phl.
ORBITAL INTEGUMENTS INFERIORLY. n-x.
EYELIDS. arum. cb-v. cro. dig. dph. grt. irs-f. phl. vr-a.
Heat. cb-v.
Movements, Closing. arum.
Convulsions. dph. grt.
Swelling, Feeling of. cro.
UPPER EYELID. cro. vr-a.
Dryness. vr-a.
Heaviness. cro.
LOWER EYELID. phl.
FORWARDS. val.
Eyeball, Pressing. val.
RIGHT. dig. irs-f. mg-ca. n-x. na-sa. ner. ol-a. phl.
Sight Impaired. ner.
Eyeball, Itching. mg-ca.
Lachrymation. na-sa. ol-a.
Orbital Integuments Superiorly, Tearing. phl.
Orbital Integuments Inferiorly, Movements, Convulsions. n-x.
Eyelids, Movements, Closing. dig.
Upper Eyelid, Shooting. irs-f.
LEFT. lyc. ol-a. phl.
Eyeball, Shooting. ol-a.
Tearing. ol-a.
Undefined. lyc.
Lower Eyelid, Tearing. phl.

VOMITING.

aga. as-o. ca-ca. cu. eug. k-bicr. nic. sb-t. vr-v.
EYEBALL. aga. asr. ca-ca. cu. eug. k-bicr. sb-t. vr-v.
Appearance Dim. sb-t.

Color Red. (k-bicr).
Heat. eug. k-bicr.
Lachrymation. asr. ca-ca. cu. k-bicr. sb-t. vr-v.
Motion in. eug.
Rolling. eug.
Swelling, Feeling of. (aga).
EYELIDS. k-bicr.
Color Red. k-bicr.
LEFT. aga.
Eyeball, Swelling Feeling of. aga.

During STOOL.

so-t. spi.
EYEBALL. so-t. spi.
Color Red. (so-t).
Lachrymation. so-t.
Pressing. (spi).
SCLEROTIC. so-t.
Color Red. so-t.
RIGHT. spi.
Eyeball, Pressing. spi.

After STOOL.

crot. na-ca.
SIGHT IMPAIRED. crot.
EYEBALL. na-ca.
Heat. na-ca.

Before ABDOMINAL **Symptoms**.

amb. anm. (ery). eug. hyp. na-cl. narth. rn-b. sep. trg. vr-a.
OBJECTS, IMAGINARY. na-cl. vr-a.
Bright. (vr-a).
Spots. (vr-a).
Bright. (vr-a).
Zigzags. na-cl.
Bright. na-cl.
SIGHT IMPAIRED. amb. (ery). narth.

EYEBALL. anm. eug. hyp. rn-b. sep. trg.
Appearance Glassy. anm.
Staring. anm. hyp.
Wild. hyp.
Heat. eug.
Itching. rn-b.
Lachrymation. eug.
Motion in. eug.
Rolling. eug.
Pressing. sep.
Projecting. anm.
IRIS. hyp.
Pupils Dilated. hyp.
LEFT. vr-a.
Objects Imaginary, Bright. vr-a.
Spots, Bright. vr-a.

During ABDOMINAL Symptoms.

acon. æsc. æth. aga. alli. alm. anan. aps. ara. arn. art-v. as-o. asr. ast. atp. bi-na. br. bry. buf. ca-ca. cac. can. cast. cb-a. cb-v. chd. chi. chio. cic. cit-c. cld. clv. cmf. con. cop. cph. crn. cro. crot. cth. cu. cyc. dig. dor. drm. dt. dt-t. ery. eupat. (eupat-p). glo. gn-l. grc. gym. hg. hg-bicl. hg-cl. hg-s. jat. jnp-s. k-bicr. k-ca. k-i. k-na. k-o. klm. lac-f. lam. lau-c. lct. li-ca. ly-b. lyc. mg-cl. msc. mtr. myris. n-x. na-ba. na-ca. na-cl. na-sa. ner. ni-ca. nic. p. pb. pet. pip. pnc. pnx. pod. ppv. pru-l. pso. pt. pul. qu-sa. rho. rph. rn-b. s. sb-t. sep. spi. spo. srr. str. str-i. thr. thu. trg. trn. tx-b. vr-a. vr-s. vr-v. zn. zng.

OBJECTS, FALSE APPEARANCE **of.** (alm). atp. cic. hg. klm. mg-cl. nic. pb. s. spo. str. thr.
Black. hg. klm.
Blue. atp.
Bright. atp.
Green. mg-cl. nic.
Grey. atp.
Moving. spo. str.
Vertically. spo. str.
Up and Down. spo. str.
Multiplied. (alm). atp. cic. pb. **s.** spo. **thr.**
Red. atp. mg-cl.

White. atp.
Yellow. as-o. nic.
OBJECTS, IMAGINARY. atp. ca-ca. can. cyc. dt. ery. k-ca. klm. myris. na-cl. pso. pt. qu-sa. sep. str. thr. trg. tx-b.
Black. thr.
Blue. pso.
Bright. atp. cyc. ery. k-ca. klm. qu-sa. sep. thr.
Circles. tx-b.
Figures. dt. myris.
Grey. atp.
Light. qu-sa.
Mist. atp. can. k-o. pso.
Grey. atp.
Spots. atp. cyc. ery. k-ca. qu-sa.
Bright. atp. cyc. ery. k-ca. qu-sa.
Stars. pso.
Blue. pso.
Veil. dt. (na-cl).
Vibrations. atp. klm. pt. sep. thr. trg.
Black. thr.
Bright. klm. sep. thr.
Visions. dt. str.
PHOTOMANIA. dt.
PHOTOPHOBIA. acon. aps. atp. ca-ca. con. hg. k-ca. (lac-f). na-ba. thr.
SIGHT DAZZLED. (na-cl).
SIGHT IMPAIRED. alm. as-o. ast. atp. bi-na. br. buf. ca-ca. can. cb-v. chi. crot. cyc. dt. (ery). glo. gym. hg. k-bicr. k-ca. klm. lac-f. lam. na-ca. na-cl. (ner). pet. pip. pnc. pru-l. pt. pul. qu-sa. rph. sep. spo. srr. trg. trn. (vr-a).
Hemeralopia. vr-a.
EYEBALL. acon. æsc. æth. aga. alli. (alm). anan. aps. ara. art-v. as-o. asr. atp. bi-na. bry. ca-ca. cac. cast. cb-a. chd. chi. cld. clv. cmf. cof. con. cph. crn. crot. cth. cu. dig. dor. drm. dt. eug. eupat. (eupat-p). glo. gn-l. gym. hg. hg-bicl. hg-cl. hg-s. hyo. jat. jnp-s. k-bicr. k-ca. k-na. klm. lac-f. lau-c. lct. li-ca. ly-b. lyc. n-x. na-ba. na-cl. na-sa. ner. ni-ca. nic. p. pb. pet. pnx. ppv. pru-l. pt. rho. rn-b. rs. s. sb-t. sep. spi. spo. str. str-i. thr. thu. trg. trn. vp-t. vr-a. vr-s. vr-v.
Appearance Bright. (alm). atp. bry. cth. dt. eupat. pb.

Dim. ara. as-o. bry. (cu). dt. hg. k-ca. ppv. sb-t. vr-a.

Glassy. atp. bry. glo. rs.

Staring. atp. cth. (cu). dor. dt. glo. k-ca. lau-c. pru-l. (spo).

Wild. dt.

Color Dark. (as-o). (clv). (cph). (crn). (cu). (dt). (jat). (k-ca). (lyc). (mtr). (ner). (p). (pod). (rs).

Red. acon. atp. bi-na. bry. cld. con. cu. dt. (eupat). (eupat-p). hg. hyo. (k-bicr). (lac-f). na-cl. pnx. ppv. s. (spi). str. str-i. trg.

Yellow. æsc. as-o. chd. chi. con. crn. dig. (eupat). (eupat-p). hg-cl. pb. s. str. vr-a.

Drawing. aga. (chio).

False Sensations. cmf.

Sand. cmf.

Eruptions. (ca-ca). (p). (s).

Styes. (p).

Ulcers. (ca-ca). (s).

Heat. (alm). cb-a. eug. gym. k-bicr. k-na. lct. na-ba. ni-ca. pet. s. sep. thu. trg.

Heaviness. anan. hg-s. k-bicr. (k-o). ppv.

Itching. (grc). hg-bicl. (ly-b). rn-b. s.

Lachrymation. alli. aps. asr. atp. bry. ca-ca. cof. con. crot. cu. drm. (eupat-p). gn-l. k-bicr. k-ca. (lac-f). lct. nic. p. pnx. ppv. pt. s. sb-t. (spi). spo. str. vr-a. vr-s. vr-v.

Hot. (spi).

Motion in. eug.

Rolling. eug.

Movements. (alm). aps. art-v. ca-ca. cit-c. cmf. cth. cu. dig. dt. dt-t. k-o. lyc. (myris). pb. pnx. ppv. s. sep. spi. spo. vr-a.

Convulsions. art-v. cth. cu. dt. pb. ppv.

Squinting. (alm). art-v. dig. dt. (pb). s. spi.

Upwards. aps. cu.

Inwards. (alm). (pb).

Paralysis. (trg).

Pressing. (acon). aga. (chio). cmf. (con). k-ca. klm. (myris). na-ba. (na-cl). sep. (str). thu. vr-a. (zng).

Projecting. æth. atp. cu. pb. (spo). str-i.

Sensitive. (zn).

Shooting. ca-ca. cmf. hg-bicl. k-ca. klm. (lac-f). na-sa. pnx.

Smarting. asr. cast. li-ca. na-ba. trg. trn.

Sunken. as-o. clv. cu. (dt). k-ca. lau-c. p. rs. vp-t. vr-a.

Swelling. (con). dt. (k-ca). (k-i). str-i.

Feeling of. (aga). cld.

Tearing. (con). na-ba. pul.

Tensive. jnp-s. k-ca. n-x.

Throbbing. (myris). (thr). trg.

Undefined. aps. cth. (spi). thu. (trg).

Same Symptom. dt. hg-bicl. thu.

EYEBALL SUPERIORLY. cac.

Smarting. cac.

EYEBALL ROUND CORNEA. s.

Color Red. s.

SCLEROTIC. con. eupat.

Color Red. con. eupat.

Yellow. eupat.

CORNEA. ca-ca. con. s.

Eruptions, Ulcers. ca-ca. s.

Opacity. con. s.

IRIS. (alm). arn. art-v. as-o. ast. atp. (br). cic. cmf. cph. dt. glo. morph-a. msc. nic. pb. spi.

Pupils Contracted. ast. atp. dt. glo.

Dilated. (alm). art-v. as-o. atp. (br). cic. cmf. cph. dt. morph-a. msc. nic. pb. spi.

Insensible. arn. as-o. dt.

ORBIT. acon. chio. con. myris. na-cl. trg.

Pressing. acon. chio. na-cl.

Tearing. con.

Undefined. trg.

ORBIT SUPERIORLY. chio. myris.

ORBITAL INTEGUMENTS. art-v. as-o. clv. cph. crn. cu. dt. jat. k-ca. lyc. mtr. ner. p. pod. rs. sep.

Color Dark. art-v. as-o. clv. cph. crn. cu. jat. lyc. mtr. ner. p. rs.

ORBITAL INTEGUMENTS SUPERIORLY. k-ca. sep.

Movements, Convulsions. sep.

Swelling. k-ca.

ORBITAL INTEGUMENTS INFERIORLY. dt. pod.

Color Dark. dt. pod.

EYELIDS. aps. bry. cit-c. cmf. con. cop. cro. cu. dt. grc. k-bicr. k-ca. k-o. lyc. myris. p. pnx. ppv. s. sep. spo. trg. vr-a. zn.

Adhesion of. (con). (k-ca).
Color Dark. k-ca.
Red. con. cu. k-bicr.
Heat. cro.
Itching. grc.
Movements, Closing. aps. (ca-ca). cit-c. cu. dt. **k-o.** lyc. pnx. ppv. sep. spo. vr-a.
Spasmodically. ca-ca. spo.
Convulsions. cmf. cu.
Opening Wide. (dt). dt-t.
Winking. myris.
Paralysis, Opening Difficult. trg.
Swelling. con. cop. cu. k-i.
UPPER EYELID. trg.
Heat. trg.
Smarting. trg.
LOWER EYELID. bry. p.
Swelling. bry.
TARSAL EDGES. s.
Eruptions, Ulcers. s.
Swelling. s.
CANTHI. s.
EXTERNAL CANTHUS. s.
Color Red. s.
FORWARDS. sep. str.
Eyeball, Pressing. sep. str.
BACKWARDS. lac-f.
To HEAD. lac-f.
To FOREHEAD. lac-f.
To TEMPLES. lac-f.
RIGHT. (alm). as-o. chio. cmf. con. k-ca. k-o. lac-f. ly-b. na-cl. ner. pb. thr. zn.
Objects Imaginary, Veil Crooked. na-cl.
Photophobia. lac-f.
Sight Dazzled. na-cl.
Sight Impaired. na-cl. ner.
Eyeball, Color Red. as-o. con. lac-f.
Drawing. as-o.
Itching. ly-b.
Lachrymation. con. lac-f.
Movements, Squinting. (alm). pb.
Inwards. (alm). pb.
Pressing. as-o. cmf. con.

Shooting. lac-f.
Throbbing. thr.
Orbit Superiorly, Drawing. chio.
Pressing. chio.
Eyelids, Adhesion of. con.
Upper Eyelid, Heaviness. k-o.
Sensitive. zn.
Swelling. k-ca.
Backwards. Eyeball, Shooting. lac-f.
To Forehead. Eyeball, Shooting. lac-f.
Throbbing. lac-f.
To Temple. Eyeball, Shooting. lac-f.
Throbbing. lac-f.
LEFT. aga. k-ca. myris. spi. zng.
Eyeball, Color Red. spi.
Lachrymation. spi.
Hot. spi.
Pressing. zng.
Swelling, Feeling of. aga.
Undefined. spi.
Orbit Superiorly, Pressing. myris.
Throbbing. myris.
Eyelids, Adhesion of. k-ca.

After ABDOMINAL Symptoms.

cic. grp. k-bicr.
OBJECTS, IMAGINARY. k-bicr.
Veil. k-bicr.
Yellow. k-bicr.
Yellow. k-bicr.
SIGHT IMPAIRED. k-bicr.
EYEBALL. cic.
To HEAD. cic.
To OCCIPUT. cic.
Eyeball, Shooting. cic.

After URINATION.

eug.
OBJECTS IMAGINARY. eug.
Light. eug.

Before URINARY **Symptoms.**

(cu).
EYEBALL. (cu).
Movements. (cu).
Convulsions. (cu).

With URINARY **Symptoms.**

acon. æsc. (alm). anag. anm. apo. aps. atp. (br). bry. buf. ca-s. chi. clv. con. cu. dor. dt. eug. eupat. (eupat-p). grp. hg-cl. hyo. k-ca. k-i. k-o. na-ca. na-cl. pb. s. sep. spo. str. thu. trg.
OBJECTS, FALSE APPEARANCE **of.** (alm). atp. pb.
Blue. atp.
Bright. atp.
Grey. atp.
Multiplied. (alm). atp. pb.
Red. atp.
White. atp.
OBJECTS, IMAGINARY. atp.
Bright. atp.
Grey. atp.
Mist. atp.
Grey. atp.
Spots. atp.
Bright. atp.
SIGHT IMPAIRED. apo. atp. chi. grp.
EYEBALL. acon. æsc. (alm). anag. anm. aps. atp. buf. ca-s. clv. con. cu. dor. dt. eug. eupat. hg-cl. hyo. k-ca. k-o. na-ca. s. str. thu. trg.
Appearance Dim. buf. k-ca.
Bright. (alm). atp. eupat.
Glassy. anm. atp.
Staring. anm. atp. dor. dt. k-o.
Wild. dt.
Color Dark. (dt). (k-ca).
Red. atp. buf. (con). cu. dt. (eupat). (eupat-p). s. str.
White. (s).
Yellow. æsc. ca-s. (eupat). hg-cl. pb. str
Heat. eug. na-ca.

Lachrymation. (con). str.
Movements. acon. (alm). aps. atp. buf. cu. dt. (k-o). (pb). (sep). (trg).
Convulsions. acon. atp. buf. (cu). dt. (sep). (trg).
Squinting. (alm). aps. atp. (pb).
Upwards. aps. buf. cu.
Inwards. (alm). (pb).
To Left. buf.
Pressing. anag. (con). (na-cl). thu.
Projecting. anm. atp. hyo. (spo).
Shooting. anag.
Sunken. clv.
Swelling. (bry). (eupat-p). (k-i).
SCLEROTIC. eupat.
Color Red. eupat.
Yellow. eupat.
CORNEA. s.
Color Red. s.
White. s.
IRIS. (alm). aps. atp. (br). buf. dt. na-ca. pb.
Pupils Contracted. atp. dt.
Dilated. (alm). aps. atp. (br). buf. dt. na-ca. pb.
Insensible. buf.
ORBIT. na-cl.
Pressing. na-cl.
ORBITAL INTEGUMENTS. dt. sep.
ORBITAL INTEGUMENTS SUPERIORLY, sep.
Movements, Convulsions. sep.
ORBITAL INTEGUMENTS INFERIORLY. dt.
Color Dark. dt.
EYELIDS. aps. bry. buf. con. cu. (dt). k-ca. k-i. k-o. sep. trg.
Adhesion of. (con).
Color Dark. k-ca.
Movements, Closing. aps. (buf). cu. k-o. sep.
Convulsions. cu.
Opening Wide. (dt).
Swelling. k-i.
LOWER EYELID. bry.
Swelling. bry.
RIGHT. (alm). con. pb.

Eyeball, Color Red. con.
Lachrymation. con.
Movements, Squinting. (alm). pb.
Inwards. (alm). pb.
Pressing. con.
Eyelids, Adhesion of. con.
LEFT. buf. trg.
Eyeball, Movements, Convulsions. trg.
Eyelids, Movements, Closing. buf.
Convulsions. trg.

Before MENSES.

atp. hg. lyc. si-x.
OBJECTS, FALSE APPEARANCE **of.** si-x.
White. si-x.
SIGHT IMPAIRED. atp.
EYEBALL. hg. si-x.
Pressing. hg. si-x.
IRIS. lyc.
Pupils Dilated. lyc.

At Commencement of MENSES.

br.
EYEBALL. br.
Pressing. br.
FORWARDS. br.
Eyeball, Pressing. br.

During MENSES.

br. ca-ca. cast. (chi). grp. hg-s. li-ca. ly-b. lyc. mg-ca. n-x. ni-ca. p. pnx. pul. sang. sep. si-x. str. zn.
OBJECTS, FALSE APPEARANCE **of.** li-ca.
Part Visible. li-ca.
SIGHT IMPAIRED. grp. hg-s. li-ca. pul. sep.
EYEBALL. br. ca-ca. cast. (chi). hg-s. mg-ca. n-x. ni-ca. (str). zn.
Color Red. zn.
Cutting. (hg-s).
Discharge. ca-ca. (mg-ca).

Dryness. mg-ca.
Heat. mg-ca. n-x. ni-ca.
Lachrymation. ca-ca. (chi).
Movements. (chi). (hg-s). (p).
Convulsions. (chi).
Paralysis. mg-ca.
Projecting. (chi).
Pressing. (br). (hg-s). (sang). (str).
Shooting. ca-ca.
Smarting. cast.
Undefined. ca-ca. mg-ca.
IRIS. lyc.
Pupils, Contracted. lyc.
ORBIT. hg-s.
ORBIT SUPERIORLY. hg-s.
Cutting. hg-s.
EYELIDS. ca-ca. hg-s. mg-ca. p.
Adhesion of. ca-ca. mg-ca. p.
Movements, Closing. hg-s. p.
Convulsions. (chi).
UPPER EYELID. hg-s.
Heaviness. hg-s.
CANTHI. mg-ca.
EXTERNAL CANTHUS. mg-ca.
Discharge. mg-ca.
FORWARDS. br. sang. str.
Eyeball, Pressing. br. sang. str.
BACKWARDS. hg-s.
Eyeball, Pressing. hg-s.
OUTWARDS. hg-s.
Orbit Superiorly, Cutting. hg-s.

After MENSES.

hg-s.
SIGHT IMPAIRED. hg-s.
EYEBALL. hg-s.
Heaviness. hg-s.
Smarting. (hg-s).
Sunken Feeling. hg-s.
Swelling, Feeling of. (hg-s).
ORBIT. hg-s.

ORBIT, SUPERIORLY. hg-s.
Smarting. hg-s.
Swelling, Feeling of. hg-s.

EMISSIONS.

dt.
OBJECTS, IMAGINARY. dt.
Veil. dt.
SIGHT IMPAIRED. dt.

SEXUAL EXCESSES.

p.
SIGHT IMPAIRED. p.

PREGNANCY.

art-v. atp. au. ca-ca. chi. cic. cyc. gel. hyo. k-o. myris. na-cl. p. pul. s.
OBJECTS, FALSE APPEARANCE **of.** atp. au. chi. gel. hyo.
Confused. chi.
Outlines. chi.
Inverted. atp.
Large. hyo.
Moving. cic.
Multiplied. atp. gel.
Part Visible. au.
Horizontal. au.
Red. hyo.
White. chi.
OBJECTS, IMAGINARY. ca-ca. chi. cyc. k-o. p. pul. s.
Bright. cyc.
Grey. p.
Halo. chi. s.
White. chi.
Mist. ca-ca. k-o. pul.
Spots. cyc.
Bright. cyc.
Veil. p.
Grey. p.

White. chi.
SIGHT IMPAIRED. art-v. atp. ca-ca. cyc. gel. k-o. pul. s.
EYEBALL. atp. hyo.
Color Red. atp.
Movements. hyo. (k-o.) (myris). na-cl.
Convulsions. (hyo).
Squinting. hyo.
EYELIDS. hyo. k-o. myris. na-cl. str.
Movements, Closing. k-o. (na-cl).
Spasmodically. na-cl.
Convulsions. hyo.
Winking. myris.
UPPER EYELID. k-o. str.
Heaviness. k-o. str.

PARTURITION.

au-cl.
SIGHT IMPAIRED. au-cl.

With SEXUAL Symptoms.

anag. ara. atp. (br). cap. chi. cmf. cyc. dt. euphr. gel. hpm. hyo. k-o. lyc. myris. na-ca. pul. sep. si-x. str. thu. trg. trn. tss. vr-a.
OBJECTS, FALSE APPEARANCE **of**. atp.
Blue. atp.
Bright. atp.
Grey. atp.
Multiplied. atp.
Red. atp.
OBJECTS, IMAGINARY. atp. cyc.
Grey. atp.
Mist. atp. cyc.
Grey. atp.
Visions. atp.
Horrible. atp.
SIGHT IMPAIRED. atp. cap. chi. cyc. gel. hyo. si-x. (vr-a).
Hemeralopia. vr-a.

EYEBALL. anag. ara. atp. cmf. euphr. myris. na-ca. pul. str. thu. trg. trn. tss.
Appearance Dim. ara.
Color Dark. (myris).
Green. (myris).
Red. atp. euphr. pul. tss.
Dryness. myris. (thu).
False Sensations. cmf.
Sand. cmf.
Heat. na-ca. (thu).
Heaviness. (k-o).
Lachrymation. euphr.
Movements. (cmf). (hyo). (k-o). (sep).
Convulsions. (cmf). (hyo). (sep).
Paralysis. (myris).
Pressing. anag. cmf. (str).
Shooting. anag. cmf.
Smarting. trn.
Throbbing. trg.
Undefined. (trg).
LENS. lyc.
Cataract. lyc.
IRIS. atp. (br). dt.
Pupils Contracted. atp.
Dilated. atp. (br). dt.
ORBIT. trg.
Undefined. trg.
ORBITAL INTEGUMENTS. myris. sep.
Color Dark. myris.
Green. myris.
ORBITAL INTEGUMENTS SUPERIORLY. sep.
Movements, Convulsions. sep.
EYELIDS. cmf. hpm. hyo. k-o. myris. sep. thu.
Movements, Closing. k-o. sep.
Convulsions. cmf. hyo.
Paralysis, Closing Difficult. myris.
UPPER EYELID. k-o.
Heaviness. k-o.
TARSAL EDGES. hpm. thu.
Heat. hpm.
LOWER TARSAL EDGE. thu.
FORWARDS. str.
Eyeball, Pressing. str.

RIGHT. thu.
Eyeball, Dryness. thu.
Lower Tarsal Edge, Heat. thu.

COUGHING.

acon. art-v. atp. cof. (eupat). grp. k-ca. k-cla. p. par. ppv. pul. spo. vr-s.
OBJECTS, IMAGINARY. k-ca. k-cla. par.
Bright. k-ca. k-cla. par.
Spots. k-ca. k-cla. par.
Bright. k-ca. k-cla. par.
EYEBALL. acon. art-v. atp. (eupat). grp. p. ppv. spo. vr-s.
Color Red. atp.
Lachrymation. acon. art-v. (eupat). grp. p. ppv. vr-s.
Projecting. atp.
Throbbing. spo.

SPEAKING.

p-x.
SIGHT IMPAIRED. p-x.
Myopia. p-x.

Before CHEST **Symptoms.**

art-v. cu.
EYEBALL. art-v. cu.
Appearance Staring. art-v.
Movements, Convulsions. cu.

With CHEST **Symptoms.**

acon. æth. ag-na. al-o. alli. (alm). amm-ca. anm. aps. ara. arn. art-v. as-o. atp. bi-na. br. bry. buf. ca-ca. ca-s. cac. cast. cb-a. cb-v. chd. chi. cic. cld. clv. cof. cph. crb-x. cu. cu-ca. dl-s. dor. dph. dro. dt. dt-t. ery. eupat. (eupat-p). euph. euphr. fe. gel. glo. glp. gym. hg. hpm. hyo. i. k-bicr. k-ca. k-cla. k-i. klm. kre. lau-c. lct. lyc. mgs. morph-a. msc. mtr. myris. n-x. na-ba. na-cl. na-sa. os. p. p-x. par. pb. pnx. pod. pol. ppv. pru-l. pul. qu-sa. rn-b. rs. s. s-x. sep. smb. sn. spi. spo. spo-f. str. te. thu. trg. trn. urg. vr-a. vr-s.

OBJECTS, FALSE APPEARANCE **of.** (alm). amm-ca. atp. cb-v. cic. gel. glo. myris. pb.

Black. amm-ca.
Blue. atp.
Bright. atp.
Far. myris.
Grey. atp.
Inverted. glo.
Moving. amm-ca.
Multiplied. (alm). atp. cic. gel. pb.
Red. atp.
Small. cb-v.
White. atp.

OBJECTS, IMAGINARY. atp. cb-v. (cu). dt. (ery). k-ca. k-cla. par. pru-l. qu-sa. sep. str.

Black. dt. (ery).
Bright. atp. dt. k-ca. k-cla. par. qu-sa. sep.
Figures. (cu). dt.
Grey. atp.
Light. qu-sa.
Mist. atp. (ery).
  Black. (ery).
  Grey. atp.
  Red. (ery).
Red. (ery).
Spirits. (cu).
Spots. atp. dt. k-ca. k-cla. par. qu-sa. sep. str.
  Black. dt.
  Bright. atp. dt. k-ca. k-cla. par. qu-sa. sep. str.
Veil. pru-l.
Vibrations. sep.
  Bright. sep.
Visions. cb-v. str.
  Horrible. cb-v.

PHOTOMANIA. dt.

PHOTOPHOBIA. acon. alli. aps. atp. euph. hg. na-ba.

SIGHT IMPAIRED. amm-ca. as-o. atp. au-cl. bi-na. ca-ca. cof. dt. (ery). gel. klm. myris. pul. s.

EYEBALL. acon. æth. aga. al-o. alli. (alm). anm. aps. ara. arn. art-v. as-o. atp. bi-na. br. bry. buf. ca-ca. ca-s. cac. cast. cb-v. chd. chi. cic. cld. clv. cph. cu. cu-ca. dl-s. dor. dph. dt. (ery). eupat. (eupat-p). euph. euphr. glo. glp. gym. hg. hyo. hyp. i. k-bicr. k-ca. k-i. kre. lau-c. lct. mgs.

morph-a. mtr. myris. na-ba. na-cl. na-sa. p. p-x. pb. pnx. pol. ppv. pru-l. pul. rn-b. rs. s. sep. sn. spi. spo. str. te. thu. trg. trn. urg. vp-t. vr-a. vr-s.

Appearance Bright. acon. (alm). atp. dt. eupat.

Dim. ara. as-o. buf. (cu). dt. k-ca. ppv. sn. vr-a.

Glassy. atp. glo. rs.

Staring. æth. as-o. atp. chi. (cu). dor. dt. glo. hyp. mgs. (spo). urg.

Wild. (alm). cu-ca. dt. hyp. pb.

Color Dark. (art-v). (cph). (cu). (dro). (lyc). (n-x). (p). (p-x). (s). (sn). (spo-f). (trg). (vr-a).

Green. (vr-a).

Red. acon. alli. arn. atp. bi-na. buf. ca-s. cld. clv. cph. cu. cu-ca. dt. (eupat). (eupat-p). euph. euphr. hg. k-bicr. morph-a. mtr. myris. pnx. pol. ppv. pul.

Yellow. as-o. (eupat). i. (n-x) (spi). vr-a.

Dryness. ca-ca. (mtr). s.

Eruptions. k-bicr.

Blisters. k-bicr.

Hæmorrhage. cb-v. (ery). mtr. str.

Heat. br. lct. mtr. na-ba. (na-cl). pol. sep. thu.

Lachrymation. acon. al-o. alli. aps. art-v. atp. br. bry. ca-ca. ca-s. cb-v. chd. cph. dl-s. dph. (ery). (eupat). euph. euphr. grp. hg. k-ca. kre. lct. mgs. na-cl. (na-sa). pnx. ppv. pul. rs. s. spi. spo. te. trg. urg. vr-a. vr-s.

Hot. bry. euph. euphr. hg. kre. na-cl.

Movements. æth. (alm). anm. aps. art-v. (br). buf. cic. cu. (dph). dt. (dt-t). (glp). hyo. (lau-c). mtr. (na-cl). (pb). (pnx). (pod). ppv. (smb). spi. (spo). (trg). vr-a.

Convulsions. anm. art-v. (br). buf. cic. cu. dt. hyo. lau-c. mtr. vr-a.

Squinting. æth. (alm). aps. art-v. (pb). spi.

Upwards. aps. buf. (cu). ppv. vr-a.

Downwards. æth. (na-cl).

Inwards. (alm). (pb).

To Left. buf.

Paralysis. (cb-a). (trg).

Pressing. atp. gym. na-ba. (na-cl). p. pol. sep.

Projecting. atp. ca-s. cu. dro. hyo. myris. pru-l. spi. (spo).

Sensitive. (na-cl). (spo-f). thu.

Shooting. br. k-ca. pnx. sep.

Smarting. bry. (cac). cast. na-ba. trn.
Sunken. ag-na. as-o. chi. clv. (cu). dl-s. (dt). k-ca. p. p-x. rs. s. sn. vp-t.
Swelling. (bry). (eupat-p). (k-ca). (k-i). (p).
Feeling of. cld.
Tensive. k-ca. trg.
Tearing. pul. str.
Throbbing. (na-cl). (s-x). spo.
Undefined. k-bicr. k-ca. k-i. rn-b. thu. trg.
Same Symptom. br. gym.
EYEBALL SUPERIORLY. cac.
Smarting. cac.
EYEBALL INTERNALLY. k-bicr.
Eruptions, Blisters. k-bicr.
SCLEROTIC. eupat.
Color Red. eupat.
Yellow. eupat.
IRIS. acon. æth. (alm). aps. art-v. as-o. atp. (br). buf. ca-ca. cic. crb-x. (cu). dt. glo. hyp. msc. myris. nic. pb. pnx. ppv. pru-l. spi. str. trg.
Pupils Contracted. atp. crb-x. glo. pnx.
Dilated. acon. æth. (alm). aps. art-v. as-o. atp. (br). buf. ca-ca. cic. dt. hyp. msc. myris. nic. pb. ppv. pru-l. spi. str. trg.
Insensible. æth. as-o. buf. crb-x. (cu). dt. myris. ppv.
Irregular. trg.
ORBIT. na-cl.
ORBIT SUPERIORLY. na-cl.
ORBITAL INTEGUMENTS. art-v. cph. cu. fe. lyc. myris. n-x. p. p-x. rs. s. sn. spi. spo-f. trg. vr-a.
Color Dark. art-v. cph. cu. lyc. n-x. p. p-x. s. sn. spo-f. trg. vr-a.
Green. vr-a.
Yellow. n-x. spi.
Swelling. fe. rs.
ORBITAL INTEGUMENTS INFERIORLY. myris. p.
Color Dark. myris.
Swelling. p.
EYELIDS. aps. atp. br. bry. buf. cb-a. clv. cu. dph. dro. dt. dt-t. (ery). glp. hpm. k-ca. k-i. mtr. na-cl. pnx. pod. ppv. smb. spo. spo-f. trg. trn. vr-a.

Adhesion of. k-ca.
Color Dark. clv. dro. k-ca. ppv.
Red. cu.
Dryness. mtr.
Hæmorrhage. (ery).
Movements, Closing. aps. atp. (br). cu. dt. glp. pnx. pod. ppv. smb. spo.
Spasmodically. br. spo.
Convulsions. cu. dph.
Opening Wide. (cu). dt-t. ppv. (spo).
Paralysis, Opening Difficult. cb-a. trg.
Sensitive. spo-f.
Smarting. trn.
Swelling. clv. cu. k-i.
UPPER EYELID. bry. k-ca. na-cl. vr-a.
Movements, Convulsions. vr-a.
Swelling. bry. k-ca.
LOWER EYELID. bry.
Swelling. bry.
TARSAL EDGES. hpm.
Heat. hpm.
FORWARDS. atp. na-cl. p. pol. trg.
Eyeball, Pressing. atp. p. pol. trg.
RIGHT. (alm). as-o. na-cl. na-sa. pb. s-x.
Eyeball, Color Red. as-o.
Drawing. as-o.
Lachrymation. na-cl. na-sa.
Movements, Squinting. (alm). pb.
Inwards. (alm) pb.
Pressing. as-o.
Throbbing. s-x.
Orbit Superiorly, Heat. na-cl.
Pressing. na-cl.
Sensitive. na-cl.
Throbbing. na-cl.
Upper Eyelid, Heat. na-cl.
Movements, Hanging down. na-cl.
Forwards. Orbit Superiorly, Pressing. na-cl.
LEFT. buf. trg.
Eyeball, Movements, Convulsions. trg.
Eyelids, Movements, Closing. buf.
Convulsions. trg.

Before BACK **Symptoms.**

alm.
SIGHT IMPAIRED. alm.
EYEBALL.
Movements. (alm).
EYELIDS. alm.
Movements, Closing. alm.

With BACK **Symptoms.**

acon. æsc. (alm). as-o. atp. au. bry. ca-ca. cast. cic. co. con. cro. cu. dig. dor. dt. eupat. (eupat-p). gel. grp. hg-bicl. k-ca. kre. lct. led. lyc. mn-ca. msc. myris. n-x. na-cl. ni-ca. pb. pnx. pru-l. s. sa-l. se. (spo). thu. trg. trn.

OBJECTS, FALSE APPEARANCE **of.** (alm). cic. gel. pb.

Multiplied. (alm). cic. gel. pb.

OBJECTS IMAGINARY. cro. myris.

Figures. myris.

Mist. cro.

PHOTOPHOBIA. acon. atp. au. ca-ca. (dt).

SIGHT IMPAIRED. atp. cro. (dt). gel. grp. lyc. msc. na-cl. pru-l.

EYEBALL. acon. æsc. (alm). as-o. atp. au. bry. ca-ca. cast. cic. co. cro. cu. dor. dt. eupat. (eupat-p). hg-bicl. k-ca. lct. led. msc. n-x. ni-ca. pb. s. sa-l. se. (spo). thu. trg. trn.

Appearance, Bright. atp. bry. dt. eupat. trg.
Dim. bry. k-ca.
Glassy. bry.
Staring. atp. cic. dor. msc.

Coldness. (sa-l).

Color Dark. (k-ca).
Red. acon. atp. (au). bry. (cu). (eupat). (eupat-p). led. s.
White. (hg-bicl).
Yellow. æsc. (eupat). s.

Cutting. au.

Discharge. (hg-bicl).
Pus. (hg-bicl).

Drawing. (se).

Eruptions. (ca-ca). (hg-bicl).
Ulcers. (ca-ca). (hg-bicl).
Heat. ca-ca. lct. n-x. (na-cl). ni-ca. s. thu.
Itching. ca-ca. s.
Lachrymation. (au). cro. lct. se.
Hot. au.
Appearance of. bry.
Feeling of. cro.
Movements. as-o. atp. (ca-ca). (hg-bicl). (kre). (na-cl). trg.
Convulsions. as-o. atp. trg.
Squinting. atp.
Paralysis. (trg).
Pressing. (na-cl). (se).
Projecting. atp. cu. (spo).
Sensitive. (na-cl).
Shooting. ca-ca. (sa-l). (se).
Cold. sa-l.
Smarting. cast. cro. trn.
Swelling. (cu). (eupat-p). hg-bicl.
Feeling of. cro.
Tearing. (con).
Throbbing. (na-cl).
Undefined. bry. co. cro. (s).
Same Symptom. ca-ca. co. (con). (s).
SCLEROTIC. eupat.
Color Red. eupat.
Yellow. eupat.
CORNEA. au. ca-ca. hg-bicl.
Color Red. au.
White. hg-bicl.
Eruptions, Ulcers. ca-ca. hg-bicl.
CHAMBERS **of** EYE. hg-bicl.
Discharge, Pus. hg-bicl.
IRIS. (alm). atp. cic. dt. mn-ca. msc. pb. pnx.
Pupils Contracted. mn-ca. msc.
Dilated. (alm). atp. cic. dt. pb. pnx.
ORBIT. con. na-cl.
Pressing. na-cl.
Tearing. con.
Same Symptom. con.
ORBIT SUPERIORLY. na-cl.

EYELIDS. au. ca-ca. cu. dig. hg-bicl. k-ca. kre. na-cl. trg.
Adhesion of. au. k-ca.
Color Dark. k-ca.
Red. cu.
Movements, Closing. (ca-ca). (dig). (hg-bicl). kre. (na-cl).
Spasmodically. ca-ca. hg-bicl.
Paralysis, Opening Difficult. trg.
Swelling. cu.
UPPER EYELID. na-cl.
FORWARDS. na-cl.
RIGHT. (alm). dig. na-cl. pb.
Eyeball, Lachrymation. na-cl.
Movements, Squinting. (alm). pb.
Inwards. (alm). pb.
Orbit Superiorly, Heat. na-cl.
Pressing. na-cl.
Sensitive. na-cl.
Throbbing. na-cl.
Eyelids, Movements, Closing. dig. na-cl.
Upper Eyelid, Heat. na-cl.
Forwards. Orbit, Pressing. na-cl.
LEFT. s. se.
Eyeball, Drawing. se.
Pressing. se.
Shooting. se.
Undefined. s.
Same Symptom. s.

RAISING ARMS.

ba-ca.
OBJECTS, FALSE APPEARANCE **of.** ba-ca.
Moving. ba-ca.
Circularly. ba-ca.

Before ARM **Symptoms.**

na-ca. hyp.
SIGHT IMPAIRED. na-ca.

EYEBALL. hyp.
Appearance Staring. hyp.
Wild. hyp.
IRIS. hyp.
Pupils, Dilated. hyp.

With ARM Symptoms.

acon. æsc. æth. (alm). anm. apo. atp. buf. cac. cb-v. clv. cop. (cu). dt. ery. eupat. (eupat-p). grp. hg. hll. hyo. k-ca. klm. kre. lct. lyc. mgs. mph. msc. myris. na-ba. na-cl. pb. ppv. pul. s. sep. smb. (spo). str. thr. thu. trg. trn. vr-a.

OBJECTS, FALSE APPEARANCE **of.** (alm). cb-v. pb. thr.
Multiplied. (alm). pb. thr.
Small. cb-v.
OBJECTS IMAGINARY. cb-v. thr. trg.
Black. thr.
Bright. thr.
Vibrations. thr. trg.
Black. thr.
Bright. thr.
Visions. cb-v.
Horrible. cb-v.
PHOTOPHOBIA. acon. (dt). hg. na-ba. str. thr.
SIGHT IMPAIRED. (alm). apo. atp. (dt). grp. msc. spo.
EYEBALL. acon. æsc. æth. (alm). anm. atp. buf. clv. cu. dt. ery. eupat. (eupat-p). hg. hll. hyo. k-ca. klm. lct. lyc. mgs. mph. msc. na-ba. pb. pul. s. (spo). thu. trg. vr-a.
Appearance Bright. (alm). dt. eupat. mgs.
Dim. (alm). buf. (cu). dt. vr-a.
Glassy. anm.
Staring. æth. anm. (cu). dt. ery. msc. (spo).
Downwards. ery.
Wild. dt.
Color Dark. (cu). (dt).
Red. acon. buf. (eupat-p). hg. hyo.
Yellow. æsc. vr-a.
Heat. lct. lyc. mgs. mph. na-ba. thu.
Heaviness ppv.

Itching. (trn).
Lachrymation. dt. (eupat-p). lct. vr-a.
Movements. acon. æth. (alm). atp. buf. con. cu. dt. hll. (kre). (myris). pb. pul. (s). (smb). (trg). (vr-a).
Convulsions. acon. atp. buf. cu. dt. pul. (trg).
Squinting. æth. (alm). hll. pb.
Upwards. buf. con. (cu).
Downwards. æth.
Inwards. (alm). (pb).
To Left. buf.
Pressing. klm. (na-cl). (str).
Projecting. (spo).
Smarting. (cac). (trn).
Sunken. clv. (cu). k-ca.
Swelling. (cop).
Tensive. k-ca.
Undefined. (s).
Same Symptom. acon. dt. lyc. mgs. pul. (s).
EYEBALL, SUPERIORLY. cac.
Smarting. cac.
SCLEROTIC. eupat.
Color Red. eupat.
Yellow. eupat.
IRIS. æth. (alm). atp. buf. (cu). dt. hll. msc. pb. str.
Pupils Contracted. dt. msc.
Dilated. æth. (alm). atp. buf. dt. hll. pb. str.
Insensible. buf. (cu). dt.
ORBIT. na-cl.
Pressing. na-cl.
ORBITAL INTEGUMENTS. (cu). dt.
Color Dark. (cu).
ORBITAL INTEGUMENTS INFERIORLY. dt.
Color Dark. dt.
EYELIDS. (alm). buf. cop. (cu). dt. kre. myris. pb. s. smb. trn. vr-a.
Itching. trn.
Movements, Closing. buf. (cu). dt. kre. s. smb. vr-a.
Convulsions. trg.
Opening Wide. (alm). pb.
Winking. myris.
Smarting. trn.
Swelling. cop.
FORWARDS. str.

Eyeball, Pressing. str.
RIGHT. (alm). pb.
Eyeball, Movements, Squinting. (alm). pb.
Inwards. (alm). pb.
LEFT. s. trg.
Eyeball, Movements, Convulsions. trg.
Undefined. s. trg.
Same Symptom. s.

Before LEG Symptoms.

hyp.
EYEBALL. hyp.
Appearance, Staring. hyp.
Wild. hyp.
IRIS. hyp.
Pupils, Dilated. hyp.

With LEG Symptoms.

acon. alm. amb. anm. apo. ast. atp. buf. ca-ca. cast. ccs. cit-c. cld. clv. cop. cth. (cu). dt. eupat. (eupat-p). hg. hll. hyo. k-bicr. k-ca. klm. kre. lac-f. lct. mph. mtr. na-ba. na-cl. pb. ppv. pul. rs. sang. sep. (spo). str. thu. trg. trn. vr-a.

OBJECTS, IMAGINARY. dt. trg.
Figures. dt.
Vibrations. trg.
PHOTOPHOBIA. acon. ca-ca. (dt). hg. (lac-f). na-ba.
SIGHT DAZZLED. (na-cl).
SIGHT IMPAIRED. (alm). amb. apo. ast. atp. (dt). lac-f. na-cl. pb. sep. trn.
EYEBALL. acon. (alm). anm. atp. buf. ca-ca. cast. cit-c. cld. clv. cth. cu. dt. eupat. (eupat-p). hg. hll. hyo. k-bicr. k-ca. klm. kre. lac-f. lct. mph. mtr. na-ba. ppv. pul. rho. rs. sang. (spo). str. thu. trg. trn. vr-a.
Appearance Bright. (alm). atp. dt. eupat. trg.
Dim. (alm). buf. (cu). dt. k-ca. vr-a.
Glassy. anm. rs.
Staring. anm. atp. (cu). dt. (spo).
Wild. dt.

Color Dark. (cu). (dt). (k-ca).
Red. acon. atp. buf. (eupat). (eupat-p.) hg. hyo. **str.**
Yellow. (eupat). str. **vr-a.**
Discharge. (kre).
Gnawing. kre.
Heat. (alm). (ccs). (cit-c). **kre. lct.** mph. **mtr. na-ba.** rho. thu.
Heaviness. ppv.
Itching. (alm). kre. trg.
Lachrymation. dt. (eupat-p). k-bicr. (lac-f). lct. str. vr-a.
Movements. acon. (alm). atp. buf. ca-ca. cu. dt. hll. (pb). (vr-a).
Convulsions. acon. atp. buf. cu. dt.
Squinting. ca-ca. hll.
Upwards. acon. buf.
To Left. buf.
Paralysis. (trg).
Pressing. (cit-c). klm. (na-cl). (str).
Projecting. anm. atp. (spo).
Shooting. (cld).
Smarting. cast. k-bicr. trn.
Sunken. clv. (cu). k-ca. rs.
Swelling. (eupat-p).
Tearing. pul.
Tensive. k-ca.
Undefined. cth. (sang).
Same Symptom. acon. (alm). (ccs). (cld). dt. (sang).
SCLEROTIC. eupat.
Color Red. eupat.
Yellow. eupat.
IRIS. ast. buf. (cu). dt. hll. pul.
Pupils Contracted. ast. dt.
Dilated. buf. dt. hll. pul.
Insensible. buf. (cu). dt.
ORBIT. na-cl.
Pressing. na-cl.
ORBITAL INTEGUMENTS. (cu). dt.
Color Dark. (cu).
ORBITAL INTEGUMENTS INFERIORLY. dt.
Color Dark. dt.

EYELIDS. (alm). buf. ccs. cld. cop. cu. dt. k-ca. pb. trg. vr-a.
Color Dark. k-ca.
Heat. ccs.
Movements, Closing. cu. dt. vr-a.
Opening Wide. (alm). pb.
Paralysis, Opening Difficult. trg.
Swelling. cop.
Same Symptom. ccs.
LOWER EYELID. alm. cld.
TARSAL EDGES. alm. cld.
LOWER TARSAL EDGE. alm. cld.
CANTHI. kre.
Discharge. kre.
RIGHT **then** LEFT. alm.
Lower Eyelid, Itching. alm.
FORWARDS. str.
Eyeball, Pressing. str.
BACKWARDS. lac-f.
To HEAD. lac-f.
To FOREHEAD. lac-f.
To TEMPLE. lac-f.
RIGHT. alm. cld. lac-f.
Photophobia. lac-f.
Eyeball, Color Red. lac-f.
Lachrymation. lac-f.
Lower Tarsal Edge, Heat. alm.
Itching. alm.
Shooting. cld.
Same Symptom. alm.
Backwards. Eyeball, Shooting. lac-f.
To Forehead. Eyeball, Shooting. lac-f.
Throbbing. lac-f.
To Temple. Eyeball, Shooting. lac-f.
Throbbing. lac-f.
LEFT. alm. buf. cit-c. cld. na-cl. sang.
Sight Dazzled. na-cl.
Sight Impaired. na-cl.
Eyeball, Heat. cit-c.
Pressing. cit-c.
Shooting. cld.
Undefined. sang.
Same Symptom. cld. sang.

Eyelids, Movements, Closing. buf.
Lower Eyelid, Itching. alm.
Same Symptom. alm.

On GOING to SLEEP.

cit-c. con. lyc. na-ca.
OBJECTS, IMAGINARY. lyc.
Bright. lyc.
Vibrations. lyc.
Bright. lyc.
EYEBALL. con.
Pressing. con.
Shooting. (cit-c).
EYELIDS. cit-c.
EYELIDS, INNER SURFACE. cit-c.
LEFT. cit-c.
Eyelids Inner Surface, Shooting. cic-c.

During SLEEP.

anm. atp. bry. chi. cit-c. con. cph. cu. dt. dt-t. fe. hll. lau-c. lyc. p-x. pod. ppv. pul. rhe. s. sb-t. smb. str-i. vr-a.
OBJECTS, IMAGINARY. lau-c.
Increasing and Decreasing in Size. lau-c.
EYEBALL. anm. bry. chi. con. cu. hll. ppv. pul. vr-a.
Appearance Staring. con.
Discharge. vr-a.
Movements. anm. bry. chi. con. cu. hll. ppv. pul. (rhe).
Convulsions. anm. bry. chi. con. cu. hll. ppv. pul. (rhe).
Upwards. hll. ppv.
EYELIDS. anm. atp. bry. chi. cit-c. con. cph. cu. dt. dt-t. fe. hll. lyc. p-x. pod. ppv. pul. rhe. s. sb-t. smb. str-i. vr-a.
Movements, Convulsions. rhe.
Opening. anm. atp. bry. chi. cit-c. con. cph. cu. dt. dt-t. fe. hll. lyc. p-x. pod. ppv. pul. s. sb-t. smb. str-i. vr-a.
RIGHT. (chi). s. (str-i). (vr-a).
Eyelids, Movements, Opening. (chi). s. (str-i). (vr-a).
LEFT. (chi). (str-i). (vr-a).
Eyelids, Movements, Closing. (chi). (str-i). (vr-a).

WAKING. (**After Sleep**).

æth. ag-na. aga. al-o. amb. amm-ca. amm-cl. apo. art-v. atp. bry. ca-a. ca-ca. ca-s. ccs. chd. chi. chio. con. cro. cub. dig. dl-s. .dro. dt. elaps. ery. euph. frm. gel. hll. hydr. k-bicr. k-ca. k-o. kre. krm. lct. lyc. men. mg-ca. mg-cl. mgs. mgs-ar. mtr. n-x. na-ca. na-cl. ni-ca. ol-a. p. pb. pul. rhe. rho. rs. rs-r. rs-v. s. sb-t. sep. smi. so-d. so-t-æg. str. str-i. te. thr. thu. trg. trn. trx. vr-a. vr-s. woo. zn.

OBJECTS, FALSE APPEARANCE **of**. dig. gel. p.

Moving. p.

Vibrating. p.

Multiplied. gel.

White. dig.

OBJECTS, IMAGINARY. amm-ca. ca-s. chio. dt. k-o. lyc. na-ca. p. so-d. str-i. zn.

Bright. amm-ca. ca-s. lyc. na-ca.

Flames. ca-s.

Flashes Bright. na-ca.

Mist. chio. k-o. lyc. na-ca. p. str-i. zn.

Spirits. ca-s. so-d. trg.

Spots. amm-ca.

Bright. amm-ca.

Veil. dt. lyc. str-i.

Vibrations. lyc.

Bright. lyc.

SIGHT IMPAIRED. ca-ca. (chd). chio. con. dt. k-o. lyc. p. pul. str-i. trn. zn.

EYEBALL. ag-na. aga. al-o. amm-ca. amm-cl. art-v. ca-a. ccs. chd. cub. dl-s. dt. elaps. ery. euph. frm. kre. krm. lct. lyc. men. mg-ca. mtr. ni-ca. ol-a. p. pb. pul. rhe. rho. s. sb-t. so-t-æg. thr. trg. trn. trx. vr-s. woo. zn.

Bruised. (smi).

Color Red. (ery). (te). woo.

Contractive. trg.

Discharge. al-o. amm-cl. art-v. ca-a. (chi). (euph). krm. mtr. p. rhe. trx.

Dryness. ag-na. dl-s. elaps. lyc. (mg-cl). (mgs). (mgs-ar). p. (vr-a).

False Sensations. ccs. (trn).

Hair. ccs. (trn).

Heat. ag-na. al-o. elaps. (k-bicr). krm. ni-ca. ol-a. rho. (smi). (thr).

Heaviness. (k-bicr). (sep).
Itching. (sep). (te).
Lachrymation. al-o. cub. dt. (ery). (kre). krm. (pb). so-t-æg. zn.
Hot. kre. pb. zn.
Movements. (amb). (ca-s). (sep). trg.
As if Taken out, Squeezed, and Put back. trg.
Paralysis. (ag-na). (amm-ca). (ca-s). (cro). (dro). (k-ca). (thu).
Pressing. aga. amm-ca. dl-s. lct. sb-t. vr-s.
Shooting. trn.
Smarting. (te).
Swelling. chd. dt. (n-x). (te). woo.
Œdematous. (te).
Red. (te).
Feeling of. mg-ca. ni-ca.
Tearing. pul.
Tensive. s.
Undefined. frm. (men). (sep).
EYEBALL INTERNALLY. ery. thr.
Heat. thr.
IRIS. mtr.
Pupils, Dilated. mtr.
ORBIT. smi.
ORBIT INFERIORLY. smi.
Bruised. smi.
ORBITAL INTEGUMENTS. n-x.
Swelling. n-x.
EYELIDS. ag-na. amb. amm-ca. ca-s. chd. chi. cro dro. hydr. k-bicr. k-ca. mg-cl. mgs. mgs-ar. rs. sep. smi. te. thu. trn. vr-a. vr-s.
Adhesion of. chd. chi. hydr. k-bicr. rs. smi. trn.
Dryness. mg-cl. mgs. mgs-ar. vr-a.
Movements, Closing. (amb). ca-s. (sep).
Spasmodically. amb. sep.
Paralysis, Opening Difficult. ag-na. amm-ca. ca-s. cro. dro. k-ca. thu.
Pressing. amm-ca. vr-s.
Undefined. sep.
UPPER. EYELID. k-bicr. sep. te.
Heaviness. k-bicr. sep.
CANTHI. chi. ery. k-bicr. sep.

EXTERNAL CANTHUS. chi.
Discharge. chi.
INTERNAL CANTHUS. ery. k-bicr. sep.
Heat. k-bicr.
Itching. sep.
RIGHT. chd. ery. euph.
Sight Impaired. chd.
Eyeball, Discharge. euph.
Lachrymation. ery.
Eyeball Internally, Color Red. ery.
Internal Canthus, Color Red. ery.
LEFT. men. rs. te. trn.
Eyeball, False Sensations, Hair. trn.
Undefined. men.
Eyelids, Adhesion of. rs.
Upper Eyelid, Itching. te.
Smarting. te.
Swelling. te.
Œdematous. te.
Red. te.

Before SLEEP **Symptoms**.

jnp-s.
SIGHT IMPAIRED. jnp-s.

With SLEEP **Symptoms**.

acon. æth. ag-na. aga. al-o. (alm). amm-ca. anm. aps. arn. art-v. arum-t. as-o. ast. atp. bru. bry. c-bis. cb-a. cb-v. chd. chi. cic. cl-hx. cof. con. cph. cro. cth. cu. dl-s. dph. dt. dt-t. ery. eryn. (eupat-p). euphr. fe. fe-a. frm. gel. grc. grt. gui. gym. hg. hll. hyo. k-ca. kre. lch. led. li-ca. lyc. mg-sa. mgs-ar. mn-ca. mph. mtr. myris. na-ca. na-cl. ol-a. os. ox-x. p. p-x. pb. phl. ppv. pru-l. pt. pul. qu-sa. rho. rn-b. rs. s. sb-t. spi. spo. sr-ca. str-i. thu. trg. trn. trx. vi-o. vi-t. vr-a. vr-s. vrb. zn. zng.

OBJECTS, FALSE APPEARANCE **of.** al-o. (alm). atp. gel. pb.
Black. al-o.
Bright. atp.
Grey. atp.

Multiplied. (alm). atp. gel. pb.
Red. atp.
White. atp.
Yellow. atp.
OBJECTS IMAGINARY. al-o. atp. cof. cro. dt. hg. k-ca. led. mtr. myris. na-ca. p. p-x. qu-sa. rs. sb-t. spo. sr-ca. thu. zn.
Blue. zn.
Bright. k-ca. qu-sa. srr.
Circles. zn.
Blue. zn.
Green. zn.
Yellow. zn.
Figures. dt. myris.
Flames. spo.
Green. zn.
Grey. atp.
Light. qu-sa.
Mist. atp. cro. k-ca.
Grey. atp.
Spots. k-ca. qu-sa. sr-ca.
Bright. k-ca. qu-sa. sr-ca.
Veil. dt.
Visions. al-o. atp. cof. dt. hg. led. mtr. na-ca. p. p-x. rs. sb-t. spo. thu.
PHOTOMANIA. dt.
PHOTOPHOBIA. cb-a. con. hg. k-ca. zng.
SIGHT IMPAIRED. aga. al-o. as-o. ast. atp. cro. dt. gel. k-ca. mg-sa. ol-a. os. qu-sa.
EYEBALL. ag-na. (alm). aps. art-v. as-o. atp. bru. bry. chi. con. cph. cro. cth. cu. dph. dt. ery. (eupat-p). euphr. fe-a. grc. gui. gym. hg. hll. k-bicr. k-ca. krc. lyc. mg-sa. mn-ca. mph. myris. ox-x. p. pb. ppv. pru-l. pt. rho. rn-b. rs. s. spi. spo. str-i. trg. trn. vr-a. vr-s. zn.
Appearance Bright. (alm). atp.
Dim. bry. cu. mg-sa. spo.
Glassy. atp.
Staring. dt. ery. k-ca. pru-l.
Color Dark. (art-v). (cu).
Red. (as-o). atp. con. (cu). (eupat-p). hg. (k-bicr). vr-a. zn.
Yellow. chi. pb.
Cutting. s.
Drawing. (as-o). dph.

Dryness. cph. grc. myris. (pul). spi. zn.
Gnawing. ox-x.
Heat. (cb-v). (cro) gym. kre. mph. pru-l. pt. rho.
Heaviness. (c-bis). (cro). (frm). p.
Itching. rn-b.
Lachrymation. bru. con. cro. (eupat-p). fe-a. k-bicr. k-ca. mph. str-i. vr-s. (zn).
Hot. zn.
Feeling of. cro.
Movements. (æth). (alm). (amm-cl). aps. art-v. (c-bis). cu. dt. (dt-t). (ery). hll. (lch). (myris). (pb). ppv. trg.
Convulsions. art-v. cu. dt. trg.
Squinting. (alm). art-v. hll. (pb).
Upwards. aps. ppv.
Paralysis. (cb-v). (hyo). (li-ca).
Pressing. (as-o). (dt). ery. euphr. k-ca. kre. lyc. mn-ca. (myris). (na-cl). p. rn-b. (rs). s.
Projecting. cu.
Feeling of. gui.
Shooting. k-ca.
Smarting. cro. cth. ox-x. trn.
Strained. dph.
Sunken. ag-na. k-ca.
Feeling. zn.
Swelling. (con). (cu). (dt). (eupat-p). spo.
Feeling of. cro. gui.
Tearing. (pb).
Tensive. k-ca. ox-x.
Undefined. cro. zn.
SCLEROTIC. con.
Color Red. con.
CORNEA. con.
Opacity. con.
IRIS. (alm). arn. art-v. as-o. ast. atp. dt. ery. hll. pb.
Pupils Contracted. ast. atp.
Dilated. (alm). arn. art-v. as-o. atp. dt. ery. hll. pb.
Insensible. as-o.
ORBIT. k-ca. na-cl. zn.
Pressing. k-ca. na-cl.
ORBIT SUPERIORLY. zn.
Undefined. zn.
ORBITAL INTEGUMENTS. art-v. cu. ox-x. spo.

Color Dark. art-v. cu.
Swelling. spo.
ORBITAL, INTEGUMENTS SUPERIORLY ox-x.
Gnawing. ox-x.
Smarting. ox-x.
Tensive. ox-x.
EYELIDS. æth. amm-cl. aps. c-bis. cb-v. chi. con. cph. cro. cth. cu. dt. dt-t. ery. frm. grt. hyo. k-bicr. k-ca. kre. lch. li-ca. myris. pb. ppv. pul. s. trx. vi-t. vr-s. zn.
Adhesion of. kre.
Color Red. con. cu. k-bicr. zn.
Dryness. cph. pul.
Heat. cb-v. cro.
Heaviness. c-bis. cro. frm.
Movements, Closing. æth. amm-cl. aps. c-bis. chi. cth. cu. ery. grt. lch. myris. ppv. s. trx. vi-t. vr-s.
Spasmodically. myris.
Opening Wide. (cu). dt-t.
Winking. myris.
Paralysis, Opening Difficult. cb-v. hyo. li-ca.
Pressing. dt.
Swelling. con. cu. dt.
Feeling of. cro.
Tearing. pb.
UPPER EYELID. k-ca.
Swelling. k-ca.
FORWARDS. rs.
Eyeball, Pressing. rs.
BACKWARDS. dph.
Eyeball, Drawing. dph.
RIGHT. (alm). as-o. pb.
Eyeball, Color Red. as-o.
Drawing. as-o.
Movements, Squinting. (alm). pb.
Inwards. (alm). pb.
Pressing. as-o.

Before CHILLS.

na-cl.
OBJECTS, IMAGINARY. na-cl.
Bright. na-cl.
Zigzag. na-cl.
Bright. na-cl.

With CHILLS.

acon. ag-na. alm. anm. aps. as-o. atp. bry. buf. ca-ca. ca-s. cap. cast. cb-a. chi. cic. cit-c. cld. clv. cn-sa. cph. crb-x. cro. cth. cu. cy-hx. dig. dph. dt. ery. eupat. (eupat-p). fe. gel. grp. hg. hyo. jnp-s. k-bicr. k-ca. k-i. kre. lct. led. lyc. mgs-au. msc. mtr. myris. na-ba. na-cl. nic. p. pol. pru-l. pul. qu-sa. rho. s. sep. spi. (spo). srr. str. str-i. thr. trg. trn. vr-a. vr-s.

OBJECTS, FALSE APPEARANCE **of.** atp. dt. gel. thr.

Blue. atp.

Bright. atp.

Grey. atp.

Large. dt.

Multiplied. atp. gel. thr.

Red. atp.

White. atp.

OBJECTS IMAGINARY. atp. cic. cro. (cu). cy-hx. dt. hyo. jnp-s. k-ca. kre. led. lyc. mtr. pru-l. sep. str. thr. trg. vr-s.

Black. thr.

Bright. atp. hyo. k-ca. led. lyc. mtr. sep. thr.

Figures. (cu). dt.

Flames. atp. hyo.

Grey. atp.

Mist. atp. cro. cy-hx. k-ca. pru-l.

  Grey. atp.

Spirits. (cu).

Spots. k-ca.

  Bright. k-ca.

Veil. kre.

Vibrations. cic. jnp-s. led. lyc. mtr. sep. thr. trg. vr-s.

  Black. thr.

  Bright. led. lyc. mtr. sep. thr.

Visions. dt. str.

PHOTOPHOBIA. acon. aps. as-o. atp. ca-s. (dt). hg. k-ca. kre. lyc. mtr. na-ba. pol. rs. sep. str. thr.

SIGHT DAZZLED. (na-cl).

SIGHT IMPAIRED. alm. atp. ca-ca. chi. cic. cy-hx. dig. (dt). gel. grp. hyo. jnp-s. k-ca. kre. lyc. mgs-au. msc. mtr. na-cl. pru-l. qu-sa. srr. trg. trn.

EYEBALL. acon. ag-na. anm. aps. as-o. atp. bry. buf. ca-ca. cap. cast. cic. cit-c. cld. clv. cth. cu. dig. dph. dt. ery.

eupat. (eupat-p). hg. hyo. k-bicr. k-ca. kre. lct. led. lyc. msc. mtr. na-ba. na-cl. p. pol. pul. rho. rs. s. sep. (spo). str. trg. trn. vr-a.

Appearance Bright. atp. dt. eupat. mtr. sep. trg. trn.

Dim. as-o. buf. (cu). dt. k-ca. mtr. vr-a.

Glassy. anm. atp.

Staring. acon. anm. cic. (cu). k-ca. msc. (spo).

Color Dark. (cu). (k-ca). (myris). p.

Red. acon. atp. buf. cu. eupat. (eupat-p). hg. kre. na-cl. rs. str.

Yellow. as-o. eupat. (eupat-p). (spi). str. vr-a.

Dryness. (rs).

Heat. (acon). (aps). (atp.) cro. k-bicr. (kre). lct. mtr. na-ba. pol. rho. (rs). sep.

Itching. (trn).

Lachrymation. ag-na. aps. atp. bry. dph. (enpat-p). k-bicr. k-ca. kre. lct. rs. str. vr-a.

Hot. bry. kre.

Movements. (acon). buf. (ca-ca). cu. dig. dt. (kre). (mtr). (myris). (rs). (trg). (vr-a).

Convulsions. cu. dt. (trg).

Squinting. dig.

Upwards. buf. (cu).

To Left. buf.

Pressing. (cit-c). ery. k-ca. kre. lyc. (na-cl). p. rs. s. sep. (str).

Projecting. anm. (spo).

Shooting. acon. aps. cit-c. k-ca. na-ba. rs.

Smarting. bry. cast. k-bicr. trn.

Stiffness. acon. atp. cic. hyo. trg.

Sunken. as-o. clv. (cu). k-ca. p.

Swelling. (aps). (fe). (k-ca). (k-i). (rs).

Tearing. pul.

Tensive. k-ca.

Undefined. acon. aps. atp. ca-ca. cap. cit-c. cld. cth. dph. kre. led. lyc. mtr. na-ba. pol. rho. rs. sep. trg.

SCLEROTIC. eupat.

Color Red. eupat.

Yellow. eupat.

IRIS. acon. aps. atp. buf. ca-ca. cap. cb-a. cic. cph. crb-x. cro. (cu). dig. dph. dt. hyo. msc. mtr. myris. p. s. sep. si-x. str. str-i. vr-a.

Pupils Contracted. acon. atp. cap. crb-x. dig. dt. msc. mtr. s. sep. si-x. str. vr-a.

Dilated. aps. atp. buf. ca-ca. cb-a. cic. cph. cro. dph. dt. hyo. mtr. myris. nic. ppv. str-i. trg.

Insensible. acon. buf. crb-x. (cu). myris. ppv.

Irregular. trg.

ORBIT. cit-c. na-cl.

Pressing. cit-c. na-cl.

ORBITAL INTEGUMENTS. (cu). myris. p. spi.

Color Dark. (cu). p.

Yellow. spi.

ORBITAL, INTEGUMENTS INFERIORLY. myris.

Color Dark. myris.

EYELIDS. acon. aps. atp. ca-ca. cro. cu. dig. fe. k-ca. kre. myris. rs. trn. vr-a.

Color Dark. k-ca.

Dryness. rs.

Heat. acon. aps. atp. cro. kre. rs.

Itching. trn.

Movements Closing. (buf). cu. (dig). dt. kre. mtr. vr-a.

Convulsions. ca-ca. cu. rs.

Opening Wide. acon.

Winking. myris.

Smarting. trn.

Swelling. aps. fe. k-i. rs.

UPPER EYELID. k-ca.

Swelling. k-ca.

FORWARDS. p. s. str.

Eyeball, Pressing. p. s. str.

RIGHT. dig.

Eyelids, Movements, Closing. dig.

LEFT. buf. na-cl. trg.

Sight Dazzled. na-cl.

Sight Impaired. na-cl.

Eyeball, Movements, Convulsions. trg.

Eyelids, Movements, Closing. buf.

Convulsions. trg.

After CHILLS.

cic. ni-ca. pet.

EYEBALL. ni-ca. pet.

Discharge. ni-ca.
Heat. pet.

Before HEAT.

str.
EYEBALL. str.
Pressing. str.
FORWARDS. str.
Eyeball, Pressing. str.

With HEAT.

acon. alm. aps. art-v. as-o. asr. atp. au. bi-na. buf. ca-ca. ca-s. cb-a. chi. cic. cit-c. con. cph. cth. (cu). dig. dor. dt. eupat. (eupat-p). fe. glo. hg. hyo. i. k-ca. k-i. k-o. lch. lct. led. ly-b. lyc. mn-ca. mtr. myris. na-ba. na-ca. na-cl. p. p-x. pet. pol. ppv. pul. qu-sa. rho. rs. rut. s. sep. smb. spi. str. trg. trn. val. vr-a. vr-s.
OBJECTS, FALSE APPEARANCE **of**. atp. cb-v. cic. i.
Blue. atp. i.
Bright. atp.
Grey. atp.
Multiplied. atp. cic.
Red. atp.
Small. cb-v.
White. atp.
OBJECTS IMAGINARY. atp. au. ca-ca. cb-a. cb-v. chi. dt. hyo. k-ca. ppv. pul. sep.
Bright. atp. au. cb-a. hyo. k-ca. ppv. sep.
Figures. dt.
Flames. atp. ppv.
Flashes Bright. hyo.
Green. chi.
Grey. atp.
Mist. atp. k-ca. sep.
Grey. atp.
Spots. atp. au. cb-a. k-ca. ppv.
Bright. atp. au. cb-a. k-ca. ppv.
Vibrations. sep.
Bright. sep.
isions. ca-ca. cb-v. (dt). ppv. pul.
Horrid. cb-v. (dt).

PHOTOPHOBIA. acon. aps. atp. ca-s. con. k-ca. na-ba. s. str.

SIGHT IMPAIRED. atp. bi-na. cb-v. (dt). hg. k-ca. k-o. mtr. na-cl. pul. qu-sa. sep.

EYEBALL. acon. aps. art-v. as-o. asr. atp. bi-na. buf. ca-ca. ca-s. cb-a. cb-v. chi. cic. cit-c. cph. cth. (cu). dig. dor. dt. eupat. (eupat-p). hyo. hyp. k-ca. lch. lct. led. ly-b. lyc. mtr. na-ba. na-ca. na-cl. p. p-x. pet. pol. ppv. pul. rho. rs. rut. s. sep. spi. str. trg. trn. val. vr-a. vr-s.

Appearance Bright. atp. dt. eupat. lch. lyc. mtr. trg. trn.

Dim. buf. dt.

Glassy. atp. glo.

Staring. atp. chi. dor. dt. glo. hyp. lyc.

Wild. dt. hyp.

Color Dark. (art-v). (dt). (fe).

Red. acon. atp. bi-na. buf. dt. (eupat-p). hyo. na-cl. (vr-a).

Yellow. (eupat).

Dryness. spi.

Heat. cb-a. k-ca. lct. na-ba. pet. rho. sep. spi. vr-a.

Itching. (ly-b).

Lachrymation. aps. atp. dt. (eupat-p). k-ca. lct.

Movements. (alm). aps. art-v. buf. (cu). (dt). (lyc). (mtr). (smb). (vr-a).

Convulsions. art-v. (cu).

Squinting. aps. art-v.

Upwards. aps. buf.

To Left. buf.

Paralysis. na-cl.

Pressing. k-ca. (myris). na-ba. (na-cl). sep.

Projecting. atp. spi.

Shooting. k-ca.

Smarting. asr. na-ba. trn.

Sunken. k-ca.

Swelling. (fe). (k-ca). (k-i).

Tensive. k-ca.

Throbbing. (myris).

Undefined. acon. aps. as-o. atp. ca-ca. ca-s. cb-a. cb-v. cic. cit-c. cph. cth. dig. dt. hyo. led. lyc. na-ba. na-cl. p-x. pol. ppv. pul. rho. rs. rut. s. sep. spi. str. trg. val. vr-a. vr-s.

SCLEROTIC. eupat.

Color Red. eupat.
Yellow. eupat.
IRIS. acon. aps. art-v. atp. buf. cic. dt. glo. hyp. lyc. mn-ca. mtr. str.
Pupils Contracted. acon. atp. glo. mn-ca. mtr.
Dilated. aps. art-v. atp. buf. cic. dt. hyp. lyc. str.
Insensible. buf. dt.
ORBIT. myris. na-cl. val.
Pressing. na-cl.
Undefined. val.
ORBIT SUPERIORLY. myris.
ORBITAL INTEGUMENTS. art-v. dt. fe.
Color Dark. art-v. fe.
Swelling. fe.
ORBITAL INTEGUMENTS INFERIORLY. dt.
Color Dark. dt.
EYELIDS. alm. aps. buf. dt. k-ca. k-i. lyc. smb. vr-a.
Movements, Closing. alm. aps. (buf). dt. lyc. smb. vr-a.
Opening Wide. (dt). lyc. mtr.
Swelling. k-i.
UPPER EYELID. k-ca.
Swelling. k-ca.
RIGHT. ly-b. vr-a.
Eyeball, Color Red. vr-a.
Itching. ly-b.
LEFT. buf. myris.
Orbit Superiorly, Pressing. myris.
Throbbing. myris.
Eyelids, Movements, Closing. buf.

After HEAT.

au-cl. bry. lyc. spo.
SIGHT. IMPAIRED. au-cl.
EYEBALL. spo.
Shooting. (spo).
Swelling. (bry).
Tearing. (spo).
LENS. lyc.
Cataract. lyc.
EYELIDS. bry.

LOWER EYELID. bry.
Swelling. bry.
LEFT. spo.
Eyeball, Shooting. spo.
Tearing. spo.

Before SWEAT.

narth.
SIGHT IMPAIRED. narth.

With SWEAT.

acon. ag-na. alm. anm. aps. arn. art-v. as-o. atp. au-cl. bry. buf. ca-ca. ca-s. cap. cb-v. chi. cl-hx. cld. con. crb-x. crot. cth. (cu). dl-s. dph. dt. grp. hg. hll. hyo. hyp. k-bicr. k-ca. k-o. lau-c. led. lyc. mtr. myris. na-ca. na-cl. na-sa. nic. ox-x. p. p-x. ppv. pul. qu-sa. rho. rs. s. sep. si-x. spi. (spo). str. thu. vr-a.
OBJECTS, FALSE APPEARANCE **of**. atp. cb-v.
Blue. atp.
Bright. atp.
Grey. atp.
Multiplied. atp.
Red. atp.
Small. cb-v.
White. atp.
OBJECTS, IMAGINARY. as-o. atp. ca-ca. cb-v. (cu). dl-s. (dt). grp. k-ca. k-o. lyc. mtr. na-cl. pul. sep. spi. str.
Bright. atp. ca-ca. dl-s. grp. k-ca. k-o. lyc. mtr. na-cl. pul. sep. spi. str.
Figures. (cu).
Flames. atp. k-ca. k-o. na-cl. pul. spi. str.
Grey. atp.
Mist. atp.
Grey. atp.
Spirits. (cu).
Vibrations. dl-s. grp. k-o. lyc. mtr. sep. str.
Bright. dl-s. grp. k-o. lyc. mtr. sep. str.
Visions. as-o. cb-v. (dt).
Horrid. cb-v. (dt).

PHOTOPHOBIA. acon. aps. arn. as-o. atp. bry. ca-ca. ca-s. chi. dt. grp. hg. lyc. mtr. p-x. pul. rs. s. sep. str.

SIGHT IMPAIRED. ag-na. alm. anm. atp. au-cl. ca-ca. ca-s. cb-v. con. crot. dt. hg. hyo. k-o. na-cl. ox-x. p. p-x. qu-sa. s. si-x.

EYEBALL. acon. anm. aps. arn. as-o. atp. bry. buf. ca-ca. ca-s. cld. con. cth. (cu). dt. hg. hll. hyp. k-bicr. k-o. led. lyc. mtr. na-ca. na-sa. p. ppv. pul. rho. rs. s. sep. si-x. spi. (spo). str. thu. vr-a.

Appearance Bright. acon. atp. dt.

Dim. as-o. buf. vr-a.

Glassy. anm. atp.

Staring. anm. as-o. (cu). dt. hyp. (spo).

Wild. dt. hyp.

Color Dark. (cu).

Red. atp. buf. cld. (con). (cu). dt. s.

Yellow. as-o. vr-a.

Eruptions. (ca-ca).

Ulcers. (ca-ca).

Heat. dt.

Heaviness. (crot). ppv.

Lachrymation. aps. bry. (con). k-bicr. (na-sa). vr-a.

Hot. bry.

Movements. acon. buf. (ca-ca). (cu). dt. hll. (myris). (ppv). (vr-a).

Convulsions. buf.

Squinting. hll.

Upwards. acon. buf.

To Left. buf.

Pressing. (con). (na-cl). s.

Projecting. anm. (cu). (spo).

Shooting. ca-ca.

Smarting. bry. k-bicr.

Sunken. as-o. (cu).

Swelling, Feeling of. cld.

Tearing. pul.

Undefined. acon. arn. as-o. atp. bry. ca-ca. ca-s. cth. (cu). hg. k-o. led. lyc. mtr. na-ca. p. pul. rho. rs. s. sep. si-x. spi. str. thu. vr-a.

CORNEA. ca-ca.

Eruptions, Ulcers. ca-ca.

IRIS. anm. art-v. atp. buf. ca-ca. ca-s. cap. cl-hx. crb-x. dph. dt. hll. hyo. hyp. lau-c. mtr. nic. p-x. ppv. pul. s. sep. si-x. spi. thu. vr-a.

Pupils Contracted. anm. atp. cap. cl-hx. crb-x. dph. lau-c. mtr. p-x. pul. s. sep. si-x. thu. vr-a.

Dilated. anm. art-v. atp. buf. ca-ca. ca-s. dt. hll. hyo. hyp. nic. ppv. spi.

Insensible. buf. crb-x. dt.

ORBIT. crot. na-cl.

Heaviness. crot.

Pressing. na-cl.

ORBITAL INTEGUMENTS. (cu).

Color Dark. (cu).

EYELIDS. buf. ca-ca. con. crot. myris. ppv. vr-a.

Adhesion of. (con).

Movements, Closing. (buf). (ca-ca). vr-a.

Spasmodically. ca-ca.

Opening Wide. ppv.

Winking. myris.

UPPER EYELID. crot.

Heaviness. crot.

RIGHT. con. na-sa.

Eyeball, Color Red. con.

Lachrymation. con. na-sa.

Pressing. con.

Eyelids, Adhesion of. con.

LEFT. buf.

Eyelids, Movements, Closing. buf.

After SWEAT.

cb-v.

EYEBALL. cb-v.

Heat. cb-v.

Before CONVULSIONS.

hyo. si-x.

OBJECTS, IMAGINARY. hyo.

Bright. hyo.

Spots. hyo.

Bright. hyo.

EYEBALL. si-x.

Lachrymation. si-x.

With CONVULSIONS.

acon. æth. aga. (alm). amm-ca. anm. apo. aps. art-v. as-o. ast. atp. buf. cic. cmf. crb-x. cth. cu. dol. dt. glo. glp. hll. hyo. k-o. lau-c. mtr. phy. ppv. pul. s. si-x. thr. trg. trn. vr-a.

OBJECTS, FALSE APPEARANCE **of**. amm-ca. cic. dt. hyo.

Black. amm-ca.

Large. dt.

Moving. amm-ca.

Multiplied. cic. hyo.

OBJECTS, IMAGINARY. (dt). hyo. thr.

Bright. hyo.

Flashes Bright. hyo.

Vibrations. thr.

Visions. (dt).

Horrid. (dt).

PHOTOPHOBIA. hyo.

SIGHT IMPAIRED. amm-ca. apo. ast. atp. dt. k-o. s.

EYEBALL. acon. æth. (alm). anm. aps. art-v. as-o. atp. buf. cic. cmf. cth. cu. dol. dt. glo. hll. hyo. k-o. lau-c. mtr. phy. ppv. pul. s. si-x. trg. trn.

Appearance Bright. (alm). cmf. cth. dt.

Dim. buf. dt. mtr. phy.

Glassy. anm.

Staring. æth. anm. atp. cic. cth. (cu). dol. dt. k-o. mtr. s. si-x.

Wild. dt.

Color Dark. (art-v). (cu). (dt).

Red. (aga). buf. cu. dt. hyo. ppv.

Heaviness. ppv.

Itching. (cu).

Movements. acon. æth. (aga). aps. art-v. as-o. atp. buf. cic. cth. cu. dol. dt. glo. glp. hyo. k-o. lau-c. mtr. (ppv). pul. si-x. trg. (vr-a).

Convulsions. acon. æth. aps. art-v. as-o. atp. buf. buf. cic. cth. cu. dt. glo. k-o. lau-c. mtr. pul. si-x. trg.

Squinting. æth. aps. art-v. atp. hll.

Upwards. acon. buf. cic. cu. glo.

Downwards. æth.

Outwards. glo.

To Left. buf.
Projecting. anm. hyo.
Smarting. trn.
Sunken. (cu). (dt).
Undefined. (cu).
IRIS. æth. anm. aps. art-v. ast. atp. cic. cu. dt. hll. mtr. phy. ppv.
Pupils Contracted. ast. crb-x.
Dilated. æth. anm. aps. art-v. atp. cic. dt. hll. mtr. phy. ppv.
Insensible. æth. atp. (cu). dt. ppv.
ORBITAL INTEGUMENTS. art-v. (cu). dt.
Color Dark. art-v. (cu).
ORBITAL INTEGUMENTS INFERIORLY. dt.
Color Dark. dt.
EYELIDS. aga. atp. buf. cu. dol. dt. glp. hyo. k-o. mtr. ppv. pul. vr-a.
Itching. (cu).
Movements, Closing. acon. (buf). cu. dt. glp. k-o. mtr. ppv. pul. vr-a.
Convulsions. atp. cu. hyo. mtr.
Opening Wide. (buf). dol. (dt). ppv.
Winking. aga.
CANTHI. aga.
INTERNAL CANTHUS. aga.
Color Red. aga.
RIGHT. buf. trg.
Eyelids, Movements, Convulsions. trg.
Opening Wide. buf.
LEFT. buf.
Eyelids, Movements, Closing. buf.

After CONVULSIONS.

bru. hyo. s.
EYEBALL. hyo. s.
Lachrymation. s.
Movements. (bru).
Tearing. (hyo).
Throbbing. (hyo).
EYELIDS. bru.
Movements, Closing. bru.

RIGHT. hyo.
Eyeball, Tearing. hyo.
Throbbing. hyo.

With EMACIATION.

cap. (dt). na-ca.
SIGHT IMPAIRED. cap.
EYEBALL. (dt).
Sunken. (dt).
IRIS. (dt). na-ca.
Pupils Dilated. (dt). na-ca.

With FAINTING.

acon. alm. amb. atp. buf. ca-ca. can. chd. chi. crot. (cu). dor. dt. fe-a. frm. gel. glo. k-na. ly-b. lyc. mg-cl. morph-a. myris. na-ba. pb. pet. s-x. str. trg. vr-a. vr-v.
OBJECTS, FALSE APPEARANCE **of.** (dt). gel. ly-b. mg-cl.
Black. (dt).
Green. mg-cl.
Inverted. ly-b.
Multiplied. gel.
Red. mg-cl.
OBJECTS, IMAGINARY. can. (cu). glo. pet. vr-a.
Black. glo.
Bright. (vr-a).
Figures. (cu).
Mist. can.
Spirits. (cu).
Spots. glo. (vr-a).
Black. glo.
Bright. (vr-a).
Veil. pet.
SIGHT IMPAIRED. alm. amb. ca-ca. can. chd. chi. dor. dt. fe-a. frm. gel. glo. lyc. myris. pb. pet. s-x. trg. vr-v.
EYEBALL. atp. buf. crot. k-na. na-ba. str.
Appearance Staring. atp.
Color Dark. (myris).
Red. crot.

Heat. crot. k-na.
Movements. buf.
Convulsions. buf.
Pressing. na-ba. (str).
Smarting. na-ba.
IRIS. acon. (dt). morph-a.
Pupils Dilated. acon. (dt). morph-a.
Insensible. (dt).
ORBITAL INTEGUMENTS. myris.
ORBITAL INTEGUMENTS INFERIORLY. myris.
Color Dark. myris.
FORWARDS. str.
Eyeball, Pressing. str.
LEFT. vr-a.
Objects Imaginary, Bright. vr-a.
Spots Bright. vr-a.

With HEAVINESS **of Body**.

aga. myris.
OBJECTS, FALSE APPEARANCE **of.** myris.
Far. myris.
EYEBALL. aga.
Drawing. aga.
Pressing. aga.

With NUMBNESS **of Body**.

grp.
SIGHT IMPAIRED. grp.

With SMARTING **of Body.**

EYEBALL. (eupat-p).
Color Red. (eupat-p).
Swelling. (eupat-p).

With STIFFNESS **of Body**.

acon. as-o. atp. ppv.
OBJECTS IMAGINARY. atp.
Bright. atp.

Spots. atp.
    Bright. atp.
EYEBALL. acon. as-o. ppv.
Appearance Dim. as-o.
    Staring. acon.
Color Yellow. as-o.
Movements. ppv.
    Convulsions. ppv.
Sunken. as-o.
IRIS. acon.
Pupils Contracted. acon.
    Insensible. acon.
EYELIDS. acon.
Movements, Opening Wide. acon.

With SWELLING of Body.

acon.
EYEBALL. acon.
Projecting. acon.

Before WEAKNESS.

(cu). thr.
OBJECTS, FALSE APPEARANCE **of.** thr.
Far. thr.
OBJECT IMAGINARY. thr.
Bright. thr.
Veil. thr.
Vibrations. thr.
    Bright. thr.
SIGHT IMPAIRED. thr.
EYEBALL. (cu).
Movements. (cu).
    Convulsions. (cu).

With WEAKNESS.

acon. alm. amm-ca. anm. aps. as-o. atp. cast. cb-v. cic. cl-hx. clv. cof. cth. cu. dro. dt. ery. eupat-p. euph-a. grp. grt. hg. hyo. k-ca. k-na. kre. lac-f. mg-cl. myris. na-ba. ni-ca. os. pb. ppv. qu-sa. rho. rs. s. si-x. smi. so-d. spo. sr-ca. str. thr. trg. trn. vr-a. vr-s. zn.

OBJECTS, FALSE APPEARANCE **of.** (alm). amm-ca. cic. mg-cl. pb. thr.

Far. thr.
Green. mg-cl.
Moving. amm-ca.
Multiplied. (alm). cic. pb.
Red. mg-cl.

OBJECTS IMAGINARY. as-o. atp. ery. hyo. k-ca. smi. sr-ca. thr. trg.

Black. (ery).
Bright. atp. ery. hyo. k-ca. sr-ca. thr.
Flashes Bright. hyo.
Mist. (ery). k-ca. smi.
  Black. (ery).
  Red. (ery).
Red. (ery).
Serpentine Bodies. ery.
  Bright. ery.
Spots. atp. ery. k-ca. sr-ca.
  Bright. atp. k-ca. sr-ca.
  White. ery.
Veil. thr.
Vibrations. thr. trg.
  Bright. thr.
Visions. as-o.
White. ery.

PHOTOPHOBIA. acon. hg. k-na. (lac-f). na-ba.

SIGHT IMPAIRED. alm. amm-ca. as-o. atp. cb-v. (ery). euph-c. grp. k-ca. lac-f. os. pb. qu-sa. smi. so-d. thr. trn. zn.

EYEBALL. acon. (alm). anm. aps. as-o. cast. clv. cof. cth. cu. dro. dt. ery. eupat-p. hg. hyo. k-ca. k-na. kre. lac-f. na-ba. ni-ca. pb. ppv. rho. rs. s. si-x. spo. str. trg. trn. vr-a. zn.

Appearance Bright. (alm). dt.
  Dim. as-o. cu. dt. ery. spo. trg. vr-a.
  Glassy. rs.
  Staring. as-o. dt. eupat-p. k-ca.
Color Dark. (ery).
  Red. acon. (as-o). (cu). hg. hyo. (lac-f) ppv. s.
  Yellow. as-o. pb. s. vr-a.
Drawing. (as-o).
Hæmorrhage. (ery).

Heat. k-na. kre. na-ba. ni-ca. rho. s.
Heaviness. (cro). ppv.
Itching. s.
Lachrymation. cof. dt. k-ca. (lac-f). ppv. spo. (trg). vr-a.
Movements. (alm). anm. aps. (cl-hx). cu. dt. (grt). (myris). (pb). ppv. (spo). trg. (vr-s).
Convulsions. anm. cu. dt. ppv. trg.
Squinting. (alm). aps. (pb).
Inwards. (alm). (pb).
Paralysis. (dro).
Pressing. (as-o). k-ca. (str).
Projecting. (cu).
Shooting. k-ca. (lac-f).
Smarting. cast. trn.
Sunken. as-o. clv. cu. dro. ery. rs.
Feeling. zn.
Swelling. (k-ca). (spo).
Feeling of. (cro).
Tensive. si-x.
Throbbing. (lac-f).
Undefined. cth. ery.
IRIS. (alm). anm. aps. as-o. atp. cic. cu. dt. pb.
Pupils Contracted. dt.
Dilated. (alm). anm. aps. as-o. atp. cic. cu. dt. pb.
Insensible. as-o. dt.
ORBITAL INTEGUMENTS. ery. spo.
Color Dark. ery.
Swelling. spo.
EYELIDS. (alm). anm. cl-hx. cro. cu. dro. dt. grt. k-ca. myris. pb. spo. trg. vr-s.
Movements, Closing. anm. cl-hx. cu. dt. grt. myris. (spo). vr-s.
Spasmodically. spo.
Convulsions. (cu).
Opening Wide. (alm). dt. pb.
Paralysis, Opening Difficult. dro.
Swelling. spo.
Feeling of. cro.
UPPER EYELID. cro. k-ca.
Heavy. cro.
Swelling. k-ca.

FORWARDS. str.
Eyeball, Pressing. str.
BACKWARDS. lac-f.
To HEAD. lac-f.
To FOREHEAD. lac-f.
To TEMPLE. lac-f.
RIGHT. (alm). as-o. lac-f. pb.
Photophobia. lac-f.
Eyeball, Color Red. as-o. lac-f.
Drawing. as-o.
Lachrymation. lac-f.
Movements, Squinting. (alm). pb.
Inwards. (alm). pb.
Pressing. as-o.
Backwards. Eyeball, Shooting. lac-f.
To Forehead. Eyeball, Shooting. lac-f.
Throbbing. lac-f.
To Temple. Eyeball, Shooting. lac-f.
Throbbing. lac-f.
LEFT. trg.
Eyeball, Lachrymation. trg.
Movements, Convulsions. trg.
Eyelids, Movements, Convulsions. trg.

After WEAKNESS.

as-o. con.
OBJECTS IMAGINARY. con.
Bright. con.
Vibrations. con.
Bright. con.
PHOTOPHOBIA. as-o.
SIGHT IMPAIRED. con.
EYEBALL. as-o.
Color Red. as-o.
Heat. as-o.
Lachrymation. as-o.

With GLANDULAR **Symptoms.**

au. ca-ca. con. hg-bicl. rs. s. trn.
OBJECTS, FALSE APPEARANCE **of.** s.

Multiplied. s.
PHOTOPHOBIA. au. ca-ca. con.
EYEBALL. au. ca-ca. con. s.
Color Red. (au). (con). (s).
White. (hg-bicl).
Cutting. au.
Eruptions. (ca-ca). (hg-bicl). (rs). (s).
Pimples. (rs).
Ulcers. (ca-ca). (hg-bicl). (rs).
Vesicles. (rs).
Itching. (trn).
Lachrymation. (au) con.
Hot. au.
Movements. (ca-ca). (hg-bicl).
Shooting. ca-ca.
Smarting. (trn).
Swelling. (con). (hg-bicl). (rs).
Undefined. (s).
Same Symptom. (s).
EYEBALL, ROUND CORNEA. s.
Color Red. s.
SCLEROTIC. con.
Color Red. con.
CORNEA. au. ca-ca. con. hg-bicl. rs. s.
Color Red. au.
White. hg-bicl.
Eruptions, Pimples. rs.
Ulcers. ca-ca. hg-bicl. s.
Vesicles. rs.
Opacity. con. (hg-bicl). s.
CHAMBERS **of** EYE. hg-bicl.
Discharge, Pus. hg-bicl.
EYELIDS. au. ca-ca. con. hg-bicl. s. trn.
Adhesion of. au.
Color Red. con.
Itching. trn.
Movements, Closing. (ca-ca). (hg-bicl).
Spasmodically. ca-ca. hg-bicl.
Smarting. trn.
Swelling. con. hg-bicl.
TARSAL EDGES. s.
Eruptions, Ulcers. s.
Swelling. s.

CANTHI. s.
EXTERNAL CANTHUS. s.
Color Red. s.
LEFT. s.
Eyeball, Undefined. s.
Same Symptom. s.

With JOINTS **Symptoms.**

(eupat-p).
EYEBALL. (eupat-p).
Color Red. (eupat-p).
Swelling. (eupat-p).

With SKIN **Symptoms.**

acon. æsc. (alm). atp. ca-ca. ca-s. cic. clv. cop. cu. dt. ery. hg. hg-cl. morph-a. pb. s. sa-l. str.
OBJECTS, FALSE APPEARANCE **of.** (alm). cic. pb. s.
Multiplied. (alm). cic. pb. s.
OBJECTS, IMAGINARY. (dt).
Figures. (dt).
PHOTOPHOBIA. ca-ca. hg.
EYEBALL. acon. æsc. (alm). ca-ca. ca-s. clv. cu. dt. ery. hg. hg-cl. morph-a. pb. s. sa-l. str.
Appearance Dim. ery.
Coldness. (sa-l).
Color Dark. (cu). (ery).
Red. (cu). dt. hg. morph-a. (s). str.
Yellow. æsc. ca-s. hg-cl. s. str.
Eruptions. (s).
Ulcers. (s).
Lachrymation. str.
Movements. (alm). ca-ca. cu. (pb). s.
Convulsions. cu.
Squinting. (alm). ca-ca. (pb). s.
Projecting. acon. cu.
Shooting. sa-l.
Cold. sa-l.
Sunken. clv. (cu). (dt). ery.

Swelling. (cop). (cu). (s).
EYEBALL ROUND CORNEA. s.
Color Red. s.
CORNEA. s.
Eruptions, Ulcers. s.
Opacity. s.
IRIS. (alm). atp. cic. dt. pb.
Pupils Dilated. (alm). atp. cic. dt. pb.
ORBITAL INTEGUMENTS. cu. ery.
Color Dark. cu. ery.
EYELIDS. cop. cu. s.
Color Red. cu.
Movements, Closing. cu.
Swelling. cop. cu.
TARSAL EDGES. s.
Eruptions, Ulcers. s.
Swelling. s.
CANTHI. s.
EXTERNAL CANTHUS. s.
Color Red. s.
RIGHT. (alm). pb.
Eyeball, Movements, Squinting. (alm). pb.
Inwards. (alm). pb.

ERUPTIONS, **Suppressed.**

atp. k-o. mg-ca. s. si-x. smi.
SIGHT IMPAIRED. atp. s.
EYEBALL. k-o. smi.
Color Red. k-o. smi.
LENS. mg-ca. s. si-x.
Cataract. mg-ca. s. si-x.

GONORRHŒA, **Suppressed**.

pul. sb-s.
EYEBALL. pul. sb-s.
Color Red. pul. sb-s.

GOUT.

bry. dig.
EYEBALL. bry. dig.
Color Red. bry. dig.

SCROFULA.

ca-ca. chi. cis. cle. con. dig.
PHOTOPHOBIA. con.
EYEBALL. chi. cis. cle. con. dig.
Color Red. chi. cle. con. dig.
Motion in. cis.
Passing Round, like something. cis.
Shooting. cis.
LENS. ca-ca.
Cataract. ca-ca.

SWEAT of FEET, Suppressed.

si-x.
LENS. si-x.
Cataract. si-x.

SYPHILIS.

ca-s. n-x.
EYEBALL. ca-s. n-x.
Color Red. ca-s. n-x.

LOSS of FLUIDS.

art-v. au-cl. cb-v. chi. dt. p. vr-v.
OBJECTS, IMAGINARY. dt. vr-v.
Circles. vr-v.
Green. vr-v.
Red. vr-v.
Green. vr-v.
Red. vr-v.
Veil. dt.
SIGHT IMPAIRED. art-v. au-cl. cb-v. chi. dt. p. vr-v.
EYEBALL. chi.
Color Red. chi.
Itching. chi.

INJURIES.

acon. (alm). con. cro. cyc. euphr. n-x. s.
SIGHT IMPAIRED. con.
EYEBALL. cro. cyc. euphr. n-x.
Color Red. euphr.
Lachrymation. n-x.
  Hot. n-x.
Movements. (cyc).
  Squinting. (cyc).
  Inwards. (cyc).
Shooting. cro.
IRIS. (alm).
Prolapsus. (alm).
LENS. con.
Cataract. con.
RIGHT. con.
Sight Impaired. con.
Lens, Cataract. con.
LEFT. cyc.
Eyeball, Movements, Squinting. cyc.
  Inwards. cyc.

ALCOHOL.

sb-t. str. zn.
SIGHT IMPAIRED. str.
EYEBALL. sb-t.
Color Red. sb-t.
Eruptions. sb-t.
  Blisters. sb-t.

BEER.

sb-t.
EYEBALL. sb-t.
Color Red. sb-t.
Eruptions. sb-t.
  Blisters. sb-t.

CAMPHOR, **Smell of.**

k-na.
SIGHT IMPAIRED. k-na.

COFFEE.

alli.
EYEBALL.
Itching. (alli).
EYELIDS. alli.
UPPER EYELID. alli.
LEFT. alli.
Upper Eyelid, Itching. alli.

LEMONADE.

dt.
IRIS. dt.
Pupils Contracted. dt.

MERCURY.

au. ca-s.
PHOTOPHOBIA. au.
EYEBALL. au. ca-s.
Color Red. au. ca-s.
Cutting. au.
Eruptions. (ca-s).
  Ulcers. (ca-s).
Lachrymation. (au).
  Hot. au.
CORNEA. au.
Color Red. au.
Eruptions, Ulcers. au.
EYELIDS. au.
Adhesion of. au.

SILVER, **Nitrate of.**

na-cl.
EYEBALL. na-cl.
Color Red. na-cl.
Discharge. na-cl.
    Excoriating. na-cl.
    Thin. na-cl.

TOBACCO.

asc. cld.
SIGHT IMPAIRED. asc.
EYEBALL. cld.
Pressing. cld.

VINEGAR.

dt.
OBJECTS, FALSE APPEARANCE **of.** dt.
Small. dt.
SIGHT IMPAIRED. dt.
Myopia. dt.
IRIS. dt.
Pupils Contracted. dt.
    Insensible. dt.

WINE.

zn.

II. B. AMELIORATIONS.

BED.

smc.
EYEBALL.
Boring. (smc).
Throbbing. (smc).
ORBIT. smc.
ORBIT SUPERIORLY. smc.
RIGHT. smc.
Orbit Superiorly, Boring. smc.
Throbbing. smc.

COLD.

ag-na. al-o. alli. amm-ca. asr. k-na. k-o. mg-ca. ni-ca. ox-x. p. thu.

SIGHT IMPAIRED. al-o. amm-cl. k-o. ni-ca.

EYEBALL. ag-na. al-o. alli. amm-cl. asr. mg-ca. ni-ca. ox-x. thu.

Color Red. ag-na.
Drawing. (alli).
Gnawing. ox-x.
Heat. al-o. amm-cl. (thu).
Lachrymation. al-o.
Hot. (al-o).
Pressing. (p).
Smarting. al-o. ox-x.
Swelling, Feeling of. ni-ca.
Tearing. mg-ca.
Tensive. ox-x.
Undefined. ag-na. asr. ni-ca.
ORBITAL INTEGUMENTS. ox-x.
ORBITAL INTEGUMENTS SUPERIORLY. ox-x.
Gnawing. ox-x.
Smarting. ox-x.
Tensive. ox-x.

EYELIDS. mg-ca. p.
Adhesion of. mg-ca.
UPPER EYELID. p.
Pressing. p.
RIGHT. thu.
Eyeball, Heat. thu.
LEFT. al-o. alli.
Eyeball, Drawing. alli.
Heat. al-o.
Lachrymation. al-o.
Hot. al-o.
Smarting. al-o.

COVERING.

thu.
EYEBALL. thu.
Undefined. thu.

HEAT.

eryn. zn.
EYEBALL. zn.
Heat. zn.
Smarting. zn.
Undefined. zn.

OPEN AIR.

ag-na. alli. amb. cit-c. cl-hx. cof. cro. dig. grc. grt. hæm. hg. hyo. jcr. jnp-s. k-o. lau-c. lyc. ox-x. p. phy. pol. pt. pul. rs. sep. smi. trg.
OBJECTS, FALSE APPEARANCE **of**. grt. hæm. jnp-s.
Confused. hæm.
Moving. grt. jnp-s.
Circularly. grt.
Vibrating. jnp-s.
OBJECTS, IMAGINARY. hæm. jnp-s. trg.
Bright. jnp-s. trg.
Mist. hæm. jnp-s.
Vibrations. jnp-s. trg.
Bright. jnp-s. trg.

SIGHT IMPAIRED. cof. hæm. hg. jnp-s. k-o.

EYEBALL. ag-na. alli. cit-c. cro. dig. grc. lyc. ox-x. phy. rs. sep. smi.

Color Red. ag-na.

Drawing. (alli).

False Sensations. smi.

Sand. smi.

Gnawing. ox-x.

Heat. grc.

Itching. (alli). (grc).

Lachrymation. cro. (dig). (grc). phy. rs.

Hot. dig. grc. rs.

Movements. (sep).

Pressing. (p). (pol). (rs).

Shooting. (lau-c). smi.

Smarting. cit-c. ox-x.

Swelling, Feeling of. (rs).

Tearing. lyc.

Tensive. ox-x.

Throbbing. (trg).

Undefined, ag-na. cit-c. (jcr).

ORBIT. jcr. lau-c. pol.

Pressing. pol.

Shooting. lau-c.

ORBIT SUPERIORLY. jcr.

Undefined. jcr.

ORBITAL INTEGUMENTS. ox-x.

ORBITAL INTEGUMENTS SUPERIORLY. ox-x.

Gnawing. ox-x.

Smarting. ox-x.

Tensive. ox-x.

EYELIDS. alli. p. rs. sep.

Movements, Closing. sep.

UPPER EYELID. alli. p. rs.

Pressing. p.

CANTHI. grc.

INTERNAL CANTHUS. grc.

Itching. grc.

RIGHT. jcr. rs. trg.

Eyeball, Throbbing. trg.

Orbit Superiorly, Undefined. jcr.

Upper Eyelid. Pressing. rs.

Swelling, Feeling of. rs.

LEFT. alli. sep.
Eyeball, Drawing. alli.
Eyelids, Movements, Closing. sep.
Upper Eyelid, Itching. alli.

ROOM, In.

al-o. amm-cl. con. k-o. men. rut. s. s-x. zn.
OBJECTS, FALSE APPEARANCE **of.** k-o.
Large. k-o.
Moving. k-o.
Circularly. k-o.
SIGHT IMPAIRED al-o. amm-cl. con.
EYEBALL. rut. s. s-x. zn.
False Sensations. (s-x).
Sand. (s-x).
Heat. s-x. zn.
Lachrymation. rut.
Pressing. s-x.
Smarting. zn.
Tensive. s.
EYEBALL ANTERIORLY. s-x.
Heat. s-x.
Pressing. s-x.
CANTHI. s-x.
EXTERNAL CANTHUS. s-x.
RIGHT. s-x.
External Canthus, False Sensations, Sand. s-x.

WASHING.

al-o. amm-cl. asr. chd. cl-hx. cld. dl-s. frm. k-na. k-o. mg-ca. na-ca. na-sa. ni-ca. p. pru-l. thu.
OBJECTS IMAGINARY. amm-cl. k-o. na-sa.
Leaf. (na-sa).
White. (na-sa).
Mist. amm-cl. k-o.
White. (na-sa).
SIGHT IMPAIRED. al-o. amm-cl. chd. k-o. ni-ca.
EYEBALL. al-o. amm-cl. frm. k-na. mg-ca. na-ca. na-sa. ni-ca. pru-l. thu.
Color Red. ni-ca.

Discharge. (na-sa). pru-l.
Pus. (na-sa).
Heat. al-o. amm-cl. asr. k-na. (thu).
Itching. na-ca.
Lachrymation. al-o. asr. mg-ca.
Hot. (al-o).
Pressing. (p).
Smarting. al-o. na-ca.
Swelling, Feeling of. ni-ca.
Tearing. mg-ca.
Undefined. frm. ni-ca.
EYELIDS. chd. mg-ca. na-sa. p.
Adhesion of. chd. mg-ca. (na-sa).
UPPER EYELID. p.
Pressing. p.
RIGHT. na-ca. na-sa. thu.
Objects Imaginary, Leaf White. na-sa.
White. na-sa.
Eyeball, Heat. thu.
Itching. na-ca.
Shooting. na-ca.
LEFT. al-o. na-sa.
Eyeball, Discharge, Pus. na-sa.
Heat. al-o.
Lachrymation. al-o.
Hot. al-o.
Smarting. al-o.
Eyelids, Adhesion of. na-sa.

LYING.

cb-a. lyc. smc. spo. str.
OBJECTS, FALSE APPEARANCE **of.** cb-a. spo. str.
Moving. cb-a. spo. str.
Vertically. spo. str.
Up and Down. spo. str.
Multiplied. spo.
SIGHT IMPAIRED. spo.
EYEBALL. lyc.

Boring. (smc).
Tearing. lyc.
Throbbing. (smc.)
ORBIT. smc.
ORBIT SUPERIORLY. smc.
RIGHT. smc.
Orbit Superiorly, Boring. smc.
Throbbing. smc.

REST.

cmc.
EYEBALL. cmc.
Pressing. cmc.
Undefined. cmc.
EYEBALL POSTERIORLY. cmc.
FORWARDS. cmc.
Eyeball, Pressing. cmc.
DOWNWARDS. cmc.
Eyeball, Pressing. cmc.
To HEAD. cmc.
To OCCIPUT. cmc.
Eyeball Posteriorly, Undefined. cmc.

SITTING.

acon. ara-d. arn. asr. led. s.
OBJECTS, FALSE APPEARANCE **of.** acon. arn.
Moving. acon. arn.
Circularly. acon. arn.
EYEBALL. ara-d. asr. led. s.
Heat. ara-d. asr.
Lachrymation. asr.
Tearing. led.
Tensive. s.

PRESSURE.

al-o. amm-cl. atp. bry. ca-ca. cac. hll. k-o. men. mn-ca. na-cl. ppv. ptv. pul. trn. vr-a.

EYEBALL. al-o. atp. ca-ca. k-o. men. mn-ca. na-cl. ppv. ptv. trn. vr-a.

Bruised. (ptv). vr-a.
Drawing. mn-ca.
Dryness. ppv.
False Sensations. ppv.
Sand. ppv.
Heat. atp. (bry).
Itching. atp.
Movements. al-o.
Convulsions. al-o.
Pressing. (cac). (hll). k-o. (na-cl).
Like a Nail. (hll).
Shooting. (trn).
Tearing. (amm-cl).
Undefined. (men). na-cl.

EYEBALL EXTERNALLY. vr-a.
Bruised. vr-a.

ORBIT. amm-cl. cac. hll. mn-ca.
Drawing. mn-ca.

ORBIT SUPERIORLY. amm-cl. cac. hll.

ORBITAL INTEGUMENTS. bry.

ORBITAL INTEGUMENTS SUPERIORLY. bry.
Heat. bry.

CANTHI. vr-a.

EXTERNAL CANTHUS. vr-a.

FORWARDS. na-cl.
Eyeball, Pressing. na-cl.

To HEAD. trn.

To SIDE OF HEAD. trn.

RIGHT. amm-cl. cac. ptv. vr-a.
Eyeball, Bruised. ptv.
Orbit Superiorly, Pressing. cac.
Tearing. amm-cl.
External Canthus, Bruised. vr-a.

LEFT. al-o. hll. men. trn.
Eyeball, Movements, Convulsions. al-o.
Undefined. men.
Orbit Superiorly, Pressing. hll.
Like a Nail. hll.

To Side of Head. Eyeball, Shooting. trn.

PRESSURE CONTINUED

amm-cl.
EYEBALL.
Tearing. (amm-cl).
ORBIT. amm-cl.
ORBIT SUPERIORLY. amm-cl.
RIGHT. amm-cl.
Orbit Superiorly, Tearing. amm-cl.

PRESSURE UPWARDS.

atp.
EYEBALL. atp.
Heat. atp.
Itching. atp.

RUBBING.

aga. al-o. alli. amm-ca. amm-cl. aps. art-v. atp. bar. ca-a. ca-ca. ca-o. cap. cb-a. ccs. chd. co. cro. cth. dl-s. dt. eupat-p. euph. f-hx. grc. grt. gym. hyo. ind. jat. jnc. k-bicr. k-i. k-o. kre. krm. lam. lct. ly-b. mg-ca. mg-cl. mll. mrl. msc. na-ba. na-ca. na-cl. na-sa. ol-a. os. p. p-x. pb. phl. phy. ppv. pru-l. pt. pul. rn-b. rs. s. s-x. se. smr. sn. spi. spo. sr-ca. str. thu. trg. trn. tx-b. urt. vi-t. vtx. zn. zng.
OBJECTS, FALSE APPEARANCE **of**. cro.
White. cro.
OBJECTS IMAGINARY. al-o. art-v. cro. kre. krm. (ly-b). p. pb. pul. trg.
Feathers. al-o. kre.
Mist. al-o. art-v. cro. (ly-b). (p). pb. pul. trg.
Spots. krm.
White. krm.
Threads. al-o.
White. krm.
SIGHT IMPAIRED. al-o. art-v. cap. cro. (k-o). (ly-b). mll. na-ca. p. p-x. pb. pul. trg.
EYEBALL. aga. amm-ca. amm-cl. ca-o. cb-a. ccs. chd. co. cro. dt. eupat-p. k-i. k-o. mg-ca. mg-cl. msc. na-ba. na-cl. na-sa. ol-a. p. phl. ppv. pru-l. pt. rn-b. sn. spi. sr-ca. str. trn. tx-b. vtx. zng.

Crampy. (msc).
Creeping. atp. (na-sa). (pt).
Discharge. aga.
Drawing. tx-b.
Dryness. ppv.
False Sensations. atp. ca-o. (cb-a). ccs. (co). (dt). (k-o). mg-cl. na-ba. p. ppv. rn-b. (trn). zng.
Hair. ccs. (trn).
Pellicle. (k-o).
Sand. atp. (cb-a). (co). (dt). mg-cl. na-ba. p. ppv. rn-b. zng.
Splinter. ca-o.
Heat. cro. ol-a. (phl). (spi). (tx-b).
Itching. aga. (alli). amm-ca. (art-v). (atp). (bar). (ca-a). cb-a. (chd). (dl-s). (dt). (euph). (f-hx). (grt). (hyo). (jat). (jnc). k-o. (lam). (mg-ca). (mg-cl). msc. na-cl. ol-a. (os). p. phl. (phy). pru-l. pt. (rs). (se). (sn). (spi). (spo). str. tx-b. (vi-t).
Lachrymation. eupat-p. (na-sa).
Movements. amm-cl. (hyo).
Convulsions. amm-cl.
Paralysis. (mrl).
Pressing. atp. (chd). cro. mg-cl. na-sa. (ol-a).
Shooting. (atp). (ca-a). (cb-a). (grt). (ind). (ol-a). phl. (spo). (vi-t).
Smarting. amm-ca. (cb-a). (grc). (hyo). (ind). (jat). (k-i). (k-o). (lct). (mg-ca). (phl). (rs). (s-x). smr. (sr-ca) (vtx). (zn).
Tearing. (hyo).
Tensive. (k-o).
Throbbing. (chd).
Tingling. (art-v).
EYEBALL SUPERIORLY. co.
False Sensations, Sand. co.
ORBITAL INTEGUMENTS. f-hx. na-cl. ol-a. pru-l. spi. spo. vi-t.
ORBITAL INTEGUMENTS SUPERIORLY. f-hx. na-cl. ol-a. pru-l. spi. vi-t.
Itching. f-hx. na-cl. pru-l.
Shooting. ol-a.
ORBITAL INTEGUMENTS INFERIORLY. spo.
EYELIDS. alli. art-v. chd. dl-s. euph. grt. jat. jnc. lam. mrl. ol-a. phl. pru-l. rs. s-x. se. tx-b.

Heat. tx-b.
Itching. grt. tx-b.
Tingling. art-v.
UPPER EYELID. alli. chd. dl-s. mrl. pru-l. rs.
Itching. pru-l.
Paralysis, Opening Difficult. mrl.
LOWER EYELID. euph. lam. ol-a. phl. s-x.
Itching. euph. lam. ol-a.
Smarting. s-x.
TARSAL EDGES. dl-s. jat. jnc. grt. se.
Itching. jat.
Smarting. dl-s.
UPPER TARSAL EDGE. dl-s.
Itching. dl-s.
CANTHI. art-v. atp. bar. ca-a. cb-a. dl-s. euph. grc. grt. hyo. ind. k-o. lam. lct. mg-ca. mg-cl. msc. os. phl. phy. pru-l. pt. zn.
Crampy. msc.
Creeping. pt.
Itching. art-v. hyo. k-o. lam.
Movements, Convulsions. hyo.
Smarting. hyo. lct.
EXTERNAL CANTHUS. ca-a. euph. grc. ol-a.
Shooting. ca-a.
Smarting. grc.
INTERNAL CANTHUS. atp. bar. ca-a. cb-a. dl-s. grt. ind. mg-ca. mg-cl. os. phl. phy. pru-l. zn.
Heat. phl.
Itching. atp. bar. ca-a. dl-s. grt. mg-ca. phl. pru-l.
Shooting. atp. ca-a. grt. ind. phl.
Smarting. cb-a. ind. zn.
RIGHT. chd. dt. k-i. k-o. mg-ca. mg-cl. na-sa. ol-a. rs. sr-ca. spi. vtx.
Sight Impaired. k-o.
Eyeball, False Sensations, Pellicle. k-o.
Sand. dt.
Itching. chd. dt. ol-a.
Lachrymation. na-sa.
Smarting. k-i. mg-ca. sr-ca. vtx.
Tensive. k-o.
Orbital Integuments Superiorly, Heat. spi.
Itching. spi.
Pressing. ol-a.

Upper Eyelid, Itching. rs.
Smarting. rs.
External Canthus, Heat. ol-a.
Throbbing. chd.
Internal Canthus, Itching. mg-cl.
Smarting. mg-ca.

LEFT. alli. cb-a. chd. euph. lct. ly-b. mg-ca. na-sa. ol-a. os. p. pru-l. sn. spi. spo. trn. vi-t. zng.

Objects Imaginary, Mist. ly-b.
Sight Impaired. ly-b.
Eyeball, Creeping. na-sa.
False Sensations, Hair. trn.
Sand. cb-a. p. zng.
Itching. mg-ca. ol-a. sn. spi.
Shooting. ol-a.
Smarting. mg-ca. zn.
Orbital Integuments Superiorly, Itching. pru-l. vi-t.
Shooting. vi-t.
Orbital Integuments Inferiorly, Itching. spo.
Shooting. spo.
Upper Eyelid, Itching. alli. chd.
Lower Eyelid, Smarting. phl.
Canthus, Smarting. lct.
External Canthus, Itching. euph.
Internal Canthus, Itching. os.
Smarting. cb-a.

TOUCH.

gui. hyo. k-o. men. spo. thu.

EYEBALL.

Gnawing. (hyo).
Heat. (men).
Pressing. (hyo).
Shooting. (spo).
Smarting. (thu).
Tearing. (thu).
Tensive. (men). (spo).

ORBITAL INTEGUMENTS. gui. hyo. thu.

ORBITAL INTEGUMENTS SUPERIORLY. hyo. thu.

Gnawing. hyo.
Pressing. hyo.
Smarting. thu.
EYELIDS. men.
UPPER EYELID. men.
CANTHI. spo.
EXTERNAL CANTHUS. spo.
LEFT. men. spo. thu.
Orbital Integuments Superiorly, Tearing. thu.
Upper Eyelid, Heat. men.
Tensive. men.
External Canthus, Shooting. spo.
Tensive. spo.

RISING. (**Generally**).

atp. au. cb-v. glo. ol-a. p. rn-b. rs. str.
OBJECTS, FALSE APPEARANCE **of**. au.
Moving. au.
Circularly. au.
EYEBALL. glo. ol-a. rs.
Heat. ol-a. rs.
Pressing. glo. rs.

RISING **from** LYING.

atp. cb-v. glo. ol-a. p. rn-b. rs. str.
EYEBALL. glo. ol-a. rs.
Heat. ol-a. rs.
Pressing. glo. rs.

RISING **from** STOOPING.

au.
OBJECTS, FALSE APPEARANCE **of**. au.
Moving. au.
Circularly. au.

STOOPING.

acon. arn. ba-ca.
OBJECTS, FALSE APPEARANCE **of**. arn.

Moving. arn.
  Circularly. arn.
EYEBALL. acon.
Bursting. (acon).
Pressing. (ba-ca).
Undefined. (acon).
EYEBALL SUPERIORLY. acon.
Bursting. acon.
Undefined. acon.
ORBIT. ba-ca.
Pressing. ba-ca.

WALKING.

acon. amb. bry. grc. hyo. na-cl. ol-a. ox-x. pul. trg.
OBJECTS, FALSE APPEARANCE **of**. acon. bry.
Moving. acon. bry.
  Circularly. acon. bry.
OBJECTS IMAGINARY. trg.
Bright. trg.
Vibrations. trg.
  Bright. trg.
SIGHT IMPAIRED. na-cl.
EYEBALL. grc. ol-a. ox-x.
Gnawing. ox-x.
Heat. grc. ol-a.
Smarting. ox-x.
ORBITAL INTEGUMENTS. ox-x.
ORBITAL INTEGUMENTS SUPERIORLY. ox-x.
Gnawing. ox-x.
Smarting. ox-x.
Tensive. ox-x.

EFFORT **of** WILL.

atp. gel.
OBJECTS, FALSE APPEARANCE **of**. atp. gel.
Moving. atp.
  Undulating. atp.
Multiplied. atp. gel.
SIGHT IMPAIRED. atp.

MENTAL EXERTION.

p.
EYEBALL.
Pressing. (p).
EYELIDS. p.
UPPER EYELID. p.
Pressing. p.

MOVING HEAD BACKWARDS.

atp. pol.
OBJECTS, FALSE APPEARANCE **of**. pol.
Multiplied. pol.
SIGHT IMPAIRED. atp.

MOVING HEAD ROUND **to** RIGHT.

ca-ca.
SIGHT IMPAIRED. ca-ca.

DARKNESS.

atp. dt. k-i. myris. p. s. si-x.
SIGHT IMPAIRED. (atp). dt. myris. p. s. si-x.
LEFT. atp.
Sight Impaired. atp.

LIGHT, **Artificial**.

ag-na. amm-cl. (atp).
SIGHT IMPAIRED. ag-na. (atp).
EYEBALL. amm-cl.
Heat. amm-cl.
LEFT. atp.
Sight Impaired. atp.

LIGHT, **Natural**.

(dt). srr.
SIGHT IMPAIRED. (dt). srr.

When FIRST LOOKING.

con.
OBJECTS, FALSE APPEARANCE **of.** con.
Multiplied. con.

LOOKING FIXEDLY. (**Long**).

al-o. bap. cb-v. con. drm. dt. eug. lac-c. lct. li-ca. p-x. pet. smc.
OBJECTS, FALSE APPEARANCE **of.** eug. li-ca. smc.
Moving. smc.
  Vibrating. smc.
Multiplied. eug.
Part Visible. li-ca.
OBJECTS, IMAGINARY. dt. lac-c.
Figures. lac-c.
  Side of Visual Ray, at. lac-c.
Side of Visual Ray, at. lac-c.
Vibrations. dt.
SIGHT IMPAIRED. bap. con. drm. dt. eug. lct. p-x.
Presbyopia. dt.

LOOKING **through a** DOUBLE CONVEX LENS.

atp.
SIGHT IMPAIRED. atp.
Presbyopia. atp.

LOOKING **through a** PIN-HOLE.

atp.
SIGHT IMPAIRED. atp.
Presbyopia. atp.

LOOKING UP.

cast.
OBJECTS, IMAGINARY. cast.
Veil. cast.

LOOKING DOWN.

ba-a. vr-s.
EYEBALL. ba-a. vr-s.
Pressing. ba-a. vr-s.

LOOKING SIDEWAYS.

ca-ca. mg-cl. qu-sa. s.
OBJECTS IMAGINARY. mg-cl.
High up. mg-cl.
Mist. mg-cl.
Rocks. mg-cl.
  High up. mg-cl.
SIGHT IMPAIRED. ca-ca. qu-sa. s.

LOOKING STRAIGHT.

gel. pol.
OBJECTS, FALSE APPEARANCE **of**. gel.
Multiplied. gel.
OBJECTS, IMAGINARY. pol.
Bright. pol.
Spots. pol.
  Bright. pol.

LOOKING at DISTANT Objects.

dt.
OBJECTS, IMAGINARY. (dt).
Figures. (dt).
SIGHT IMPAIRED. dt.
Presbyopia. dt.

LOOKING at SMALL Objects.

ca-ca. ca-s. cof. dt. mgs-au.
OBJECTS, FALSE APPEARANCE **of**. dt.
Oblique. dt.
SIGHT IMPAIRED. ca-ca. cof. mgs-au.

LOOKING AWAY for a MOMENT.

p-x.
SIGHT IMPAIRED. p-x.
Presbyopia. p-x.

HOLDING FINGER VERTICALLY before NOSE.

gel.
SIGHT IMPAIRED. gel.

LACHRYMATION.

ca-ca. p-x. snp. spi.
OBJECTS, IMAGINARY. ca-ca. spi.
Bright. spi.
Feathers. ca-ca.
Flames. spi.
Veil. ca-ca.
SIGHT IMPAIRED. ca-ca. p-x. spi.
EYEBALL. snp.
Shooting. (snp).
LEFT. snp.
Eyeball, Shooting. snp.

MOVING EYES.

cit-c. n-x. p.
OBJECTS, IMAGINARY. cit-c. n-x. p.
Bright. cit-c.
Circle. p.
  Variegated. p.
Cobweb. n-x.
Spots. cit-c.
  Bright. cit-c.
Variegated. p.

MOVING EYELIDS.

sn.
EYEBALL. sn.
Scraping. sn.

OPENING EYELIDS.

ag-na. asr. si-x. spo.
OBJECTS, FALSE APPEARANCE **of**. si-x.
Moving. si-x.
Circularly. si-x.
OBJECTS, IMAGINARY. spo.
Bright. spo.
Flames. spo.
SIGHT IMPAIRED. ag-na.
EYEBALL.
Movements. (asr).
Convulsions. (asr).
EYELIDS. asr.
UPPER. EYELID. asr.
LEFT. asr.
Upper Eyelid, Movements, Convulsions. asr.

CLOSING EYELIDS.

al-o. anan. asr. au. ba-a. chd. cic. cmc. cro. cth. dt. gel. grt. hpm. k-o. lyc. myris. n-x. narth. p-x. pol. pt. sep. snp-n. spi. str.
OBJECTS, FALSE APPEARANCE **of**. pol. str.
Moving. str.
Vertically. str.
Up and Down. str.
Multiplied. pol.
OBJECTS, IMAGINARY. n-x.
Cobweb. n-x.
PHOTOPHOBIA. k-o.
SIGHT IMPAIRED. anan. asr. cro. grt.
EYEBALL. au. ba-a. chd. dt. gel. hpm. k-o. p-x. pt. snp-n. spi.
Dryness. spi.
False Sensations. chd. (dt).
Sand. chd. (dt).
Heat. pt. spi.
Movements. gel.
Convulsions. gel.
Paralysis. (myris).
Pressing. ba-a. (cic). k-o. snp-n.

Shooting. (p-x).
Tensive. au.
Undefined. chd. snp-n.
EYEBALL SUPERIORLY. p-x.
Shooting. p-x.
EYEBALL EXTERNALLY. dt.
EYELIDS. myris.
CANTHI. cic. p-x. snp-n.
INTERNAL CANTHUS. cic. p-x. snp-n.
Heat. p-x.
Pressing. snp-n.
DOWNWARDS. snp-n.
Internal Canthus, Pressing. snp-n.
RIGHT. cic. myris.
Eyelids, Paralysis, Opening Difficult. myris.
Internal Canthus, Pressing. cic.
RIGHT. dt.
Eyeball Externally, False Sensations, Sand. dt.

CLOSING ONE EYE.

ca-ca. gel. p. pol.
OBJECTS, FALSE APPEARANCE **of**. ca-ca. pol.
Multiplied. ca-ca. pol.
SIGHT IMPAIRED. gel.

CLOSING LEFT EYE.

pol.
OBJECTS, FALSE APPEARANCE **of**. pol.
Multiplied. pol.

BLOWING NOSE.

(au).
EYEBALL. (au).
Undefined. (au).

DISCHARGE **from** NOSE.

k-i. mgs.
SIGHT IMPAIRED. k-i.
EYEBALL. k-i.
Dryness. (mgs).

Smarting. k-i.
EYELIDS. mgs.
Dryness. mgs.

HÆMORRHAGE. from NOSE.

br.
EYEBALL. br.
Undefined. br.

SNEEZING.

mgs.
EYEBALL.
Dryness. (mgs).
EYELIDS. mgs.
Dryness. mgs.

EATING.

chi. fe-mgs. li-ca. men. smc. snp-s.
OBJECTS, IMAGINARY. fe-mgs.
Blue. fe-mgs.
Bright. fe-mgs.
Circles. fe-mgs.
  Blue. fe-mgs.
  Bright. fe-mgs.
  Red. fe-mgs.
  Zigzags. fe-mgs.
Red. fe-mgs.
Zigzags. fe-mgs.
SIGHT IMPAIRED. fe-mgs.
EYEBALL. men. snp-s.
Boring. (smc).
Movements. (men).
  Convulsions. (men).
Pressing. men. snp-n.
Throbbing. (smc).
Undefined. snp-n.
ORBIT. chi. li-ca. smc.
Undefined. li-ca.
ORBIT SUPERIORLY. chi. smc.
Undefined. chi.

EYELIDS. men.
Movements, Convulsions. men.
DOWNWARDS. snp-n.
Eyeball, Pressing. snp-n.
RIGHT. smc.
Orbit Superiorly, Boring. smc.
Throbbing. smc.
LEFT. li-ca.
Orbit, Undefined. li-ca.

FLATUS, **Emission of.**

ca-a.
OBJECTS, FALSE APPEARANCE **of.** ca-a.
Strange. ca-a.
PHOTOMANIA. ca-a.

VOMITING.

rph.
SIGHT IMPAIRED. rph.

URINATING.

gel.
SIGHT IMPAIRED. gel.

SPEAKING.

lac-d.
EYEBALL. lac-d.
Undefined. lac-d.

On GOING **to** SLEEP.

smc.
EYEBALL.
Boring. (smc).
Throbbing. (smc).
ORBIT. smc.
ORBIT SUPERIORLY. smc.
RIGHT. smc.
Orbit Superiorly, Boring. smc.
Throbbing. smc.

WAKING.

ca-ca. chi. cro.
SIGHT IMPAIRED. chi.

SWEAT.

rho.
EYEBALL. rho.
Heat.. rho.

TOUCHING the OBJECT.

pru-l.
OBJECTS, FALSE APPEARANCE **of**. pru-l.
Large. pru-l.

COFFEE.

trg.
EYEBALL. trg.
Itching. trg.
Pressing. trg.

TOBACCO.

ara-d.
EYEBALL. ara-d.
Heat. ara-d.

WINE.

aga.
EYEBALL. aga.
Contractive. (aga).
Lachrymation. (aga).
Movements. (aga).
  Convulsions. (aga).
Smarting. (aga).
CHANGING CHARACTER **or** PLACE. aga.

Eyeball, Contractive then Lachrymation. (aga).
„ **then Smarting.** (aga).
Lachrymation then Movements, Convulsions. (aga).
Smarting then „ (aga).
RIGHT **then** LEFT. aga.
Eyeball, Movements, Convulsions. aga.
Right Eyeball Contractive, then Left Eyeball Movements, Convulsions. aga.
Lachrymation, then „ aga.
Smarting, then „ aga.
RIGHT. aga.
Eyeball, Contractive. aga.
Lachrymation. aga.
Movements, Convulsions. aga.
Smarting. aga.
Changing. Eyeball Contractive then Lachrymation. aga.
„ „ **then Smarting.** aga.
LEFT. aga.
Eyeball, Movements, Convulsions. aga.

APPENDIX.

In the Rubric **Changing Character or Place,** at page 62, the collectives of the varieties of Change, either of Character or Place, were omitted. As they are rather numerous, to give them as **addenda** would confuse; I have therefore here reprinted the entire Rubric in its complete form. A strict arrangement would also require a similar change to be made in the Rubric **Alternating in Character or Place** at page 65, but as the symptoms in this Rubric are very few, I have not thought it necessary to make any alteration.

CHANGING CHARACTER or PLACE in EYES.

aga. amb. atp. ba-ca. ber. bru. ca-a. ca-ca. ca-s. can. cb-a. ccs. chd. chio. cic. cl-hx. con. cot. cro. crot. cu. cy-hx. dl-s. dt. (ery). eryn. f-hx. gn-l. grp. jnp-s. k-bicra. k-ca. k-o. kre. lam. lau-c. men. mg-ca. mgs. mgs-ar. msc. n-x. na-ba. na-cl. na-sa. ner. p. p-x. pb. phy. pnx. pol. pru-l. pul. qu-sa. s. sb-t. sep. si-x. smb. smc. smi. sn. spi. spo. sr-ca. str-i. thu. trg. trn. trx. u-na.

OBJECTS, FALSE APPEARANCE of. **Blue then Grey.** atp.

Blue then White. atp.

Bright then Red. atp.

Red then Blue. atp.

OBJECTS IMAGINARY. **Bright then White.** p-x.

Bright then Red. f-hx.

Mist then Bright. (na-sa).

„ **then Green.** (na-sa).

„ **then Stars.** (na-sa).

„ **then** „ **Bright Green Yellow Near Eye.** (na-sa).

„ **then Yellow.** (na-sa).

Plain White then Bright. p-x.

Spots Bright then White. p-x.

Vibrations then Flames. f-hx.

„ **Bright Red then** „ **Red.** f-hx.

White then Bright. p-x.

SIGHT IMPAIRED. **Presbyopia then Myopia.** dt. phy.

EYEBALL. **Coldness then False Sensations, Sand.** f-hx.

„ **then Shooting.** mgs-ar.

Color Red then Discharge, Pus. (eryn).

„ **then Itching.** (bru).

„ **then Lachrymation.** grp.

Contractive then Lachrymation. (aga).

„ **then Smarting.** (aga).

Drawing then Lachrymation. grp.

„ **then Pressing.** (rho).

Eruptions, Blisters then Granulations. sb-t.

False Sensations, Hairs then Pressing. (ccs).

Pellicle then Shooting. (k-o).

Wind (cold) then Sand. f-hx.

Gnawing then Discharge. (kre).

Heat then Coldness. chd.

„ **then Color Red.** sr-ca.

„ **then Discharge.** (kre).

„ **then Pressing.** (atp).

„ **then Shooting.** sr-ca.

Itching then Color Red. kre.

„ **then Discharge.** (kre).

„ **then False Sensations, Sand.** kre.

„ **then Heat.** cb-a. k-bicra. kre.

„ **then Lachrymation.** cb-a. k-o.

„ **then Pressing.** ca-ca. cb-a. kre. (pru-l). trg.

„ **then Smarting.** kre.

„ **then Undefined.** k-bicra.

Lachrymation then Dryness. s.

„ **then Movements, Convulsions.** (aga).

Motion in then Sensitive. (cb-a).

Movements, Convulsions then Itching.

Pressing then Color Red. kre.

„ **then Discharge, Pus.** (eryn).

„ **then Lachrymation.** ca-s. grp. kre.

„ **Hot.** grp. kre.

„ **then Shooting.** k-ca.

Sensitive then Drawing. (ber).

„ **then Pressing.** (na-sa).

„ **then Shooting.** (gn-l).

„ **then Throbbing.** (ber).

Shooting then Color Red. n-x.
" **then Drawing.** (mgs).
" **then Heat.** (p-x).
" **then Lachrymation.** (snp).
Feeling of. (ba-ca).
" **then Numbness.** (s).
" **then Pressing.** (ba-ca). (na-sa). spo.
Smarting then Dryness. (s).
" **then Lachrymation.** s.
" **then Movements, Convulsions.** (aga).
Softness, Feeling of, then Pressing. (na-sa).
Swelling then Color Red. (chio).
" **then Discharge, Pus.** (eryn).
" **then Eruptions, Pustules.** (chio).
" **then Itching.** (chio).
" **then Wrinkled.** (chio).
Tearing then Lachrymation. mg-ca.
" **then Shooting.** (thu).
Tensive then Shooting. (k-o).
Throbbing then Pressing. (amb).
" **then Sensitive.** (thu).
Tingling then Drawing. (ber).
" **then Pressing.** (amb).
" **then Throbbing.** (ber).
Undefined then Color Red. crot.
" **then Shooting.** (gn-l).

IRIS. **Pupils Contracted then Dilated.** aga-p. atp. can. cic. cl-hx. cu. dl-s. jnp-s. k-o. lam. lau-c. men. pb. pnx. pol. pul. smb. smc. sn. trx.

Dilated then Contracted. aga. atp. ca-a. cy-hx. ner. p-x. qu-sa.

ORBIT. **Shooting then Pressing.** ba-ca.

TARSAL EDGES. **Sensitive then Drawing.** ber.
" **then Throbbing.** ber.
Tingling then Drawing. ber.
" **then Throbbing.** ber.

EYELIDS, INNER SURFACE. **Smarting then Dryness.** s.

CANTHI. **Color Red then Itching.** bru.

OBJECTS, IMAGINARY **then** SIGHT IMPAIRED. p.

OBJECTS, IMAGINARY **then** EYEBALL. (ery). na-sa. spi.

Flames Red then Lachrymation. spi.
Mist Red then Lachrymation. (ery).
Red then Lachrymation. (ery). spi.
OBJECTS, IMAGINARY **then** IRIS. spi.
Flames Red then Pupils Dilated. spi.
Red then Pupils Dilated. spi.
SIGHT IMPAIRED **then** OBJECTS IMAGINARY. na-sa.
SIGHT IMPAIRED **then** SIGHT DAZZLED. na-cl.
SIGHT IMPAIRED **then** EYEBALL. ca-ca. dt. kre. p-x. spi.
„ **then Appearance Dim.** dt.
„ **then Color Red.** kre.
„ **then Lachrymation.** ca-ca. dt. kre. p-x. spi.
Hot. kre.
„ **then Pressing.** dt.
„ **then Smarting.** dt.
SIGHT IMPAIRED **then** IRIS. spi.
„ **then Pupils Dilated.** spi.
EYEBALL **then** OBJECTS IMAGINARY. k-ca. spi.
Heat, then Flames Red. spi.
„ **then Red.** spi.
Shooting then Mist. k-ca.
EYEBALL, **then** SIGHT IMPAIRED. cic. con. cro. k-ca. msc. sep. spi.
Appearance Staring, then „ cic. msc.
Heat, then „ spi.
Lachrymation, then „ cro.
Pressing, then „ cro. (sep).
Shooting, then „ k-ca.
Undefined, then „ con. cro.
EYEBALL, **then** CORNEA. phy.
Color Red, then Opacity. phy.
EYEBALL, **then** IRIS. msc.
Appearance Staring, then Pupils Contracted. msc.
EYEBALL, **then** LENS. atp. n-x.
Color Red, then Cataract. atp. n-x.
EYEBALL, **then** ORBIT. cb-a.
EYEBALL, **then** EYELIDS. eryn. gn-l. k-bicra. u-na.
Itching, then Adhesion of. k-bicra.
EYEBALL, **then** UPPER EYELID. gn-l.

Sensitive, then Shooting. gn-l.
Undefined, then „ gn-l.
EYEBALL, **then** CANTHI. cot. kre.
Gnawing, then Discharge. kre.
Heat, then „ kre.
Itching, then „ kre.
EYEBALL, **then** EXTERNAL CANTHUS. cot.
ORBIT, **then** EYEBALL. ba-ca.
Shooting, then Lachrymation, Feeling of. ba-ca.
ORBIT, **then** ORBIT SUPERIORLY. chio.
Pressing, then Downwards Pressing. chio.
ORBIT, **then** EYELIDS. ba-ca.
EYELIDS, **then** OBJECTS IMAGINARY. spi.
Movements, Closing, then Flames Red. spi.
„ **then Red.** spi.
EYELIDS, **then** SIGHT IMPAIRED. spi.
Movements, Closing then „ spi.
EYELIDS, **then** EYEBALL. f-hx. lau-c. smi. str-i.
Adhesion, then Lachrymation. smi. str-i.
Movements, Closing, then Appearance Staring. lau-c.
„ **then** „ **Upward Looking.** lau-c.
„ **Opening Spasmodically, then False Sensations, Sand.** f-hx.
EYELIDS, **then** ORBIT. cb-a. na-ba.
UPPER EYELID, **then** ORBIT. cb-a.
CANTHI, **then** EYELIDS. k-bicra. pul.
EXTERNAL CANTHUS, **then** EYELIDS. pul.
Pressing, then Adhesion. pul.
INTERNAL CANTHUS, **then** LOWER EYELID. k-bicra.
Heat, then Heat. k-bicra.
EYEBALL **to** JAW, **then** EYEBALL **to** ABDOMEN. mgs.
„ **then** „ **to** CHEST. mgs.
„ **then** „ **to** BACK. mgs.
„ **then** „ **to** LEGS. mgs.

ERRATA.

All through the volume make the following corrections :—

For	ara.	*read*	ara-d.
„	hg-bi.	„	hg-bini.
„	k-bicr.	„	k-bicra.
„	lac-ac.	„	lac-cg.
„	pru.	„	pru-sp.
„	so-t.	„	so-t-æg.

Page 9, line I2, *for* clf. *read* clv.

Page 16, line 4 from bottom, *for* (pb). *read* (pul).

Page 21, line 5, *for* (Al-o). *read* (al-o).

Page 60, line 9, *for* fc-mgs. *read* fe-mgs.

Page 75, lines 11 to 13, *for* **Black.** **Moving.** **Moving.** *read* **Black.** **Moving.** **Moving.**

lines 13 and 14 from bottom, *for* **Near Eye.** **Yellow.**

read—**Near Eye.** **Yellow.**

Page 120, line 4 from bottom, *for* na-sa. *read* (na-sa).

Page 130, *Heading*, *for* POSTURE, *read* SITUATION.

Page 269, line 2 from bottom, *for* **isions** *read* **Visions.**

INDEX.

—o—

SYMPTOMS PP. 1–99.

CONDITIONS PP. 100–312.

OPINIONS OF THE PRESS, &c.

"Carefully arranged."——"A valuable Repertory."—*(Hahnemannian Monthly*, 1869, p. 344).

"This work is rapidly making its way into favor as its character and scope become more developed. We have received numerous letters from our subscribers, who are delighted with it, and who are looking forward to the publication of 'The Head Chapter.' "—*(Hahnemannian Monthly*, 1869, p. 479.)

"Those who have made use of it pronounce it the most perfect and useful Repertory for the Head and Eye thus far published. It makes a book of 220 pages, which will often be consulted by those who are desirous to make exact prescriptions for affections of the eyes and head."—*(Hahnemannian Monthly*, 1871, p. 230.)

"*It is the only complete one we have; it is the clearest and best arranged;* and it will enable us to do twice as much as formerly in diseases of the eyes."——"Those who do not like to be fed by what others have chewed for them, will be glad to have it."—(*Constantine Hering, M.D.*, 1869.)

"Whenever I have used your Repertory, I have found it very complete."—
(A. Lippe, M.D., 1870.)

"Your work is practical, and a safe guide into that vast labyrinth of our Materia Medica"——"I am well aware that the getting up of such a work requires a peculiar tact and considerable lexicographical talent, which you (to me) seem to possess."—*(B. Fincke, M.D.*. 1870.)

"I am glad your complete Repertory is about to be published. Through your kindness I have used a MS. copy of it for some time, and have found it most useful in the elucidation of the Eye cases that have come under my care. I have been repeatedly directed to medicines which would never have suggested themselves, but for the aid supplied by the Repertory. For completeness and fulness of symptoms it seems to me unique,—and the arrangement both of symptoms and conditions is as nearly perfect as the present state of our knowledge admits. I believe it will become indispensible to every medical man who desires to practice with scientific accuracy and precision, and I hope it will encourage others to take up other regions of the body to make Repertories of them with equal earnestness and perseverance."—
(R. M. Theobald, M.A., M.R.C.S., 1873.)

BY THE SAME AUTHOR,

THE PATHOGENETIC RECORD;

An Arrangement of the Physiological and Toxicological Effects of Drugs, collected from Medical and General Literature.

Now being published as an Appendix to the British Journal of Homœopathy.

In course of Preparation (arranged like the present Volume),

DISEASES OF THE HEAD AND MIND.

DISEASES OF THE EARS.

DISEASES OF THE ABDOMEN.

DISEASES OF THE CHEST.

www.ingramcontent.com/pod-product-compliance
Lightning Source LLC
LaVergne TN
LVHW010201110826
845151LV00002B/576

* 9 7 8 1 4 2 5 5 3 6 0 6 0 *